Gender, Physical Activity, and Aging

GENDER, PHYSICAL ACTIVITY, AND AGING

Edited by

ROY J. SHEPHARD

CRC Press
Taylor & Francis Group
Boca Raton London New York

CRC Press is an imprint of the
Taylor & Francis Group, an **informa** business

CRC Press
Taylor & Francis Group
6000 Broken Sound Parkway NW, Suite 300
Boca Raton, FL 33487-2742

First issued in paperback 2019

ISBN-13: 978-0-8493-1027-0 (hbk)
ISBN-13: 978-0-367-39701-2 (pbk)
Library of Congress Card Number 2001035596

Library of Congress Cataloging-in-Publication Data

Gender, physical activity, and aging / edited by Roy J. Shephard.
p. cm.
Includes bibliographical references and index.
ISBN 0-8493-1027-X (alk. paper)
1. Aging--Sex differences. 2. Aging--Physiological aspects. 3. Exercise--Physiological aspects--Sex differences. I. Shephard, Roy J.

QP86 .G388 2001
612.6′7--dc21 2001035596

Visit the Taylor & Francis Web site at
http://www.taylorandfrancis.com

and the CRC Press Web site at
http://www.crcpress.com

Preface

As in most areas of human biology, traditional texts examining physical activity and aging have drawn largely upon research conducted with male subjects, since almost no experimental data has compared the course of aging, in general, and effort tolerance, in particular, between women and men. There seem to be several reasons for the gender bias in published research information. Until recently, investigators in human biology were usually men; subjects were often recruited from fellow workers, and constraints of modesty made it easier to examine those of the same sex, rather than to recruit, chaperone, and test female volunteers. Thus, little research was conducted on women. The past decade has seen vigorous efforts to redress this imbalance in many areas of human biology, but there is still a need to examine critically the respective contributions of constitution, environment, and sociocultural influences to observed gender differences in human performance at various ages. Vigorous discussion continues between those who regard the gender gap as determined largely by inherent constitutional factors, and those who hold that it is mainly a manifestation of male exploitation of women, and a related lack of opportunities for women to develop and sustain their physical potential over the life course.

Critical evaluation of the extent and causation of gender differences has particular practical importance when considering issues of aging, physical activity, and health. A large proportion of those who reach an advanced age are women,[4] and typically, it is frail elderly women who find difficulty in undertaking the activities of daily living during their final years of life. Does ownership of paired X chromosomes confer more prolonged survival on females, or is the gender difference in life expectancy a cumulative consequence of differing life experiences for women and men? Do women have some lifestyle secret that could be adopted by their male peers in quest of a longer life? And is the apparent success of the female in part an illusion, with the benefits of greater longevity currently offset by a much longer period when physical weakness deteriorates into prolonged disability and institutional residence?[3] One study found that, in extreme old age, there were gender differences in 13 of 28 measures of personality, social relationships, habitual activity, and reported well-being.[5] Is a poor quality of life during the final ten years of survival an inevitable consequence of the aging process, or could it be averted by genetic manipulation or adoption of a physically more active lifestyle at an earlier age? Are women forever destined to experience several more years of poor quality life than their male counterparts? How far is the greater prevalence of disability among elderly women a consequence of social disadvantages relative to their male peers (for instance, lesser availability of paid work, lower wages, greater contribution to household labor, less leisure, and less sleep[2])? Could the disturbing current economic projections of the prevalence of extended disability and associated social costs soon be invalidated by genetic therapy or changes in current patterns of living?[1]

Sometimes, beliefs concerning these issues are themselves influenced by gender.[6] In order to avoid this dilemma, this book seeks objective rather than doctrinaire answers to the important questions just raised through a critical examination of available literature that has explored interactions between the aging process, gender, and physical activity. In the past few years, research on age-related changes in biological function, physical capacity, and the training responses of women has grown. The time is thus opportune to present a succinct summary of these investigations, exploring the interesting issues of potential gender differences in both the course of aging and responses of the elderly to physical activity. This book undertakes this task, drawing upon the knowledge of leading experts in exercise gerontology.

A necessary starting point for the book is a brief review of the technical problems that arise when attempting to equate biological data between men and women in the face of constitutionally determined differences of size and body composition. Gender comparisons between women and men are often confounded by discrepancies of size, body composition, and fitness between the sexes. Aging also leads to a decrease in stature, complicating analyses of the influence of aging upon various body functions. The opening chapter examines the extent of these two problems and their influence upon published data. It also reviews proposed ways of circumventing problems due to interindividual differences in body size and body composition. An optimal approach is suggested that allows gender comparisons of the aging process and its modification by regular physical activity, with minimal effects from differences in body size and composition.

There is substantial evidence that, in general, both women and men become physically less active as they become older. The second chapter thus examines details of these age-related changes, comparing the activity profiles of women and men, and exploring reasons why habitual physical activity diminishes with age. The contribution of diminished physical activity to the overall loss of functional capacity is discussed, and appropriate gender-specific tactics to motivate women and men to higher levels of physical activity are proposed.

The question arises whether gender-related differences in the rate of aging and interactions with physical activity are a consequence of genetically coded sex differences, or whether they are an expression of socioculturally conditioned differences in lifestyle (particularly physical activity) operating from an early age. Likewise, do genes, environment, or sociocultural factors explain apparent differences in the rate of functional loss and overall longevity between ethnic groups? The next chapter explores the extent to which gender and ethnic differences in the aging process and its interaction with physical activity have an immutable genetic basis, and how far these differences are an expression of potentially modifiable differences in physical environment, lifestyle, and sociocultural factors.

The distinguished panel of contributors continues with a systems approach, exploring the impact of gender and habitual physical activity upon specific physiological, biochemical, and pathological features of the aging process important to physical performance, independence, and quality of life for the old and very old. Age-related cardiorespiratory losses are first examined from this perspective. In most cultures, women live several years longer than men, but this apparent advantage is offset by a longer period of chronic disability, so there is little gender difference in the quality-adjusted life span. One chapter explores why women live longer than men, discussing and comparing factors that lead to loss of independence and poor quality of life in the two sexes. Based on these data, an assessment is made of what changes in lifestyle (particularly an increase of physical activity) could contribute to a reduced risk of chronic disability in both sexes.

Attention is then directed to neuromuscular function, the molecular basis of sarcopenia, and the relative risks of overtraining at various ages. A section on deterioration in metabolic regulation looks at such issues as the effects of gender, physical activity, and aging upon obesity, as well as the prevalence of diabetes mellitus, the weakening and deterioration of bone and joint structures, and alterations in immune and humoral responses among older women and men.

A final chapter considers some implications of the existing situation for health policy, and makes recommendations for change. The growing number of old and very old people, particularly women, in most developed societies poses major problems for support services. The personal, social, and economic costs imposed by likely changes in the numbers and physical abilities of elderly men and women are examined, together with the potential for alleviating such costs by encouraging acceptance of the active lifestyle seen in individuals who age most successfully.

This book should be of interest to all who are concerned with the process of human aging, from physiologists and biochemists and their colleagues in gerontology and geriatric departments to inquiring individuals who sense the advancing hand of time reducing their own functional capacity. The primary readership of this volume will be the growing population of investigators concerned with gerontology and geriatric medicine. However, the topic should also appeal to a broader range of applied scientists interested in the interactions between aging and physical activity, and to those interested in whether current gender differences in human performance have a genetic, constitutional basis, or are attributable largely to sociocultural differences that afford men greater opportunities for physical activity and a satisfying life course.

Roy J. Shephard
Toronto, 2001

References

1. Banks, D.A. and Fossel, M., Telomeres, cancer and aging: altering the human life span, *JAMA*, 278, 1345–1348, 1997.
2. Bird, C.E. and Fremont, A.M., Gender, time use and health, *J. Health Soc. Behav.*, 32, 114–129, 1991.
3. Murtaugh, C.M., Kemper, P., and Spillman, B.C., The risk of nursing home use in later life, *Med. Care*, 28, 952–962, 1990.
4. Shephard, R.J., *Aging, Physical Activity and Health*, Human Kinetics Publishers, Champaign, IL, 1997.
5. Smith, J. and Baltes, M.M., The role of gender in very old age: profiles of functioning and everyday life patterns, *Psychol. Aging*, 13, 676–695, 1998.
6. Wallace, J.E., Gender differences in beliefs of why women live longer than men, *Psychol. Rep.*, 79, 587–591, 1996.

About the Editor

Roy J. Shephard, M.D., Ph.D., D.P.E., is presently professor emeritus of applied physiology in the Faculty of Physical Education and Health and the Department of Public Health Sciences, Faculty of Medicine, University of Toronto. He was director of the School of Physical and Health Education at the University of Toronto for 12 years (1979–1991), and director of the University of Toronto Graduate Programme in Exercise Sciences from 1964 to 1985.

Dr. Shephard is also a consultant to the Defence and Civil Institute of Environmental Medicine, and the Toronto Rehabilitation Centre. He has also held academic appointments in the Department of Physiology and the Institute of Medical Sciences at the University of Toronto, the Centre des Sciences de la Santé, Université de Québec à Trois Rivières, and the Hôpital Pitié Salpetrière, Université de Paris, and was Canadian Tire Acceptance Limited Resident Scholar in Health Studies at Brock University from 1994 to 1998. Prior to moving to Toronto in 1964, Dr. Shephard held appointments in the Department of Cardiology (Guy's Hospital, University of London), the R.A.F. Institute of Aviation Medicine, the Department of Preventive Medicine (University of Cincinnati), and the U.K. Chemical Defence Experimental Establishment (Porton Down, U.K.).

Dr. Shephard holds four scientific and medical degrees from London University (B.Sc., M.B.B.S., Ph.D., and M.D.) and honorary doctorates from Gent University (Belgium) and the Université de Montréal, together with the Honour Award of the Canadian Society of Exercise Physiology and the Honor Award and a Citation from the American College of Sports Medicine. He is a former president of the Canadian Association of Sport Sciences, a former president of the American College of Sports Medicine, editor-in-chief of the *Year-Book of Sports Medicine,* founding editor of the *Exercise Immunology Review,* a former editor-in-chief of the *Canadian Journal of Sport Sciences,* associate editor of the *International Journal of Sports Medicine,* and a member of the editorial board of many other journals.

His research has covered many facets of sports, fitness, exercise and environmental physiology, biochemistry and immunology, and he has been author, co-author, or co-editor of approximately 100 books and more than 1400 scientific papers on related issues.

In his leisure time, Dr. Shephard enjoys walking, cycling, gardening, choral singing, and philately.

Contributors

Barbara E. Ainsworth, Ph.D. Norman J. Arnold School of Public Health, University of South Carolina, Columbia, SC

David A. Cunningham, Ph.D. Canadian Centre for Activity and Aging, School of Kinesiology, Faculty of Health Sciences, and The Department of Physiology, Faculty of Medicine and Dentistry, University of Western Ontario, London, Ontario

Jack M. Goodman, Ph.D. Faculty of Physical Education and Health, University of Toronto, Toronto, Ontario

Wendy M. Kohrt, Ph.D. University of Colorado Health Sciences Center, Department of Medicine, Division of Geriatric Medicine, Denver, CO

Gianni Parise, Ph.D. Neuromuscular Disease Unit, McMaster University Medical Centre, Hamilton, Ontario

Donald H. Paterson, Ph.D. Centre for Activity and Aging, School of Kinesiology, Faculty of Health Sciences, University of Western Ontario, London, Ontario

Charles L. Rice, Ph.D. Canadian Centre for Activity and Aging, School of Kinesiology, Faculty of Health Science, and The Departments of Anatomy and Cell Biology, Faculty of Medicine, London, Ontario

Charlotte F. Sanborn, Ph.D. Institute for Women's Health, Texas Woman's University, Denton, TX

Roy J. Shephard, M.D., Ph.D., D.P.E. Faculty of Physical Education and Health and Department of Public Health Sciences, Faculty of Medicine, University of Western Ontario, Toronto, Ontario

Shoji Shinkai, M.D., Ph.D., M.P.H. Department of Community Health, Tokyo Metropolitan Institute of Gerontology, Tokyo, Japan

Maureen J. Simmonds, PT, Ph.D. School of Physical Therapy, Texas Woman's University, Houston, TX

Liza Stathokostas, M.Sc. Centre for Activity and Aging, School of Kinesiology, Faculty of Health Sciences, University of Western Ontario, London, Ontario

Mark A. Tarnopolsky, Ph.D. Neuromuscular Disease Unit, McMaster University Medical Centre, Hamilton, Ontario

Scott G. Thomas, Ph.D. Department of Rehabilitation Medicine, University of Toronto, Toronto, Ontario

Peter M. Tiidus, Ph.D. Department of Kinesiology and Physical Education, Wilfrid Laurier University, Waterloo, Ontario

Catrine E. Tudor-Locke, Ph.D. Norman J. Arnold School of Public Health, University of South Carolina, Columbia, SC

Sara Wilcox, Ph.D. Norman J. Arnold School of Public Health, University of South Carolina, Columbia, SC

Contents

1

Technical Problems in Comparing Data for Male and Female Subjects

Roy J. Shephard

CONTENTS

1.1 Introduction

A variety of technical considerations conspire to obscure the nature and extent of fundamental biological differences between women and men.[27] In the contexts of physical activity and aging, dominant issues include:

0-8493-1027-X/02/$0.00+$1.50

- The impact of gender and age-related differences in body size and composition upon physical performance and related measures of functional capacity,
- Gender differences in anatomy, particularly alignment of the bones and resulting differences in the mechanical efficiency of movement,
- Gender differences in physiological and biochemical characteristics, particularly hemoglobin level, and thus the oxygen-carrying capacity of the blood,
- Problems in matching habitual physical activity and initial levels of physical fitness between women and men,
- The choice between relative and absolute units when making gender comparisons of the rate of aging, and
- Nonlinearities in the aging process imposed by both female and male menopause.

This chapter briefly reviews these issues, suggesting optimal solutions to problems that they pose for the exercise gerontologist.

1.2 Effects of Body Size and Composition upon Physical Performance and Measures of Functional Capacity

The typical woman is 0.1 m (approximately 6%) shorter than the average man, and she also carries a larger and differently distributed burden of body fat. Old age, also, is associated with a decrease in stature of several centimeters. Indigenous populations often have a shorter average height than people living in developed societies; if there is rapid acculturation to a modern lifestyle, there may be important intercohort differences in stature.[31] These various factors all have a substantial influence on the performance of many physical tasks, and the magnitude of "size-standardized" measures of functional capacity. However, it remains a matter of debate how far data should be adjusted for age, gender, and ethnic differences in size and body composition before one attempts comparisons between young and old, women and men, or indigenous and modern populations.

1.2.1 Body Size

Dimensional theorists have yet to agree on the most appropriate method of allowing for the influence of interindividual differences in standing height upon various measures of human performance and function. Currently, the dominant theory-based viewpoint seems to be that two of the physiologist's most important functional indices, muscle strength and maximal aerobic power, are each proportional to the second power of an individual's standing height, whereas body volumes such as vital capacity and heart size are proportional to the third power of height.[2,34] In contrast, empirical data suggest that the impact of height upon strength and maximal aerobic power approximates to a third power relationship.[30] Depending on which viewpoint one accepts, the biologically imposed height differential would give the average man a 12% or an 18% advantage of absolute muscle strength and maximal aerobic power over a woman at any given age, age-related decreases in height would influence function by 3 to 5%, and ethnic group by 18 to 27%.

Aging is a special case, since the decrease in stature reflects a shrinking of intervertebral discs, an increasing curvature of the spine, and (in extreme age) a collapse of one or more vertebrae.[26] These changes have little influence on the function of the heart or skeletal muscles, and if muscle strength or maximal aerobic power is expressed relative to stature, scores for the elderly will be artificially inflated. Fortunately, the change in stature is slight, except in extreme old age.

Total body mass is also proportional to the third power of standing height, so that in gender and ethnic comparisons, strength and aerobic power relative to body mass are largely independent of body size. Is it then appropriate to adjust data for interindividual size differences before comparing the performance of women and men, or indigenous and modern populations? Much depends on the nature of the task to be undertaken. In some types of heavy employment (for instance, deployment of hoses and rescue of victims during fire-fighting, or lifting heavy loads in front-line military operations), a large fraction of the total mechanical work is expended external to the individual. Employees then need a specific minimum of absolute muscle strength and maximal aerobic power in order to complete their task satisfactorily and safely. Size standardization of functional capacity is inappropriate for such activities. The spread of functional capacities is such that some women will meet the minimal job requirements and some men will not; nevertheless, at any given age the average woman is less likely than the average man to meet standards specified for recruitment and continuing employment. Equally, the average individual from an indigenous or minority population will face a substantial size handicap when seeking such types of work.[15,22]

In other types of physical activity (for instance, many of the tasks performed around the home important to the "activities of daily living"), a substantial fraction of total energy consumption is expended in displacing body mass.[9] It is then appropriate to base gender comparisons on size-standardized values for strength and maximal aerobic power. Statistical purists have argued for many years[32] that any statistical adjustments for interindividual differences in body size should be based on allometric regression analysis rather than simple height or body-mass ratios. This is certainly an important issue when comparing small children with adults,[35,36] but over the range of likely size differences among adults, any errors arising from the use of simple ratios are likely to be quite small. On grounds of simplicity, it thus seems best to retain the traditional practice of expressing muscle strength and maximal aerobic power per kilogram of body mass.

1.2.2 Body Composition

The fundamental influence of body mass upon physical performance is modulated by differences in body composition related to gender, age, and ethnic group. On average, a larger fraction of total body mass is fat and bone structure is lighter in women than in men; likewise, most older individuals accumulate body fat, and in recent years many members of indigenous populations have become very obese. It is sometimes argued that the typical woman's added burden of fat reflects in part socioculturally imposed gender differences in habitual physical activity, and is thus irrelevant to a "true" gender comparison. Nevertheless, much of the extra fat is a biologically determined reserve of energy, intended to meet the needs of pregnancy and lactation,[24] and it would seem wrong to discount this in any comparison.

Gender differences in muscle strength and maximal aerobic power become much smaller if values are expressed per unit of lean body mass. A lean mass adjustment may be appropriate when comparing specific aspects of muscle and cardiac function between women and men, young and old, or indigenous and modern populations. But during most activities of normal daily life a person must displace the entire body mass rather than just lean tissue; if the type of activity to be performed requires a size adjustment, then total body mass is the most appropriate unit of reference.[25]

Gender-, age-, and ethnic group-related differences in the amount and distribution of subcutaneous fat influence the relationship between cardiovascular function and maximal power output.[24] Fat is a poor conductor of heat, and if the layer of subcutaneous fat is increased by gender, age, or ethnic group, then the person concerned must direct an increased fraction of total cardiac output to skin rather than working muscles when carrying out heavy physical work in a warm environment.[27] This reduces the external power output for a given maximal oxygen intake.

1.3 Gender Differences in the Alignment of Bones and Resulting Mechanical Efficiency

Among anatomical differences between women and men, there are gender-related differences in the alignment of the bones, particularly in parous women.[3,11,17] The broader hips of the female and other differences in skeletal anatomy affect the mechanical efficiency of movement, thus influencing energy costs of movement and maximal rate of working for a given strength and maximal aerobic power.[27] Nevertheless, inherent, anatomically determined differences in mechanical efficiency are not very large, and such influences are heavily overlaid by culturally determined differences in opportunities to practice particular skills. As a result, women tend to excel in fine motor skills, whereas men demonstrate a more efficient pattern when undertaking gross motor activities.[10]

The smaller average stature of women is a further factor limiting their efficiency of movement and thus their peak external work rate for a given strength and maximal aerobic power.[17] Their shorter limbs limit leverage when undertaking many heavy physical tasks, and influence optimal stride length when walking or running. Moreover, much current equipment is designed for male operators: both size and mass are such that the average woman can only manipulate controls with difficulty;[19] plainly, this is a culturally imposed handicap that should disappear as equipment manufacturers become more enlightened.

Finally, age may alter mechanical efficiency. One recent study of healthy women aged 69 to 82 years found the energy cost of six common physical activities was similar to that stated in the FAO/WHO/UNU norms.[33] However, increases over accepted norms of energy cost are likely in older individuals who have developed various types of musculoskeletal disability.[23] Furthermore, a frail elderly person unaccustomed to sustained walking may adopt short and hesitant steps. In such an individual, efficiency of movement can be enhanced by participation in a suitable training program.

1.4 Hemoglobin Level and Oxygen-Carrying Capacity of the Blood

From a physiological point of view, there is an important gender difference in average blood hemoglobin concentration. Whereas the hemoglobin level of adult males averages approximately 156 $g \cdot l^{-1}$, that of the typical mature female is 11 to 12% lower, at 138 $g \cdot l^{-1}$.[8] The lower average figure in females reflects mainly physiologic influences: menstrual blood loss and much lower levels of androgenic hormones; nevertheless, socioculturally imposed gender differences in diet and habitual physical activity may also make some contribution. Given the predominantly biological basis of the hemoglobin differential, the gender gap seems likely to be small after menopause;[37] at this stage, values remain relatively constant in women, but tend to decrease in men.

Hemoglobin concentration is important in terms of cardiovascular performance, and thus maximal aerobic power.[25] The maximal oxygen content of unit volume of blood is stoichiometrically related to the hemoglobin concentration.[20] Thus, for each liter of blood pumped by the heart, a woman necessarily transports approximately 10% less oxygen than a man, at least prior to menopause.

The stoichiometric relationship is distorted by exposure to carbon monoxide, whether from cigarette smoking or high concentrations of vehicle exhaust.[21] Such exposure can reduce the oxygen transporting capacity of blood by up to 10%, exacerbating or reducing inherent gender differences in hemoglobin concentration.

1.5 Matching of Habitual Physical Activity and Initial Fitness Levels between Men and Women

Feminist scholars have argued that many apparent differences in function and physical performance between men and women arise because, from an early age, females have fewer opportunities to engage in vigorous physical activity than males.[7,14] Plainly, this argument has some relevance in most countries, particularly for older members of the population.

Over a 3-month period, even a moderate training program can augment muscle strength and maximal aerobic power by 20% or more,[25,26] — equivalent to a reversal of approximately 20 years of normal aging.[26] It is thus important that any gender comparisons of the aging process be based on individuals who begin with a similar initial training status and are pursuing similar patterns of habitual physical activity.

1.5.1 Matching of Habitual Physical Activity

Current laboratory-measured indices of physical fitness (such as treadmill endurance time) bear a closer relationship to health outcomes than do questionnaire assessments of an individual's level of habitual physical activity.[4] Possibly, biological determinants of a high level of physical fitness make a contribution to health beyond that derived from associated habitual physical activity. However, an alternative explanation is that many of the physical activity questionnaires currently available have limited validity because they were devised for use with male subjects. They thus tend to focus on types of physical activity where men accumulate a substantial energy expenditure, but neglect a number of heavy physical activities (particularly the care of dependents) which form an important part of daily life for many women. Thus, attempts to match habitual physical activity between men and women in terms of responses to physical activity questionnaires are unlikely to succeed unless instruments validated in both women and men are used.

A different method of matching is to base gender comparisons either on athletes[6] or on individuals who are completely sedentary.[25] In the case of young international-level athletes, there is now little difference in the intensity of training between male and female competitors. Nevertheless, gender comparisons of physiological characteristics[28] may still be flawed because a large part of athletic achievement is genetically determined, and male competitors are drawn from a much larger fraction of the total world population than are female contestants. The male sample is thus much more likely to include anomalous individuals who have a strength or maximal aerobic power four or even five standard deviations above the population average. The problem of gender difference in size of the contestant pool becomes even more marked if conclusions about gender differences are based on the characteristics of master athletes.[29]

Gender comparisons based on individuals who report that they are totally sedentary may also be flawed because of sex differences in concepts of totally sedentary behavior. For example, women who are homemakers may consider themselves to be completely sedentary and yet be incurring substantial energy expenditures in management of their home and the care of their dependents.

1.5.2 Initial Levels of Physical Fitness

It is relatively easy to determine maximal aerobic power in the laboratory,[25] and, in principle, such observations provide opportunities to match men and women at least in terms of the aerobic component of physical fitness. However, in practice, gender comparisons remain very controversial.

Some authors have equated male and female subjects directly in terms of their relative aerobic power, expressed in $ml \cdot min^{-1}$ per kg of total body mass.[6] However, as already discussed, this seems to be an incorrect approach. Because of such biological influences as body fat content and hemoglobin levels, if women achieve the same scores as the men, one is necessarily comparing very fit women with relatively unfit men.

A more appropriate approach may be to use the individual's score for maximal aerobic power or muscular strength in order to rank him or her within gender-specific population norms. The desired variable (for example, the rate of aging of oxygen transport) can then be compared between similarly ranked men and women. The main limitation to this approach is that, as yet few reliable population norms allow implementation of such a tactic. Moreover, a fundamental problem remains because gender differences in the two extremes of the distribution curve (athletic excellence and extreme sedentariness) reflect sociocultural factors as well as any fundamental biological differences.

More work on appropriate methods of matching samples is needed. The two most promising avenues seem physical activity questionnaires that have been validated for both sexes, and comparisons based on similar fitness rankings.

1.6 Relative vs. Absolute Units When Making Gender Comparisons of the Rate of Aging

In the context of aging research, a further important issue is the method of expressing deterioration of function with time. There are at least four alternatives; for example, in the case of maximal aerobic power, one might report the

1. Decrease in relative aerobic power over a fixed time interval such as ten years ($ml \cdot kg^{-1} \cdot min^{-1}$ per decade),
2. Decrease in absolute aerobic power over a similar interval ($l \cdot min^{-1}$ per decade),
3. Percentage decrease in relative aerobic power per decade, or
4. Percentage decrease in absolute aerobic power per decade.

1.6.1 Decrease in Relative Aerobic Power

One U.S. study attributed as much as a half of variance in the age-linked decrease in relative aerobic power to a combination of a decrease in habitual physical activity and an increase in body mass.[12] In order to see the true influences of gender and aging upon the primary variable, it is thus desirable to focus attention on a population sample where habitual physical activity and body fat content have remained constant over the individual's life span. Master athletes may approximate such a sample,[29] although even in this group it is arguable that advanced age leads to a progressive attenuation of the subject pool and a decrease in the intensity of training sessions.

As discussed earlier, the decline in relative aerobic power is important when performing tasks where displacement of body mass accounts for a large fraction of total energy expenditure, including many activities of daily living. Thus this may be the approach of choice when looking at the relationship between maximal aerobic power and continued independence. However, if the task requires a large fraction of the total power output to be developed external to the body, as in heavy industrial work, then the decline in absolute power output has greater significance.

1.6.2 Decrease in Absolute Aerobic Power

Absolute aerobic power is influenced little by moderate age-related changes in body composition, although a gross loss of muscle mass[13] or a gross accumulation of body fat[5] can limit physical working capacity independently of any changes in cardiorespiratory function. On the other hand, an age-related decrease in habitual physical activity and, thus, cardiovascular function, leads to losses in both relative and absolute aerobic power.

1.6.3 Percentage Changes

It is by no means certain that aging of organ function proceeds or indeed should proceed at the same absolute rate in both sexes.[26] It seems more logical to make comparisons on the basis of anticipating a similar *percentage* decrease of function in the sexes. For example, in terms of maximal aerobic power, one might envisage an age-related deterioration amounting to 10% of the individual's initial score over each decade of life. Over a 10-year interval, women would then lose perhaps 0.22 $l \cdot min^{-1}$, or 4 $ml \cdot kg^{-1} \cdot min^{-1}$, and men 0.35 $l \cdot min^{-1}$, or 5 $ml \cdot kg^{-1} \cdot min^{-1}$; however, their relative levels of function would remain the same.

Since muscle strength and maximal aerobic power are usually less in women than in men — even as young adults — age-related losses are likely to have more serious functional consequences for women than for men. It remains a matter of discussion whether one should anticipate men and women showing similar *absolute* or *percentage* changes over a given time interval. Nevertheless, the choice of approach influences prediction of the age at which functional incapacity will develop.[26] For example, assume a similar *absolute* loss of maximal aerobic power of 5 $ml \cdot kg^{-1} \cdot min^{-1}$ per decade in both women and men, and that the threshold needed to carry out the instrumental activities of daily living is a maximal aerobic power of 18 $ml \cdot kg^{-1} \cdot min^{-1}$.[16] If the maximal aerobic power at an age of 25 years averages 40 $ml \cdot kg^{-1} \cdot min^{-1}$ in women and 50 $ml \cdot kg^{-1} \cdot min^{-1}$ in men, women would then reach the functional threshold needed to carry out activities of daily living at an age of 69 years, whereas men would not do so until they were 89 years old. In contrast, if aging proceeds with a similar *percentage* change in women and men, with a loss of 4 $ml \cdot kg^{-1} \cdot min^{-1}$ per decade in women and 5 $ml \cdot kg^{-1} \cdot min^{-1}$ per decade in men, the respective thresholds for incapacitation would be at the more realistic ages of 80 and 89 years, respectively.

1.7 Influence of Menopause, and Nonlinearities of Aging

For reasons of simplicity, the rate of aging of various physiological functions has commonly been estimated by the fitting of linear regressions. These have extended, for example, between 20 and 65 years of age. However, it has also been recognized for many years that the aging process actually shows some curvilinearity. Thus, changes in vital capacity over the span of working life are best described by a biphasic curve, with a break-point at 24 years of age.[1] In older samples of the population, analysis is complicated by further nonlinearities of aging associated with female menopause, and equivalent but less dramatic changes in the production of male sex hormones. For example, women show a sharp acceleration in the rate of bone mineral loss during the five years around the age of menopause;[18] in men, there is an accelerating loss of lean tissue after retirement, apparently associated with declining production of androgens.[29] The need to fit nonlinear functions greatly increases the volume of data needed to describe aging processes accurately, and often it is necessary to continue using a linear regression approach.

1.8 Conclusions

Currently, a variety of tactics are used to equate body size, patterns of habitual physical activity, and fitness levels between men and women, young and older individuals, and members of various ethnic groups. An understanding of the consequences of such choices may help to resolve some of the apparent differences in current conclusions about interactions among aging, gender, and habitual physical activity. Optimal methods of comparing data between male and female subjects have yet to be finalized, but the principles outlined in this chapter currently seem to be the most objective approach.

References

1. Anderson, T.W., Brown, J.R., Hall, J.W., et al., The limitations of linear regressions for the prediction of vital capacity and forced expiratory volume, *Respiration*, 25, 140–158, 1968.
2. Asmussen, E. and Christensen, E.H., *Kompendium: legemsölvernes Specielle Teori*, Kobenhavns Universitets Fond til Tilvjebringelse af Läremidler, Copenhagen, 1967.
3. Beals, R.K., The normal carrying angle of the elbow, *Clin. Orthoped.*, 119, 194–196, 1976.
4. Blair, S.N., Kohl, H.W., Paffenbarger, R.S., et al., Physical fitness and all-cause mortality: a prospective study of healthy men and women, *JAMA*, 262, 2395–2401, 1989.
5. Dempsey, J.A., Reddan, W.G., Balke, B., et al., Work capacity determinants and physiologic cost of weight-supported work in obesity, *J. Appl. Physiol.*, 21, 1815–1820, 1966.
6. Drinkwater, B., Women and exercise: physiological aspects, *Ex. Sport Sci. Rev.*, 12, 21–52, 1984.
7. Durkin, K., Social cognition and social context in the construction of sex differences, in *Sex Differences in Human Performance*, Baker, M.A., Ed., John Wiley & Sons, Chichester, U.K., 1987, 141–170.
8. Gledhill, N., Haemoglobin, blood volume and endurance, in *Endurance in Sport*, Shephard, R.J. and Åstrand, P.O., Eds., Blackwell Scientific Publications, Oxford, U.K., 2000.
9. Godin, G. and Shephard, R.J., Body weight and the energy cost of activity, *Arch. Environ. Hlth.*, 27, 289–293, 1973.

10. Greendorfer, S.L. and Brundage, C.L., Gender differences in children's motor skills, in *Sports Women*, Adrian, M.J., Ed., Karger Publications, Basel, Switzerland, 1987, 125–137.
11. Hunter-Griffin, L.Y., Orthopedic concerns, in *Women and Exercise. Physiology and Sports Medicine*, Shangold, M. and Mirkin, G., Eds., F. A. Davis, Philadelphia, PA, 1988, 195–219.
12. Jackson, A.S., Beard, E.F., Wier, L.T., et al., Changes in aerobic power of men ages 25–70 years, *Med. Sci. Sports Exerc.*, 27, 113–120, 1995.
13. Kay, C. and Shephard, R.J., On muscle strength and the threshold of anaerobic work, *Int. Z. Angew. Physiol.*, 27, 311–328, 1969.
14. Maccoby, E.E., *The Development of Sex Differences*, Stanford University Press, Stanford, CA, 1966.
15. Nottrodt, J.W. and Celentano, E.J., Use of validity measures in the selection of physical screening tests, in *Proceedings of the 1984 International Conference of Occupational Ergonomics*, Attwood, D.A. and McCann, C., Eds., Human Factors Association of Canada, Toronto, Ontario, 1984.
16. Paterson, D.H., Cunningham, D.A., Koval, J.J., et al., Aerobic fitness in a population of independently living men and women aged 55–86 years, *Med. Sci. Sports Exerc.*, 31, 1813–1820, 1999.
17. Percival, L. and Quinkert, K., Anthropometric factors, in *Sex Differences in Human Performance*, Baker, M.A., Ed., John Wiley & Sons, Chichester, U.K., 1987, 121–139.
18. Riggs, B.L. and Melton, L.J., The prevention and treatment of osteoporosis, *N. Engl. J. Med.*, 327, 620–627, 1992.
19. Shephard, R.J., *Men at Work. Applications of Ergonomics to Performance and Design*, C.C. Thomas, Springfield, IL, 1974.
20. Shephard, R.J., *Physiology and Biochemistry of Exercise*, Praeger Publications, New York, 1982.
21. Shephard, R.J., *Carbon Monoxide: The Silent Killer*, C.C. Thomas, Springfield, IL, 1983.
22. Shephard, R.J., Assessment of occupational fitness in the context of human rights legislation, *Can. J. Sport Sci.*, 14, 74–84, 1990.
23. Shephard, R.J., *Fitness in Special Populations*, Human Kinetics Publishers, Champaign, IL, 1990.
24. Shephard, R.J., *Body Composition in Biological Anthropology*, Cambridge University Press, London, 1991.
25. Shephard, R.J., *Aerobic Fitness and Health*, Human Kinetics Publishers, Champaign, IL., 1994.
26. Shephard, R.J., *Aging, Physical Activity and Health*, Human Kinetics Publishers, Champaign, IL., 1997.
27. Shephard, R.J., Exercise and training in women, Part 1. Influence of gender on exercise and training responses, *Can. J. Appl. Physiol.*, 25, 19–34, 2000.
28. Shephard, R.J. and Åstrand, P.O., *Endurance in Sport*, Blackwell Scientific Publications, Oxford, U.K., 2000.
29. Shephard, R.J., Kavanagh, T., and Mertens, D.J., Personal health benefits of master athletic competition, *Br. J. Sports Med.*, 29, 35–40, 1995.
30. Shephard, R.J., Lavallée, H., Jéquier, J.-C., et al., On the basis of data standardization in prepubescent children, in *Kinanthropometry II*, Ostyn, M., Beunen, G., and Simons, J., Eds., Karger Publications, Basel, Switzerland, 1980, 306–316.
31. Shephard, R.J. and Rode, A., *The Health Consequences of "Modernization": Evidence from Circumpolar Peoples*, Cambridge University Press, London, 1996.

32. Tanner, J.M., Fallacy of per-weight and per-surface area standards, and their relation to spurious correlation, *J. Appl. Physiol.*, 2, 1–15, 1949.
33. Visser, M., van der Horst, A., de Groot, L.C., et al., Energy cost of physical activities in healthy elderly women, *Metabolism*, 44, 1046–1051, 1995.
34. von Döbeln, W., Kroppstorlek, Energiomsättning och Kondition, in *Handbok i Ergonomi*, Luthman, G., Åberg, U., and Lundgren, N., Eds., Almqvist & Wiksell, Stockholm, Sweden, 1966.
35. Welsman, J.R. and Armstrong, N., Interpreting exercise performance data in relation to body size, in *Paediatric Exercise Science and Medicine*, Armstrong, N. and van Mechelen, W., Ed., Oxford University Press, London, 2000, 3–10.
36. Williams, J.R., Armstrong, N., Winter, E.M., et al., Changes in peak oxygen uptake with age and sexual maturation in boys: physiological fact or statistical anomaly?, in *Pediatric Work Physiology*, Coudert, J. and van Praagh, E., Eds., Masson, Paris, 1992, 35–38.
37. Wintrobe, M.M., *Clinical Hematology*, 7th Ed., Lea & Febiger, Philadelphia, 1974.

2

Physical Activity Patterns, Assessment, and Motivation in Older Adults

Sara Wilcox, Catrine E. Tudor-Locke, and Barbara E. Ainsworth

CONTENTS

0-8493-1027-X/02/$0.00+$1.50

2.1 Introduction

The projected growth in the number of older adults, combined with the age-associated increase in chronic diseases and disability, poses major health, economic, and social challenges to both developed and developing nations.[1] These factors combined with the well-documented benefits of physical activity, even into old age, underscore the importance of studying physical activity and aging.[2] In this chapter, we summarize the epidemiology of physical activity in older adults, discuss issues related to measurement of physical activity in older ages, and summarize gender and age differences in physical activity motivations. Although age and gender differences in motivations are emphasized, accurate assessment is critical for interpreting both epidemiology and motivation literatures.

2.2 Epidemiology of Physical Activity in Older Adults

The majority of national surveys in the U.S. and elsewhere have focused on *exercise,* defined as planned, structured, and repetitive bodily movement undertaken to improve or maintain one or more components of physical fitness.[3] Exercise includes activities such as deliberate walking, jogging, aerobic dance, and sport participation. Few studies in the areas of epidemiology, measurement, or motivation have focused on *physical activity,* defined as bodily movement produced by contraction of skeletal muscle that substantially increases energy expenditure.[3] Physical activity includes activities that are a part of one's daily living, such as walking to the store, cleaning one's house, yard work, or climbing stairs in a building. Because exercise is considered a subcategory of physical activity[3] these terms are used interchangeably throughout this chapter, although most research has focused on planned and structured activities.

Two robust findings from population-based surveys are that older adults are less active than younger adults, and older women are less active than older men.[3-7] However, differences in activity level within an older aged sample are rarely examined by sociodemographic factors. A study by Yusuf et al.,[4] based on the U.S. 1990 National Health Interview Survey, provides the most detailed information regarding the prevalence of physical activity in adults aged 65 years and older. Unique to this study, prevalence rates are related to sociodemographic factors. Overall, 37% of older (≥65 years) men and 23% of older women engaged in regular leisure-time physical activity (LTPA), defined in this survey as participating for 30 minutes or more at least 3 times a week during the past 2 weeks. Among middle-aged adults (45 to 64 years), the gender difference was less striking, with 37% of men and 32% of women reporting participation in LTPA. As shown in Figure 2.1, the prevalence of LTPA was lowest for both men and women among those who were oldest, were black, had less education, rated their health as fair to poor, had activity limitations, were smokers, had less exercise knowledge, and reported greater stress. Although sociodemographic patterns were similar for older men and women in this survey and are seen in younger adult samples,[8] the rates of LTPA among older women in these higher-risk groups were very low, averaging less than 15%.

Kamimoto[7] analyzed differences in the prevalence of physical inactivity among older U.S. adults by gender and race. Based on the 1994 and 1996 Behavioral Risk Factor Surveillance Survey, physical inactivity was defined as reporting no leisure-time physical activities during the past month. For white women, rates of physical inactivity were 33% at ages 55 to 64 years, 36% at ages 65 to 74 years, and 47% at ages >75 years. For black women, these rates were 49, 53, and 61%, respectively. For white men, rates of physical inactivity were 34% at ages 55 to 64 years, 31% at ages 65 to 74 years, and 37% at ages >75 years. Finally, for black men, these rates were 47, 47, and 59%, respectively. Together, these studies underscore the importance of relating the physical activity patterns of older adults to sociodemographic factors.

Although such prevalence rates are quite informative in terms of identifying groups of older adults who are at risk, the data should be interpreted cautiously. Firstly, these data speak to age *differences* in leisure-time physical activity, but they cannot be interpreted as age *changes*. Differences may result from the aging process itself, may reflect cohort differences, or a combination of the two. Secondly, most of these data have not assessed physical activity resulting from transportation, household activities, or other domestic activities such as caregiving. These activities may be particularly important and more common in the lives of women, and current population-based prevalence data may thus underestimate physical activity levels in older women.

2.3 Measurement of Physical Activity in Older Adults

Older adults, especially older women, ethnic minorities, those with lower levels of income and education, and individuals living with disabilities and chronic illnesses are the least active segments of the population.[3,9,10] Therefore, researchers studying older adults face a major challenge in attempting to determine very low levels of physical activity.[11] Methods used to infer

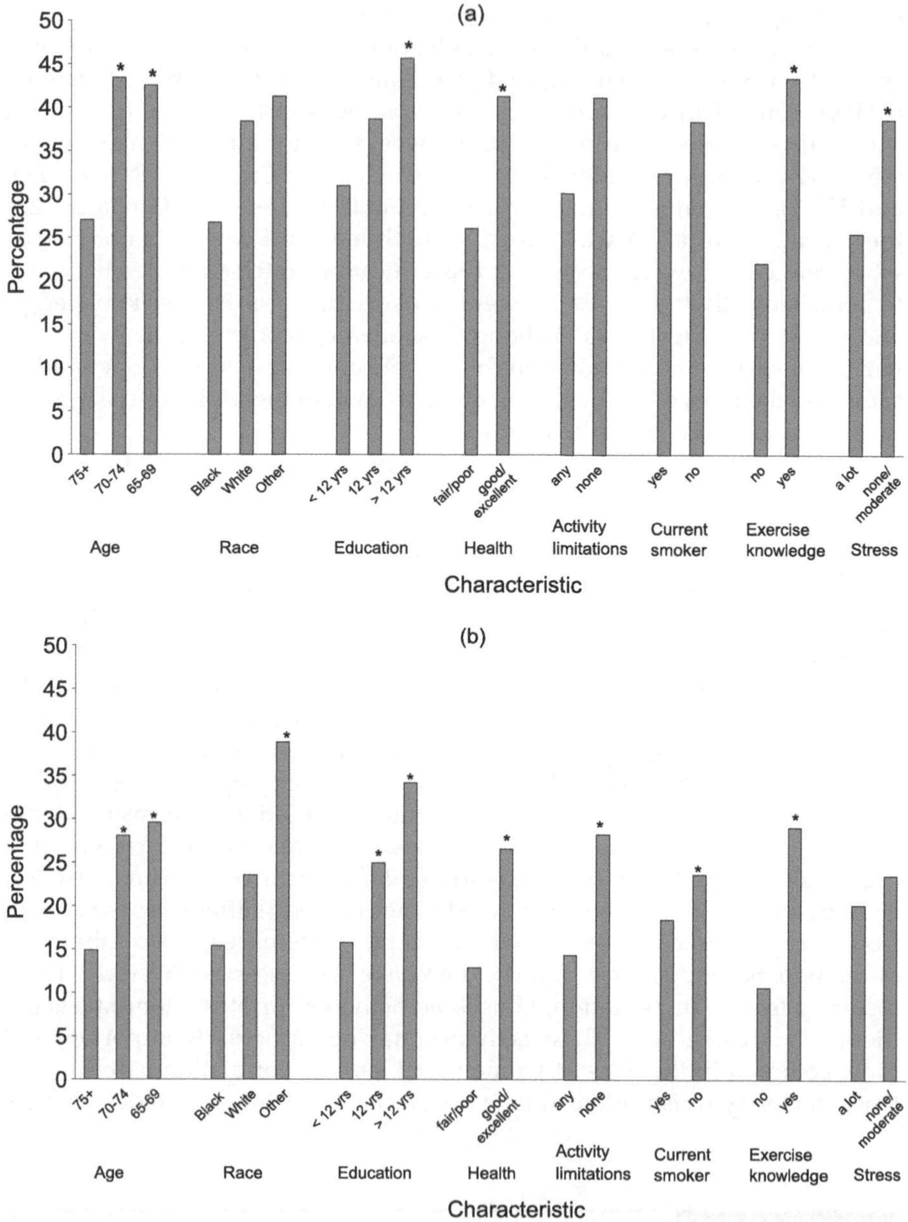

FIGURE 2.1
The percentages of men (a) and women (b) aged 65 years and older who participated in regular leisure-time physical activity, classified by sociodemographic characteristics. These data, based on the U.S. 1990 National Health Interview Survey, were extracted from Yusuf et al.[4] Asterisks indicate that the 95% confidence interval for the adjusted odds ratio (adjusted for all other characteristics) when comparing a given subgroup to the referent subgroup (always the first subgroup listed) did not contain 1.0.

physical activity behaviors in general populations have been reviewed elsewhere.[12] The purpose here is to focus on appropriate methods for describing the daily physical activity characteristics of older adult populations and to identify issues that may impact study design and instrument selection.

2.3.1 The Type and Content of Physical Activity in Older Adults

Significant gender differences in preferred physical activities persist even into the oldest old.[13] Women report spending more hours per day on physically active tasks indoors and/or domestic-related activities[13-16] including walking while shopping.[13] Although men have sometimes reported more outdoor and leisure activities,[4,13] this is not always the case.[14] Older, physically impaired community-living men have less active lifestyles (as assessed by pedometer) than do similarly impaired women.[17] Regardless of gender, a substantial amount of discretionary time is spent watching television,[18] and on the whole, older adults participate in few leisure-time physical activities.[19] Most activities are carried out alone and in the home.[18]

Despite much lower physical activity levels than those in younger age groups, there is evidence of day-to-day variability, at least in community-living older adults.[13,20] Fluctuations in fatigue, pain, medical conditions, medications, mood and depression may also impact physical activity levels acutely. It seems plausible that little variation in physical activity occurs from day to day in homebound and institutionalized older adults; however, this has yet to be examined.

2.3.1.1 The Use of Self-Report Assessment Methods

Diaries, logs, and questionnaires may be self- or interviewer-administered. Self-report methods are the most feasible approach to large population surveys and can capture important contextual information about specific activity choices. Nevertheless, such observations are liable to recall social desirability biases, and a common understanding of ambiguous terms such as "leisure," "physical activity," "moderate," and "vigorous" must be assumed.[21] Poor vision, hearing impairments, and cognitive impairments are among age-related factors that compound difficulties of measurement using these approaches.[22] Methods designed to capture the array of activities typical of young and middle-aged samples are often inappropriate for use with older people.[23] The problem is likely magnified for the study of older women: few instruments intended for general populations address household activities[24] despite evidence of the considerable proportion of time spent in such activities by older women.[13-16] Further, the metabolic cost of activities is likely lower for older adults and therefore the widespread practice of assigning MET values to reported activities using published compendiums based on values for young adults[25] is suspect.[26] At the present time, there are no similar normative data for older adults, although Stewart et al.[27] have attempted to adjust MET values to more age-appropriate estimates based on defensible assumptions. Additionally, many questionnaires suffer from "floor" effects. The lowest available score is too high for many older adults; this leaves researchers struggling to interpret the meaning of an overwhelming proportion of subjects categorized as sedentary because no activity is registered by the instrument used.[11] A high proportion of zero scores may indicate activity choice preferences rather than sedentariness.[13] The "floor" effect is only a problem, however, if the research goal is to examine the relationship of lower levels of physical activity with health outcomes, or to evaluate changes resulting from interventions.

Washburn[23] reviewed four published physical activity questionnaires designed specifically for use in older adults (including evidence of their validity). Specifically, these instruments were (1) the Modified Baecke Questionnaire for Older Adults;[28] (2) the Physical Activity Scale for the Elderly;[29,30] (3) the Yale Physical Activity Survey;[31] and (4) the Zutphen Physical Activity Questionnaire.[32] Since that time Stewart et al.[27] have published the CHAMPS Physical Activity Questionnaire for Older Adults. Each of these instruments varies with respect to recall time frame, activity components queried (typically, combinations of leisure/recreational, household and occupational activities, sport, exercise), mode of administration (interviewer- or self-administered), output (unitless score/category, energy expenditure, and/or time active), and the number of items queried (10–42 items). Each instrument has advantages and disadvantages, depending in part on the sample and study setting, testifying that no one instrument is appropriate for all circumstances and all populations of older adults.

Measurement approaches to physical activity must be both reliable and valid. To be useful, however, they must also be responsive to change with interventions over and beyond the typical day-to-day variations of everyday life. Few studies have examined the sensitivity of instruments to change in any population. Two exceptions applicable to older adults may be noted. Stewart et al.[27] reported a small- to moderate-size effect (0.38–0.64) when using a questionnaire to evaluate the change induced by a 6-month public health model physical activity promotion intervention aimed at community-living older adults. Tudor-Locke[33] reported a large-size effect (1.68) using pedometers to evaluate change resulting from a 4-week individualized walking intervention aimed at community-living older adults (average age 53 years) with type 2 diabetes. In that study, concurrent daily activity logs showed no change, possibly due to over-reporting at baseline.

2.3.1.2 The Use of Motion Sensors

Motion sensors such as accelerometers and pedometers are body-worn devices that register the wearer's movements. Depending on design, accelerometers can detect movement of the torso in up to three planes and can capture frequency of initiation of movement (from which one can infer the number of steps taken) and its acceleration (from which one can infer intensity).

Pedometers detect only movements indicative of ambulation (i.e., walking or running) and not the pattern, intensity, or type of physical activity. Ostensibly healthy community-living older adults take approximately 6000 to 8500 steps per day; individuals living with disabilities and chronic illnesses take 3500 to 5500 steps per day.[34] Accelerometers are considerably more expensive than pedometers, and the analysis of their output usually demands greater investment in terms of time, personnel, and computer expertise.[11] Data collected using both types of motion sensors are affected by the degree of subject compliance to the study protocol, including the time that the instrument is worn,[35] and subject interference. For example, cognitively impaired residents have been reported as "fiddling" with instruments.[36] Because of visual and cognitive impairments, and poor manual dexterity, research staff or caregivers may need to oversee instrument attachment, protocol compliance, and data recording. The shuffling, slow gaits characteristic of frail, institutionalized older adults may also fail to register on motion sensors designed to detect more forceful movements. Finally, accurate readings may be difficult to obtain from individuals with excessive abdominal tissue or postural deformities that interfere with recommended instrument placement.[26]

2.3.1.3 Consideration of Residential Status and Heterogeneity

Older adults are a heterogeneous population that can be classified by age groupings, disease and/or cognitive functional status, or level of independence or mobility, to name just a few approaches. Another way of classifying older adults and approaching physical activity assessment is by residential status (community living, homebound, or institutionalized). Physical inactivity reflects decreasing independence and a need for increasing care as well as increasing age.[18] A questionnaire specifically designed for community-dwelling older adults is unlikely to capture the extremely low, yet likely still varied activity levels of homebound and institutionalized older adults. The homebound elderly rarely leave their homes and often receive formal home support services.[37,38] Institutionalized older adults, ambulatory or not, spend much of their day lying or sitting.[39] It would be pointless to query these types of older adults about engagement in sports, occupational, or leisure time activities, or even about many household chores (e.g., vacuuming or scrubbing the floor). The self-report instruments reviewed by Washburn[23] and published by Stewart et al.[27] are unlikely to be appropriate for this group. In such cases, life-space diaries may prove useful. They can be self- or proxy-administered.[40,41] Such diaries identify concentric circles of "life space," for example, the bedroom, the rest of the house, the yard outside the house, the block, across the street, and beyond. Concentric circles appropriate for institutional life can also be used,[41] for example, the resident's room, the hallway, the nursing station, etc. The assumption underlying life-space diaries is that movement in greater concentric circles is indicative of increased physical activity, although this has not yet been tested empirically.

The rating of directly observed or video-recorded movements[42] is a plausible approach in institutions and for the analysis of specific times or events (e.g., the time spent at an adult day program). Time sampling (e.g., observing and recording activities every 15 minutes of an 8-hour period) has been used to classify institutionalized older adults' activity as lying, sitting, standing, walking, or propelling a wheelchair[39,43,44] and to examine the wandering or pacing behaviors characteristic of cognitively impaired residents.[36,45] Video recordings have also been used to categorize wandering behaviors.[46] Observational methods, including the time required to code and analyze data, are generally considered labor-intensive; extensive training is also required to ensure close agreement between observers.

2.3.1.4 A Combined Approach to Assessment

Although self-report methods seem the most feasible for use in large scale epidemiological studies of older adults,[23] the measurement approach is best chosen after considering the specific research question in the context of pragmatic issues including mode of administration, subject burden, and, ultimately, personnel and financial resources.[11] If resources permit, it is advisable to collect physical activity data by a combination of methods in order to understand patterns of behavior better. For example, doubly labeled water can be used to estimate changes in energy expenditure due to physical activity, a motion sensor can be worn concurrently to identify specific daily fluctuations in the volume of movement performed, and a face-to-face interview can help put these data into a realistic context. Tudor-Locke et al.[20] used a combination of activity records and pedometers to compartmentalize daily physical activity into structured or informal exercise and incidental activities comprising shopping, errands, and chores. As yet, such a combined approach has not been well exploited; concurrent measurements of physical activity by more than one measurement approach have been used primarily to support or discredit the validity of another approach.

2.3.2 The Importance of Pilot Testing in Assessment

Since few studies have examined protocols for assessing physical activity in older adults,[26] the researcher is left to decide crucial questions about study design, including the mode of administration, number of days and timing of samples, data reduction, and treatment. The measurement approach(es) and protocols selected should be appropriate for the population under study and the characteristics of the activities of interest.[47] This can best be determined by systematic pilot testing with a representative sample. Although physiological measurements (including doubly labeled water measurement of energy expenditure) can be used in most populations of older adults, motion sensors must be pilot tested to determine their acceptability and accuracy within the sample at hand. Motion sensors may be inappropriate for use in older adults with gait abnormalities including the slow and/or shuffling movements characteristic of arthritis or general frailty.[26] Pilot testing of any self-report approach is extremely important to determine the relevance of individual instrument items, "floor" effects, and acceptability of the instrument. Such preliminary studies can save much subsequent time and frustration. It is also responsible practice for researchers to publish decisions made as a result of pilot testing. For example, Hays and Clark[48] shared pilot study findings that the Physical Activity Scale for Elderly (PASE) was inappropriate for their planned study of individuals over 55 years of age with type 2 diabetes; most respondents of this type reported less than one hour of daily activity, a value less than the "floor" of the PASE.

2.3.3 Corroborative Measurements

Measurements of physical activity have been traditionally corroborated by indirect evidence. Variables or parameters known to be influenced by physical activity levels include aerobic power, muscular strength, and body composition. Such traditional indirect indicators of validity are inappropriate for many segments of the older adult population, since they are most sensitive to high intensity activities infrequently performed in older age groups.[23] In older adults, the list of corroborative measurements needs expanding to include measurements of function[26] and performance.[49-51] Physical activity is associated with physical function, even in those living with chronic disease[52] and is inversely related to disability in women.[53] A low level of physical activity is considered a risk factor for functional decline in older adults.[54,55] Inclusion of simple corroborative measurements provides valuable evidence assisting the researcher in interpreting findings.

2.4 Motivations for Physical Activity in Older Adults

Motivation of older individuals to be physically active remains an important challenge facing researchers and clinicians alike. In recent years, empirical study of motivations for and determinants of physical activity and exercise among older adults has increased. A number of comprehensive reviews have discussed determinants in older adults[56-60] and in women,[61,62] but *gender differences among older adults* have not been the focus of these reviews. This section reviews studies of gender differences in physical activity motivations among older adults. Studies that presented gender-specific analyses or included samples comprising primarily or exclusively women were included, but because sociodemographic differences in physical activity prevalence were discussed earlier, this review does not consider sociodemographic factors.

2.4.1 Theoretical Perspectives

Theories of motivations for physical activity that have received the most empirical support or have been applied most widely to physical activity in older adults are described briefly, so that later reference to constructs from these theories will be clear.

2.4.1.1 *Social Cognitive Theory*

Social cognitive theory[63] is one of the most comprehensive theories of human behavior. It posits that behavior, personal, and environmental factors interact in a reciprocal manner (*reciprocal determinism*). Outcome expectations, or beliefs that a behavior will lead to specific outcomes, are viewed as important determinants of motivation and behavior. Outcome expectations for exercise can be positive (e.g., improved physical functioning) or negative (e.g., increased risk of heart attack); clearly, both types must be considered. Self-efficacy, a belief that one is capable of engaging in or executing a behavior, even when faced with barriers, is viewed as another important determinant of motivation and behavior. Social cognitive theory has been applied successfully to physical activity in adult[8] and older adult[64] populations.

2.4.1.2 *Ecological Models of Physical Activity*

There is increasingly strong interest in the influence of physical environment and public policies upon physical activity. Ecological models of physical activity are similar to social cognitive theory, but place even greater emphasis on physical environment and public policies that impact behavior. McLeroy and colleagues[65] conceptualize behavior as determined by a combination of intrapersonal factors (e.g., attitudes, beliefs, skills), interpersonal factors (e.g., family, friends, colleagues), institutional factors (e.g., schools, worksites), community factors (e.g., neighborhoods, health care providers), and public policies (e.g., local, state, and national legislation and policies). Sallis and colleagues[66] have proposed an ecological model for physical activity that adds the physical environment (e.g., weather, sidewalks, parks) to this model.

2.4.1.3 *Stages-of-Change or Transtheoretical Model*

The stages-of-change or transtheoretical model conceptualizes behavior change as a process in which individuals progress through a series of five stages.[67] These include precontemplation (not considering making a change in the near future), contemplation (considering making a change in the future, usually defined as within the next 6 months), preparation (considering making a change in the very near future, usually defined as within the next month), action (has made a change, but has not yet maintained it for 6 months), and maintenance (has sustained a behavior change for 6 months or more). Cognitive and behavioral processes are associated with movement from one stage to the next, with cognitive processes such as awareness of the benefits of physical activity more important in the early stages of behavior adoption and behavioral processes such as enlisting social support for physical activity more important in supporting and maintaining behavioral changes. The stages-of-change theory has been widely applied to the interpretation of exercise behavior.[68]

2.4.1.4 Theory of Planned Behavior

The theory of planned behavior[69] postulates that the intention to engage in a behavior precedes the actual behavior, and that this intention is determined by a combination of *attitudes* (beliefs that the behavior will produce specified outcomes, weighted by the perceived importance of these outcomes), *subjective norms* (beliefs that important others think one should change one's behavior, weighted by one's motivation to comply with significant others), and *perceived behavioral control* (beliefs that one has personal control over behavioral outcomes). The *attitude* construct is conceptually very similar to outcome expectations in social cognitive theory, and *perceived behavioral control* is similar to self-efficacy. The theory states that attitudes and subjective norms influence behavior indirectly (i.e., through intentions), but that perceived behavioral control has both indirect and direct effects on behavior. The application of the theory of planned behavior to exercise participation has yielded significant findings.[70-72]

2.4.1.5 Personal Investment Theory

Duda and Tappe[73] argue that an understanding of the motivations for exercise among older adults requires an interactionist perspective emphasizing interplay between the characteristics of the individual and the situational factors with which he or she is faced. This perspective is exemplified in the theory of personal investment,[74] which proposes that motivation is determined by personal incentives (e.g., social and health incentives), sense of self (e.g., sense of competence, self-reliance), and perceived options (e.g., behavioral alternatives or barriers in a given situation).

2.4.1.6 Health Belief Model

The health belief model proposes that the likelihood of behavior change is increased when individuals believe they are at risk of developing a condition (*perceived susceptibility*), when they view the condition as serious (*perceived severity*), and when the perceived benefits to behavior change outweigh the perceived barriers.[75] Individual characteristics (e.g., age, gender, knowledge) and "cues to action" (e.g., symptoms, illness, media) are considered factors that modify the perceived threat of a condition.

2.4.2 Gender Differences in Motivations for Physical Activity

2.4.2.1 History and Socialization

Older women's personal histories with respect to sport, exercise, and physical activity provide a logical place from which to begin to understand gender differences in motivations for physical activity. Men and women who are now over the age of 65 years differ widely in their patterns of exposure to sport and exercise during childhood and young adulthood. Today's older women typically faced institutional and social constraints to exercise and sport in their younger years. These societal barriers are well described elsewhere.[76-80] They include historical beliefs that women who engaged in vigorous activity were not feminine, that physical energy should be saved for childbearing, and that women's anatomy and physiology prevented vigorous physical activities. Cousins[81] recently demonstrated that childhood confidence in performing six movement skills (e.g., hanging by one's knees) was a strong correlate of current exercise self-efficacy in women who averaged 77 years of age, supporting the importance of early socialization into physical activity. Similarly, Ebrahim and Rowland[82] found that prior sports participation was associated with present vigorous activities and sports in a sample of older women averaging 66 years of age. Clearly, attitudes and beliefs develop within a sociocultural context and, as will be described, early socialization of the current generation of older women has likely had a negative impact on their participation in physical activity.

2.4.2.2 Ageism

O'Brien and Vertinsky[78] provide an excellent discussion of how ageism combined with sexism, has constrained the physical activity of older women. Women may feel guilty at taking time away from family responsibilities to engage in leisure-time physical activity. In addition, society tends to have ageist views about what is "appropriate" behavior for older women. Also, for those women who married and did not work outside the home, widowhood may increase the risk of poverty, with associated poorer health and health practices. Furthermore, society tends to view aging as a time of decline, and older adults may believe that it is too late to improve their health and physical functioning. Consistent with these stereotypes, O'Neill and Reid[83] found that 14% of older adults in their sample stated that they were "too old" to exercise, and 23% said that they did not need as much physical activity now that they were older. Booth et al.[84] also reported that 20% of individuals aged 60 to 78 years stated they were "too old" to be active; similar beliefs have been reported in older African American women[85] and older adults with diabetes.[48] In addition, a number of studies have shown that older adults believe that they are already getting enough exercise[86] or that they get more exercise than their peers.[87] Thus, it appears that older adults have internalized some of the negative stereotypes of aging.

It is difficult to examine directly the influences of ageism and negative stereotypes on physical activity. However, a recent study[88] produced intriguing findings that could lead to further research. Using a reaction time paradigm common in cognitive psychology and social cognition research, Hausdorff and colleagues[88] presented older adults with words on a computer screen at speeds impossible to be perceived consciously. Participants believed that they were simply playing a computer game. Based on random assignment, participants were presented with words that reflected either positive stereotypes of aging (positive priming) or negative stereotypes (negative priming). Without the participant's knowledge, the investigators assessed gait speed immediately before and after the priming task. Participants presented with positive stereotypes of aging significantly increased their walking speed compared to those who received negative priming. The authors concluded that their results suggested that positive messages could counter the negative stereotype of aging.

2.4.2.3 Self-Efficacy and Perceived Behavioral Control

Self-efficacy, a central construct in social cognitive theory,[63] is one of the most consistently reported determinants of health behaviors,[89,90] including physical activity.[8] Bandura stated that efficacy expectations predict whether an individual will initiate a behavior, how much effort the individual will expend on the behavior, and how persistent he or she will be in spite of barriers or obstacles.[91] Bandura theorized that personal mastery or performance accomplishments are the most powerful way to increase self-efficacy. Unfortunately, older women are less likely to have past experience of physical activities upon which to draw. Further, as will be described, they are less likely to be encouraged or supported in their physical activity participation, and they may have anxieties or concerns about activity that decreases their self-efficacy.

Older women have lower self-efficacy for physical activity than younger women and older men. Self-efficacy in women is negatively associated with age.[81,92,93] For example, Wilcox and Storandt[93] found that age was a stronger negative correlate of self-efficacy than factors such as exercise participation and health status. Gender differences in self-efficacy have also been reported: self-efficacy is lower among older women than older men in a range of study populations.[48,73,94,95]

As in younger adults,[8] self-efficacy is a strong predictor of physical activity in older women and men. In older women, self-efficacy seems the strongest correlate of exercise,[96-98] explaining up to 31% of the variance in exercise participation. Cousins[99] found that self-efficacy and social support were the strongest correlates of exercise in women averaging 77 years of age. In addition, self-efficacy and perceived behavioral control are independent correlates of physical activity for both men and women.[100,101] Most studies in this area have been cross sectional, but self-efficacy and perceived behavioral control can also predict exercise participation and exercise adherence in middle-aged and older adults.[102-104] In older adults, self-efficacy appears to have a more potent role in adoption than in maintenance of physical activity.[105] This suggests that an increase of self-efficacy may be critical in increasing the likelihood that older women will initiate a physical activity program. As Bandura's theory would predict, McAuley and colleagues have shown that self-efficacy can be manipulated, with increased self-efficacy leading to greater physical activity.[102]

In summary, self-efficacy is an important physical activity motivator in older adults. However, likely due to differences in socialization, self-efficacy is lower among older women than older men and is negatively associated with age.

2.4.2.4 Social Environmental Factors

Social support is another central construct in social cognitive theory[63] (where it is conceptualized as an environmental influence), and in ecological models[65] (where it is conceptualized as an interpersonal influence). Typically, support received from family, friends, and physicians is included under the broader heading of social support. Like self-efficacy, social support has received a great deal of study in the areas of health behavior and health outcomes;[106] it is a positive correlate of participation in physical activity.[8] Chogahara et al.[60] reviewed the more limited literature on social support and physical activity in older adults. Based on seven studies that included participants over 65 years of age, they concluded that social support appears to be a *stronger* determinant of physical activity participation in older than in young adults.

Among adults in general, social support seems a stronger predictor of physical activity for women than men,[8] but gender differences have not been well studied in older ages. Hovell et al.[100] found that social support from friends for exercise was a significant independent correlate of walking in older women, but not in older men. Clark reported that lower income Caucasian and African American women were more likely to discuss the importance of social support than were their male counterparts.[107] Although social support for exercise has been associated with higher levels of physical activity in diverse samples of older adults,[99,100,108-113] there is evidence that older adults, particularly older women, receive less support for exercise than other groups. Clark and Nothwehr[94] found no gender differences in those persuaded to be physically active by family and doctors, but noted that the percentage of older individuals who received these types of support was relatively low (32% for family and 43% for doctors, respectively). When asked who would approve of their physical activity, Conn[114] found that most older women cited their family and many cited friends, but only about 50% cited their physicians. Cousins[115] also found that women did not perceive their physicians as supporting physical activity. Half of older women in her sample reported that they received positive support for exercise from friends or family, but 38% were unsure if their physician would approve of exercise, and 25% reported that their physician would strongly *disapprove* of exercise. In addition, age was negatively related to social support for exercise in this study. This perceived lack of physician support for physical activity is disturbing because physician advice has been shown to increase physical activity.[116] Older adults have an average of 11.4 contacts per year with a physician or health care provider,[1] providing an important opportunity for physical activity counseling. Further, the desire for professional advice and support for physical activity appears greatest in older adults.[84] Finally, Lee[109] found that older women generally reported high levels of social support for exercise, yet 40% said that their family would not help them so that they could exercise.

The subjective norm construct of the theory of planned behavior emphasizes the importance of significant others in behavior change. Although the attitudinal and perceived behavioral control constructs of this theory have received empirical support for their ability to explain exercise behavior in adults, the subjective norm construct has typically shown a weak or nonsignificant relationship to exercise behavior or intention.[70-72] However, consistent with the conclusion of Chogohara et al.,[60] subjective norms play a more important role in explaining exercise intention and behavior in older than in younger adults, as evidenced by significant findings in several studies of older men and women.[117,118] Brenes et al.[104] followed a sample of older adults enrolled in an exercise class, finding that, although perceived behavioral control was most predictive of exercise intentions and behavior at 1 and 3 months, the subjective norm explained 18% of exercise behavior at 1 month. In a large cross-sectional study of Canadian adults, Wankel and colleagues[101] found that attitudes, perceived behavioral control, and subjective norms were all significant predictors of exercise intention among all age and gender groups; however, subjective norms were stronger predictors of intention for adults over 60 years than for younger adults.

When asked reasons for not being physically active, lack of an exercise companion is often cited by older women,[82,119] but not by older men.[119] Satariano and colleagues[119] found that, with increasing age, lack of an exercise companion was less frequently cited as a reason for not exercising. Although women have a greater preference for group-based activities than men, studies in a wide range of older populations have indicated that around two-thirds of individuals prefer activities that can be performed outside a group format.[84,109,111,120] Booth et al.[84] found that fewer adults aged 60 to 78 years wanted to exercise in a group than did younger adults (20% vs. 40%, respectively). In the Rancho Bernardo Study, only 5% of older adults participated in organized exercise programs.[121] Furthermore, randomized controlled exercise trials with older adults have shown that exercise adherence is comparable or superior for home-based compared to group-based exercise.[122-124] These findings do not negate the importance of social support. Instead, they suggest that encouraging or assisting older adults to become more active is probably more useful than exercising with the individual or offering group-based programs. Clark's[107] study of lower income African American and Caucasian older adults further suggests that the *type* of group offered is important. Women in his sample were quite interested in exercising with others, but only with individuals similar to themselves in terms of ability and confidence; these women were not interested in established exercise programs that attracted individuals with good health and a high level of confidence.

In summary, social support is an important determinant of physical activity in older men and women. It may actually increase in importance with increasing age, and it seems a stronger determinant in older women than older men, consistent with gender differences observed in younger adults. Despite the importance of this variable, older adults, especially older women, appear to receive less support for physical activity than do younger adults. Perceptions of support from physicians are particularly low.

2.4.2.5 Physical Environmental Factors

The relationship between physical environmental factors and physical activity has been understudied in both young and older adults, but it is becoming a topic of considerable interest.[66] Older adults frequently cite poor weather as a barrier to physical activity.[92,94,107,114] Other environmental barriers cited by older adults include crime or personal safety,[94,114,125] lack of sidewalks,[94,107] lack of transportation,[82,107] lack of facilities or places to exercise,[82,86,107,125,126] the lack of places to sit down while out exercising,[94] and cost.[125] In one study, women were more likely than men to cite environmental barriers to physical activity,[94] but typically, gender differences have not been examined.

2.4.2.6 Perceived Benefits and Outcome Expectations

It is not surprising that older adults are more likely to cite the health benefits of physical activity as a motivation for exercise than are younger adults. The prevalence of chronic health conditions amenable to physical activity, such as cardiovascular disease, diabetes, and some forms of cancer, begins to increase in middle age,[1] probably serving as a "cue to action" for behavioral change.[75] Consistent with this idea, Duda and Tappe[73] found that salience of the health benefits of exercise increased with age, and wellness incentives (including psychological benefits) were more common motivators for older men and women than for younger adults. Two studies reported that younger women were more likely than their older peers to state that they exercised for weight control, whereas older women were more likely than younger women to cite health reasons for exercising.[92,127] Mental health and social affiliation are other benefits commonly cited by older adults,[83,114,126] and their importance may increase with age.[127]

As reported in younger aged samples,[8] perceived exercise benefits or outcome expectations are positively associated with physical activity participation in older women.[82,96,98,109,128] In a randomized controlled trial of exercise in older women, Caserta and Gillett[124] found that greater perceived benefits of exercise were positively related to exercise adherence at 6- and 18-month follow-up examinations. Finally, it is important that the older person's outcome expectations be realistic, as older adults who have very high expectations of exercise that are not met may be at increased risk of subsequent nonadherence.[129]

In summary, there is greater motivation to be physically active for physical and mental health benefits in the elderly than in younger adults. However, the perceived benefits of physical activity are major motivators of physical activity behavior in both younger and older adults. No clear gender differences have been reported in this area, but increasing age may be associated with decreased outcome expectancies,[94] indicating that the oldest-old segment may not expect health and wellness benefits to the same extent as younger-old adults, despite evidence to the contrary.

2.4.2.7 Perceived Barriers

Health status. Although physical and mental health benefits are major motivators for older men and women alike, poor health status is a negative determinant of physical activity in older adults,[48,82,96,98,111,126,130] and is often cited as a barrier to physical activity.[83,84,94,107,114,119,125,126] Even among disabled older women, health factors are associated with walking.[121] Arthritic pain, fatigue, and other physical symptoms seem to be key health issues that decrease motivation to be physically active in older age.[82,83,86,94,107,114,119,125] The prevalence of arthritis is higher in older women than in men;[1] this may be why older women are more likely than older men to cite pain as a barrier to physical activity,[94] especially in advanced age.[82] Unfortunately, the avoidance of exercise due to arthritic pain excludes the pain reduction and gains of physical functioning now known to result from moderate intensity aerobic and strength training in older individuals with osteoarthritis.[131]

Fear of injury. Fear of falling and fear of injury from exercise are important barriers to physical activity in older adults. Howland and colleagues[132] found that fear of falling was very common among older adults living in public housing developments, with 55% of residents reporting this fear. Furthermore, 56% of residents had curtailed their activity because of fears of falling. Women seem more likely than men to cite fear of falling as a barrier to physical activity,[94,132] and a qualitative study of older women found that this fear was one of the most commonly raised disincentives to physical activity.[114] Fear of heart attack and fear of falling were barriers frequently cited by ethnically diverse women.[125] Cousins[133] completed an in-depth analysis of the perceived risks and benefits of six fitness activities (walking, cycling, aqua activities, stretching, curl-ups, and push-ups) in women who averaged 77 years of age. Although these women recognized the benefits of physical activity, they also held strong beliefs about the associated risks, particularly those involving strength and flexibility training. Risks were often described in extreme terms, such as heart hemorrhage, muscle seizure, and death. Women reported the fewest risks for walking,[133] although the perceived risks were quite common even in this activity. The fewer perceived risks of walking relative to other exercises are consistent with women's preference[82,84,107,108,121] and self-efficacy[93,99] for walking.

Other barriers. Although lack of time is the most commonly cited barrier to physical activity in adults in general,[8] and is cited by older adults,[82,111,114,125] the importance of time as a barrier appears to decline with increasing age;[82,84,86,92] possibly, more time is available after retirement or other barriers such as health problems become more salient. "Lack of time" can mean different things to different people. Older women largely bear the burden of caring for older family members with dementia or disability, creating time and other logistical constraints to physical activity,[111,112] whereas among younger women time constraints may relate more to juggling the roles of mother, wife or partner, community member, and employee.[61] General self-motivation is associated with physical activity in women, but this construct does not appear to be more important for older women than for younger women,[93] for older adults than for younger adults,[84] or for older women than for older men.[119] Nevertheless, a lack of motivation or "willpower," not having an interest in physical activity, and not having the "discipline" to exercise have been cited as barriers to exercise by older adults.[82,83,107] When examined as a composite, perceived barriers to physical activity are consistently associated with lower levels of physical activity, both in older women and combined gender samples.[48,82,97,98,109,112]

2.4.2.8 Attitudes

Positive attitudes toward physical activity are generally associated with higher levels of physical activity participation in older men and women,[93,101,117,134] as in younger populations,[70-72] although strength of attitudes in predicting exercise intentions seems to decline with age.[101] Older sedentary women report more negative attitudes toward exercise than younger women and older active women,[93] and these attitudes may interfere with the adoption of an exercise program. Lee[109] noted that, although older Australian women generally had positive attitudes toward exercise, 34% said that they would "look silly in exercise clothes" and 29% disagreed with the statement, "I have friends of my own age who exercise."

2.4.2.9 Knowledge

Knowledge is not a consistent or strong determinant of physical activity in adult populations.[8] However, in samples where knowledge may be lower or more variable due to poor socioeconomic or educational status, knowledge may play a more important role. In these instances, knowledge regarding physical activity may be a necessary but not sufficient prerequisite to the adoption of physical activity. Dean[135] found that, among older Danish adults, knowledge regarding practices to reduce cancer, heart attacks, and hypertension was related to exercise, but only among women. Similarly, Ebrahim and Rowland[82] found that knowledge was an independent predictor of participation in vigorous activities among older women but not older men. Lee's[109] study of older Australian women found that those in the precontemplation stage of change had significantly less exercise knowledge than women in other stages of change. Other studies have reported knowledge as associated with exercise in both older men and women.[48,85] A large population-based survey of older adults in the U.S. indicated that knowledge was a significant correlate of physical activity in men and women, even after adjustment for a host of sociodemographic and health factors (adjusted odds ratio of 2.4 for men and 2.7 for women).[4]

Relative to other age groups, older adults may lack knowledge regarding exercise. Fitzgerald[85] found that both African American and Caucasian older adults overestimated the time required for exercise to be effective; this was especially true among African American women. Hays and Clark[48] reported that knowledge regarding physical activity was negatively associated with age, independent of gender. Finally, Lee[109] found that only 9% of older women responded accurately to three questions regarding the frequency, duration, and intensity of exercise needed for health benefits. Contrary to these results, Morrow et al.[136] found that awareness of the Surgeon General's Report on Physical Activity and Health increased with increasing age, and was independent of gender. Some 45% of adults over the age of 61 years stated they were aware of the Surgeon General's report, but this percentage dropped to 16% among adults aged 18 to 25 years.

2.5 Conclusions

The findings in studies of older women and in combined studies of older men and women that have examined gender differences are typically consistent with observations on younger adults. Greater exercise self-efficacy, social support for exercise, perceived benefits of exercise, positive attitudes toward exercise, and fewer perceived barriers to exercise are the major motivators for physical activity among older men and women. Yet, important age and gender differences exist. Relative to men, older women have lower exercise self-efficacy; they report greater health barriers to exercise, especially arthritic pain; they perceive greater health risks that could result from exercise; they receive less social support for exercise; they have a greater fear of falling; and they may hold more negative attitudes toward exercise. Knowledge, self-efficacy, and social support appear to be stronger determinants of physical activity in older than in younger adults, whereas attitudes may be weaker determinants. Older adults are more motivated by the health benefits of exercise than are their younger peers. These findings underscore the importance of designing interventions to target mediators of physical activity in addition to the actual behavior, especially among sedentary women who may hold beliefs precluding the initial adoption of physical activity.

Although substantial research has focused on physical activity in older adults in recent decades, studies of determinants, measurements, and epidemiology have tended to focus on well-educated, affluent, healthy individuals of Caucasian origin. Much less is known about older adults from diverse ethnic backgrounds, who are isolated, rural, disabled, institutionalized, or living in poverty, and who suffer from chronic illnesses and disabilities. Relatively few studies have examined gender differences in motivations for physical activity among older adults. Even fewer studies have examined age by gender interactions. Moreover, prevalence, measurement, and determinants research has focused largely on leisure-time physical activity; far less attention has been devoted to other types of activities that may be especially relevant for older women, such as household and caregiving activities. Finally, the influence of the physical environment on physical activity is not well understood in most age groups. Analyses of age and gender differences in these determinants of physical activity remain important challenges.

Gaining a better understanding of underserved and potentially at-risk populations, in addition to understanding gender differences within these populations, will be critical to the promotion of physical activity in all segments of the older adult population.

References

1. USDHHS, *Health, United States, 1999. Health and Aging Chartbook*, U.S. Government Printing Office, Washington, D.C., 1999.
2. American College of Sports Medicine position stand, exercise and physical activity for older adults, *Med. Sci. Sports Exerc.*, 30, 992–1008, 1998.
3. USDHHS, *Physical Activity and Health: a Report of the Surgeon General*, U.S. Department of Health and Human Services, Centers for Disease Control and Prevention, Atlanta, GA, 1996.
4. Yusuf, H.R., Croft, J.B., Giles, W.H., et al., Leisure-time physical activity among older adults, U.S., 1990, *Arch. Intern. Med.*, 156, 1321–1326, 1996.
5. Jones, D.A., Ainsworth, B.E., Croft, J.B., et al., Moderate leisure-time physical activity: who is meeting the public health recommendations? A national cross-sectional study, *Arch. Fam. Med.*, 7, 285–289, 1998.
6. Crespo, C.J., Ainsworth, B.E., Keteyian, S.J., et al., Prevalence of physical inactivity and its relation to social class in U.S. adults: results from the third national health and nutrition examination survey, 1988–1994, *Med. Sci. Sports Exerc.*, 31, 1821–1827, 1999.
7. Kamimoto, L.A., Easton, A.N., Maurice, E., et al., Surveillance for five health risks among older adults — United States, 1993–1997, *MMWR Morb. Mortal. Wkly. Rep.*, 48, 89–156, 1999.

8. Sallis, J.F. and Owen, N., Determinants of physical activity, in *Physical Activity and Behavioral Medicine*, Sage, Thousand Oaks, CA, 1999, 110–134.
9. Taylor, W.C., Baranowski, T., and Young, D.R., Physical activity interventions in low-income, ethnic minority, and populations with disability, *Am. J. Prev. Med.*, 15, 334–343, 1998.
10. King, A.C., Rejeski, W.J., and Buchner, D.M., Physical activity interventions targeting older adults. A critical review and recommendations, *Am. J. Prev. Med.*, 15, 316–333, 1998.
11. Tudor-Locke, C.E. and Myers, A.M., Challenges and opportunities for measuring physical activity in sedentary adults, *Sports Med.*, 31, 91–100, 2001.
12. Montoye, H.J., Kemper, H.C.G., Saris, W.H.M., et al., *Measuring Physical Activity and Energy Expenditure*, Human Kinetics, Champaign, IL, 1996.
13. Dallosso, H.M., Morgan, K., Bassey, E.J., et al., Levels of customary physical activity among the old and the very old living at home, *J. Epidemiol. Comm. Health.*, 42, 121–127, 1988.
14. Osler, M., de Groot, L.C., and Enzi, G., Life-style: physical activities and activities of daily living, *Eur. J. Clin. Nutr.*, 45, 139–151, 1991.
15. Schuit, A.J., Schouten, E.G., Westerkerp, K.R., et al., Validity of the physical activity scale for the elderly (PASE): according to energy expenditure assessed by the doubly labeled water method, *J. Clin. Epidemiol.*, 50, 541–546, 1997.
16. Klumb, P.L. and Baltes, M.M., Time use of old and very old Berliners: productive and consumptive activities as functions of resources, *J. Gerontol.*, 54, S271–S278, 1999.
17. Hachisuka, K., Tsutsui, Y., Furusawa, K., et al., Gender differences in disability and lifestyle among community-dwelling elderly stroke patients in Kitakyushu, Japan, *Arch. Phys. Med. Rehabil.*, 79, 998–1002, 1998.
18. Horgas, A.L., Wilms, H.U., and Baltes, M.M., Daily life in very old age: everyday activities as expression of successful living, *Gerontologist*, 38, 556–568, 1998.
19. Crespo, C.J., Keteyian, S.J., Heath, G.W., et al., Leisure-time physical activity among U.S. adults: results from the third national health and nutrition examination survey, *Arch. Intern. Med.*, 156, 93–98, 1996.
20. Tudor-Locke, C., Jones, G.R., Myers, A.M., et al., Contribution of structured exercise class participation and informal walking for exercise to daily physical activity in community-dwelling older adults, *Res. Q. Exerc. Sport*, in press.
21. Sallis, J.F. and Saelens, B.E., Assessment of physical activity by self-report: status, limitations, and future directions, *Res. Q. Exerc. Sport*, 71, 1–14, 2000.
22. Shephard, R.J., Assessment of physical activity and energy needs, *Am. J. Clin. Nutr.*, 50, 1195–1200, 1989.
23. Washburn, R.A., Assessment of physical activity in older adults, *Res. Q. Exerc. Sport*, 71, 79–88, 2000.
24. Masse, L.C., Ainsworth, B.E., Tortolero, S., et al., Measuring physical activity in midlife, older and minority women: issues from an expert panel, *J. Wom. Health*, 7, 57–67, 1998.
25. Ainsworth, B.E., Haskell, W.L., Whitt, M.C., et al., Compendium of physical activities: an update of activity codes and MET intensities, *Med. Sci. Sports Exerc.*, 32, S498–S516, 2000.
26. Rikli, R.E., Reliability, validity, and methodological issues in assessing physical activity in older adults, *Res. Q. Exerc. Sport*, 71, 89–86, 2000.

27. Stewart, A.L., Mills, K.M., King, A.C., et al., CHAMPS physical activity questionnaire for older adults: outcomes for interventions, *Med. Sci. Sports Exerc.*, in press.
28. Voorrips, L.E., Ravelli, A.C.J., Dongelmans, P.C.A., et al., A physical activity questionnaire for the elderly, *Med. Sci. Sports Exerc.*, 23, 974–979, 1991.
29. Washburn, R.A., Smith, K.W., Jette, A.M., et al., The physical activity scale for elderly (PASE): development and evaluation, *Clin. J. Epidemiol.*, 46, 153–162, 1993.
30. Washburn, R.A., McAuley, E., Katula, J., et al., The physical activity scale for the elderly (PASE): evidence for validity, *J. Clin. Epidemiol.*, 52, 643–651, 1999.
31. DiPietro, L., Williamson, D.F., Caspersen, C.J., et al., The descriptive epidemiology of selected physical activities and body weight among adults trying to lose weight: the behavioral risk factor surveillance system survey, 1989, *Int. J. Obes.*, 17, 69–76, 1993.
32. Westerterp, K.R., Saris, W.H.M., Bloemberg, B.P.M., et al., Validation of the Zutphen physical activity questionnaire for the elderly with doubly labeled water, *Med. Sci. Sports Exerc.*, 24, S68, 1992.
33. Tudor-Locke, C., A preliminary study to determine instrument responsiveness to change with a walking program: physical activity logs vs. pedometers, *Res. Q. Exerc. Sport,* in press.
34. Tudor-Locke, C.E. and Myers, A.M., Methodological considerations for researchers and practitioners using pedometers to measure physical (ambulatory) activity, *Res. Q. Exerc. Sport*, 72, 1–12, 2001.
35. Kochersberg, G., McConnell, E., Kuchibhatla, M.N., et al., The reliability, validity, and stability of a measure of physical activity in the elderly, *Arch. Phys. Med. Rehabil.*, 77, 793–795, 1996.
36. Cohen-Mansfield, J., Werner, P., Culpepper, W.J., et al., Assessment of ambulatory behavior in nursing home residents who pace or wander: a comparison of four commercially available devices, *Dement. Geriatr. Cogn. Disord.*, 8, 359–365, 1997.
37. Gilbert, G.H., Branch, L.G., and Orav, E.J., An operational definition of the homebound, *Health. Serv. Res.*, 26, 786–800, 1992.
38. Lindesay, J. and Thompson, C., Housebound elderly people: definition, prevalence and characteristics, *Int. J. Geriatr. Psychiatry,* 8, 231–237, 1993.
39. MacRae, P.G., Schnelle, J.F., Simmons, S.F., et al., Physical activity levels of ambulatory nursing home residents, *Nurs. Home Resid.*, 4, 264–278, 1996.
40. May, D., Nayak, U.S.L., and Isaacs, B., The life-space diary: a measure of mobility in old people at home, *Int. Rehabil. Med.*, 7, 182–186, 1985.
41. Tinetti, M.E. and Ginter, S.F., The nursing home life-space diameter — a measure of extent and frequency of mobility among home residents, *J. Am. Geriatr. Soc.*, 38, 1311–1315, 1990.
42. Ainsworth, B.E., Sternfeld, B., Slattery, M.L., et al., Physical activity and breast cancer: evaluation of physical activity assessment methods, *Cancer,* 83, 611–620, 1998.
43. MacRae, P.G., Asplund, L.A., Schnelle, J.F., et al., A walking program for nursing home residents: effects on walk endurance, physical activity, mobility, and quality of life, *J. Am. Geriatr. Soc.*, 44, 175–180, 1996.
44. Schnelle, J.F., MacRae, P.G., Ouslander, J.G., et al., Functional incidental training, mobility performance, and incontinence care with nursing home residents, *J. Am. Geriatr. Soc.*, 43, 1356–1362, 1995.

45. Algase, D.L., Kupferschmid, B., Beel-Bates, C.A., et al., Estimates of stability of daily wandering behavior among cognitively impaired long-term care residents, *Nurs. Res.*, 46, 172–178, 1997.
46. Martino-Saltzman, D., Blasch, B.B., Morris, R.D., et al., Travel behavior of nursing home residents perceived as wanderers and nonwanderers, *Gerontologist*, 31, 666–672, 1991.
47. LaPorte, R.E., Black-Sandler, R., Cauley, J.A., et al., The assessment of physical activity in older women: analysis of the interrelationship and reliability of activity monitoring, activity surveys, and caloric intake, *J. Gerontol.*, 38, 394–397, 1983.
48. Hays, L.M. and Clark, D.O., Correlates of physical activity in a sample of older adults with type 2 diabetes, *Diabetes Care*, 22, 706–712, 1999.
49. Keith, R.A., Granger, C.V., Hamilton, B.B., et al., The functional independence measure: a new tool for rehabilitation, *Adv. Clin. Rehabil.*, 1, 6–28, 1987.
50. Podsiadlo, D. and Richardson, S., The timed "Up and Go": a test of basic functional mobility for frail elderly persons, *J. Am. Geriatr. Soc.*, 39, 142–148, 1991.
51. Himann, J.E., D.A, C., Rechnitzer, P.A., et al., Age-related changes in speed of walking, *Med. Sci. Sports Exerc.*, 20, 161–166, 1988.
52. DiPietro, L., The epidemiology of physical activity and physical function in older adults, *Med. Sci. Sports Exerc.*, 28, 596–600, 1996.
53. Rantanen, T., Guralnik, J.M., Sakari-Rantala, R., et al., Disability, physical activity, and muscle strength in older women: the women's health and aging study, *Arch. Phys. Med. Rehabil.*, 80, 130–135, 1999.
54. Unger, J.G., Johnson, C.A., and Marks, G., Functional decline in the elderly: evidence for direct and stress-buffering protective effects of social interactions and physical activity, *Ann. Behav. Med.*, 19, 152–160, 1997.
55. Stuck, A.E., Walthert, J.M., Nikolaus, T., et al., Risk factors for functional status decline in community-living elderly people: a systematic literature review, *Soc. Sci. Med.*, 48, 445–469, 1999.
56. Rhodes, R.E., Martin, A.D., Taunton, J.E., et al., Factors associated with exercise adherence among older adults. An individual perspective, *Sports Med.*, 28, 397–411, 1999.
57. Shephard, R.J., Determinants of exercise in people aged 65 years and older, in *Advances in Exercise Adherence*, Dishman, R.K., Ed., Human Kinetics, Champaign, IL, 1994, 343–360.
58. King, A.C., Intervention strategies and determinants of physical activity and exercise behavior in adult and older adult men and women, *World. Rev. Nutr. Diet*, 82, 148–158, 1997.
59. Dishman, R.K., Motivating older adults to exercise, *South. Med. J.*, 87, S79–82, 1994.
60. Chogahara, M., Cousins, S.O.B., and Wankel, L.M., Social influences on physical activity in older adults: a review, *J. Aging Phys. Activity*, 6, 1–17, 1998.
61. Pinto, B.M., Marcus, B.H., and Clark, M.M., Promoting physical activity in women: the new challenges, *Am. J. Prev. Med.*, 12, 395–400, 1996.
62. Eyler, A.A., Brownson, R.C., King, A.C., et al., Physical activity and women in the U.S.: an overview of health benefits, prevalence, and intervention opportunities, *Wom. Health*, 26, 27–49, 1997.
63. Bandura, A., *Social Foundations of Thought and Action: A Social Cognitive Theory*, Prentice-Hall, Englewood Cliffs, NJ, 1986.

64. Dzewaltowski, D.A., A social cognitive theory of older adult exercise motivation, in *Aging and Motor Behavior*, Ostrow, A.C., Ed., Benchmark Press, Indianapolis, IN, 1989, 257–281.
65. McLeroy, K.R., Bibeau, D., Steckler, A., et al., An ecological perspective on health promotion programs, *Health Educ. Q*,. 15, 351–377, 1988.
66. Sallis, J.F., Bauman, A., and Pratt, M., Environmental and policy interventions to promote physical activity, *Am. J. Prev. Med.*, 15, 379–397, 1998.
67. Prochaska, J.O., DiClemente, C.C., and Norcross, J.C., In search of how people change. Applications to addictive behaviors, *Am. Psychol.*, 47, 1102–1114, 1992.
68. Prochaska, J.O. and Marcus, B.H., The transtheoretical model: applications to exercise, in *Advances in Exercise Adherence*, Dishman, R.K., Ed., Human Kinetics, Champaign, IL, 1994, 161–180.
69. Ajzen, I., The theory of planned behavior, *Organ. Behav. Hum. Decis. Process.*, 50, 179–211, 1991.
70. Blue, C.L., The predictive capacity of the theory of reasoned action and the theory of planned behavior in exercise research: an integrated literature review, *Res. Nurs. Health*, 18, 105–121, 1995.
71. Hausenblas, H.A., Carron, A.V., and Mack, D.E., Application of the theories of reasoned action and planned behavior to exercise behavior: a meta-analysis, *J. Sport Exerc. Psychol.*, 19, 36–51, 1997.
72. Godin, G. and Kok, G., The theory of planned behavior: a review of its applications to health-related behaviors, *Am. J. Health Promot.*, 11, 87–98, 1996.
73. Duda, J.L. and Tappe, M.K., Personal investment in exercise among middle-aged and older adults, in *Aging and Motor Behavior*, Ostrow, A.C., Ed., Benchmark Press, Indianapolis, IN, 1989, 219–238.
74. Maehr, M.L. and Braskamp, L.A., *The Motivation Factor: A Theory of Personal Investment*, Lexington Press, Lexington, MA, 1986.
75. Strecher, V.J. and Rosenstock, I.M., The health belief model, in *Health Behavior and Health Education. Theory, Research, and Practice*, Glanz, K., Lewis, F.M., and Rimer, B.K., Eds, Jossey-Bass, San Francisco, 1997, 41–59.
76. Lee, C., Factors related to the adoption of exercise among older women, *J. Behav. Med.*, 16, 323–334, 1993.
77. O'Brien, S.J. and Vertinsky, P.A., Elderly women, exercise and healthy aging, *J. Women Aging*, 2, 41–65, 1990.
78. O'Brien, S.J. and Vertinsky, P.A., Unfit survivors: exercise as a resource for aging women, *Gerontologist*, 31, 347–357, 1991.
79. Vertinsky, P.A., Stereotypes of aging women and exercise: a historical perspective, *J. Aging Phys. Activity*, 3, 223–237, 1995.
80. Cousins, S.O. and Vertinsky, P.A., Recapturing the physical activity experiences of the old: a study of three women, *J. Aging Phys. Activity*, 3, 146–162, 1995.
81. Cousins, S.O., Elderly tomboys? Sources of self-efficacy for physical activity in late life, *J. Aging Phys. Activity*, 5, 229–243, 1997.
82. Ebrahim, S. and Rowland, L., Towards a new strategy for health promotion for older women: determinants of physical activity, *Psychol. Health Med.*, 1, 29–40, 1996.
83. O'Neill, K. and Reid, G., Perceived barriers to physical activity by older adults, *Can. J. Publ. Health*, 82, 392–396, 1991.
84. Booth, M.L., Bauman, A., Owen, N., et al., Physical activity preferences, preferred sources of assistance, and perceived barriers to increased activity among physically inactive Australians, *Prev. Med.*, 26, 131–137, 1997.

85. Fitzgerald, J.T., Activity levels, fitness status, exercise knowledge, and exercise beliefs among healthy, older African American and white women, *J. Aging Health*, 6, 296–313, 1994.
86. Richter, D.L., Macera, C.A., Williams, H., et al., Disincentives to participation in planned exercise activities among older adults, *Health Values*, 17, 51–55, 1993.
87. Wilcox, S. and King, A.C., Self-favoring bias for physical activity in middle-aged and older adults, *J. Appl. Soc. Psychol.*, 30, 1773–1789, 2000.
88. Hausdorff, J.M., Levy, B.R., and Wei, J.Y., The power of ageism on physical function of older persons: reversibility of age-related gait changes, *J. Am. Geriatr. Soc.*, 47, 1346–1349, 1999.
89. Strecher, V.J., DeVellis, B.M., Becker, M.H., et al., The role of self-efficacy in achieving health behavior change, *Health Educ. Q.*, 13, 73–92, 1986.
90. Grembowski, D., Patrick, D., Diehr, P., et al., Self-efficacy and health behavior among older adults, *J. Health Soc. Behav.*, 34, 89–104, 1993.
91. Bandura, A., Self-efficacy: toward a unifying theory of behavioral change, *Psychol. Rev.*, 84, 191–215, 1977.
92. Scharff, D.P., Homan, S., Kreuter, M., et al., Factors associated with physical activity in women across the life span: implications for program development, *Wom. Health*, 29, 115–134, 1999.
93. Wilcox, S. and Storandt, M., Relations among age, exercise, and psychological variables in a community sample of women, *Health Psychol.*, 15, 110–113, 1996.
94. Clark, D.O. and Nothwehr, F., Exercise self-efficacy and its correlates among socioeconomically disadvantaged older adults, *Health Educ. Behav.*, 26, 535–546, 1999.
95. Courneya, K.S. and McAuley, E., Efficacy, attributional, and affective responses of older adults following an acute bout of exercise, *J. Soc. Behav. Personal.*, 8, 729–742, 1993.
96. Conn, V.S., Older women: social cognitive theory correlates of health behavior, *Wom. Health*, 26, 71–85, 1997.
97. Conn, V.S., Older adults and exercise: path analysis of self-efficacy related constructs, *Nurs. Res.*, 47, 180–189, 1998.
98. Ali, N.S. and Twibell, R.K., Health promotion and osteoporosis prevention among postmenopausal women, *Prev. Med.*, 24, 528–534, 1995.
99. Cousins, S.O., Exercise cognition among elderly women, *J. Appl. Sport Psychol.*, 8, 131–145, 1996.
100. Hovell, M.F., Sallis, J.F., Hofstetter, C.R., et al., Identifying correlates of walking for exercise: an epidemiologic prerequisite for physical activity promotion, *Prev. Med.*, 18, 856–866, 1989.
101. Wankel, L.M., Mummery, W.K., Stephens, T., et al., Prediction of physical activity intention from social psychological variables: results from the Campbell's survey of well-being, *J. Sport Exerc. Psychol.*, 16, 56–69, 1994.
102. McAuley, E., Lox, C., and Duncan, T.E., Long-term maintenance of exercise, self-efficacy, and physiological change in older adults, *J. Gerontol.*, 48, 218–224, 1993.
103. McAuley, E., Self-efficacy and the maintenance of exercise participation in older adults, *J. Behav. Med.*, 16, 103–113, 1993.
104. Brenes, G.A., Strube, M.J., and Storandt, M., An application of the theory of planned behavior to exercise among older adults, *J. Appl. Soc. Psychol.*, 28, 2274–2290, 1998.
105. McAuley, E., The role of efficacy cognitions in the prediction of exercise behavior in middle-aged adults, *J. Behav. Med.*, 15, 65–88, 1992.

106. Heaney, C.A. and Israel, B.A., Social networks and social support, in *Health Behavior and Health Education. Theory, Research, and Practice*, Glanz, K., Lewis, F.M., and Rimer, B.K., Eds., Jossey-Bass, San Francisco, 1997, 179–205.
107. Clark, D.O., Identifying psychological, physiological, and environmental barriers and facilitators to exercise among older low income adults, *J. Clin. Geropsychol.*, 5, 51–62, 1999.
108. Lian, W.M., Gan, G.L., Pin, C.H., et al., Correlates of leisure-time physical activity in an elderly population in Singapore, *Am. J. Publ. Health*, 89, 1578–1580, 1999.
109. Lee, C., Attitudes, knowledge, and stages of change: a survey of exercise patterns in older Australian women, *Health Psychol.*, 12, 476–480, 1993.
110. Oka, R.K., King, A.C., and Young, D.R., Sources of social support as predictors of exercise adherence in women and men ages 50 to 65 years, *Wom. Health: Res. Gender Behav. Policy*, 1, 161–175, 1995.
111. King, A.C., Castro, C., Wilcox, S., et al., Personal and environmental factors associated with physical inactivity among different racial–ethnic groups of U.S. middle-aged and older-aged women, *Health Psychol.*, 19, 354–364, 2000.
112. Wilcox, S., Castro, C., King, A.C., et al., Determinants of leisure time physical activity in rural compared with urban older and ethnically diverse women in the United States, *J. Epidemiol. Comm. Health*, 54, 667–672, 2000.
113. Eyler, A.A., Brownson, R.C., Donatelle, R.J., et al., Physical activity social support and middle- and older-aged minority women: results from a U.S. survey, *Soc. Sci. Med.*, 49, 781–789, 1999.
114. Conn, V.S., Older women's beliefs about physical activity, *Publ. Health Nurs.*, 15, 370–378, 1998.
115. Cousins, S.O., Social support for exercise among elderly women in Canada, *Health Prom. Int.*, 10, 273–282, 1995.
116. Marcus, B.H., Pinto, B.M., Clark, M.M., et al., Physician-delivered physical activity and nutrition interventions, *Med. Exerc. Nutr. Health*, 4, 325–334, 1995.
117. Courneya, K.S., Nigg, C.R., and Estabrooks, P.A., Relationships among the theory of planned behavior, stages of change, and exercise behavior in older persons over a three year period, *Psychol. Health*, 13, 355–367, 1998.
118. Michels, T.C. and Kugler, J.P., Predicting exercise in older Americans: using the theory of planned behavior, *Mil. Med.*, 163, 524–529, 1998.
119. Satariano, W.A., Haight, T.J., and Tager, I.B., Reasons given by older people for limitation or avoidance of leisure time physical activity, *J. Am. Geriatr. Soc.*, 48, 505–512, 2000.
120. Wilcox, S., King, A.C., Brassington, G.S., et al., Physical activity preferences of middle-aged and older adults: a community analysis, *J. Aging Phys. Activity*, 7, 386–399, 1999.
121. McPhillips, J.B., Pellettera, K.M., Barrett-Connor, E., et al., Exercise patterns in a population of older adults, *Am. J. Prev. Med.*, 5, 65–72, 1989.
122. King, A.C., Haskell, W.L., Young, D.R., et al., Long-term effects of varying intensities and formats of physical activity on participation rates, fitness, and lipoproteins in men and women aged 50 to 65 years, *Circulation*, 91, 2596–2604, 1995.
123. King, A.C., Pruitt, L.A., Phillips, W., et al., Comparative effects of two physical activity programs on measured and perceived physical functioning and other health-related quality of life outcomes in older adults, *J. Gerontol.*, 55, M74–M83, 2000.

124. Caserta, M.S. and Gillett, P.A., Older women's feelings about exercise and their adherence to an aerobic regimen over time, *Gerontologist,* 38, 602–609, 1998.
125. Eyler, A.A., Baker, E., Cromer, L., et al., Physical activity and minority women: a qualitative study, *Health. Educ. Behav.,* 25, 640–652, 1998.
126. Jones, M. and Nies, M.A., The relationship of perceived benefits of and barriers to reported exercise in older African American women, *Publ. Health Nurs.,* 13, 151–158, 1996.
127. Gill, K. and Overdorf, V., Incentives for exercise in younger and older women, *J. Sport Behav.,* 17, 87–97, 1994.
128. Schneider, J.K., Self-regulation and exercise behavior in older women, *J. Gerontol.,* 52, P235–P241, 1997.
129. Neff, K. and King, A.C., Exercise program adherence in older adults: the importance of achieving one's expected benefits, *Med. Exerc. Nutr. Health,* 4, 355–362, 1995.
130. Elward, K., Larson, E., and Wagner, E., Factors associated with regular aerobic exercise in an elderly population, *J. Am. Board Fam. Pract.,* 5, 467–474, 1992.
131. Ettinger, W.H., Jr., Burns, R., Messier, S.P., et al., A randomized trial comparing aerobic exercise and resistance exercise with a health education program in older adults with knee osteoarthritis. The fitness, arthritis, and seniors trial (FAST), *JAMA,* 277, 25–31, 1997.
132. Howland, J., Lachman, M.E., Peterson, E.W., et al., Covariates of fear of falling and associated activity curtailment, *Gerontologist,* 38, 549–555, 1998.
133. Cousins, S.O., "My heart couldn't take it": Older women's beliefs about exercise benefits and risks, *J. Gerontol.,* 55B, P283–P294, 2000.
134. Courneya, K.S., Understanding readiness for regular physical activity in older individuals: an application of the theory of planned behavior, *Health Psychol.,* 14, 80–87, 1995.
135. Dean, K., Relationships between knowledge and belief variables and health maintenance behaviors in a Danish population over 45 years of age, *J. Aging. Health,* 3, 386–406, 1991.
136. Morrow, J.R., Jr., Jackson, A.W., Bazzarre, T.L., et al., A one-year follow-up to physical activity and health. A report of the surgeon general, *Am. J. Prev. Med.,* 17, 24–30, 1999.

3

Constitution or Environment? The Basis of Regional and Ethnic Differences in the Interactions among Gender, Age, and Functional Capacity

Roy J. Shephard

CONTENTS

0-8493-1027-X/02/$0.00+$1.50

3.1 Introduction

The preventive and therapeutic advances of recent years have shifted the causes of morbidity and mortality in most developed societies from early problems of acute infection to chronic disease in old age, a process that has been termed a "squaring" of the mortality curve. Determinants of susceptibility to chronic disease include genetic factors, environment, and personal lifestyle, as well as the intrinsic aging process.[76] Substantial regional and ethnic differences remain in the overall course of aging and in the apparent impact of gender, environment, and personal lifestyle upon morbidity and mortality as age advances. Such differences offer a potential window through which one may examine the intriguing question of whether gender differences in susceptibility to chronic disease and the preventive action of regular physical activity (Chapter 11) are entirely the expression of immutable, genetically coded constitutional differences, or whether the choice of a particular environment or lifestyle can optimize the aging process for men or women.

The ecological/anthropological/evolutionary argument is that humans have adapted to the lifestyle of the "primitive" hunter-gatherer or agriculturalist over the course of many centuries. Part of this adaptation has been cultural, but through the process of natural selection there has also been a substantial genetic adaptation. Thus, neolithic patterns of physical activity (long periods of moderately intense exercise during at least the first half of adult life) may be optimal for human health and survival.[212] In apparent support of this hypothesis, an abnormally large proportion of centenarians was reported among certain isolated populations where "primitive" patterns of agriculture persisted. These groups including the Vilcabambans (in the Ecuadorian Andes), the Hunza community in the Himalayas, and inhabitants of the mountainous regions of rural Georgia.[128]

In principle, any regional, ethnic, or gender-related differences in morbidity and mortality seem likely to reflect the influence of both genes and environment, together with interactions between these two factors. Nevertheless, the genetically vulnerable tend to die prematurely, so the relative importance of environment increases with age.[82] The respective impacts of genetic and environmental influences upon the aging process will be reviewed, and some reported regional and ethnic differences in gender-specific rates of aging will then be examined.

3.2 Genetic Factors Influencing the Aging Process

The adaptive value of aging, gender differences in longevity, formal studies of twins and other family members, and the identification of aging genes all point to a substantial impact of constitution upon aging, quality of life, and longevity. Comparative studies show a rapid increase of life span as organisms move through the evolutionary scale. Based on the rapidity of this change, it has been suggested that the number of genes regulating the overall process is relatively small.[83] Presumably, the role of these genes is to moderate and synchronize the pace of decay in key biological systems vital to survival of the organism.

3.2.1 Adaptive Value of Aging

Evolutionary principles suggest that the emergence of a particular characteristic depends upon its adaptive value to a species. Some authors argue that prolonged survival is a negative adaptation and, for this reason, development through natural selection is unlikely. Particularly in "primitive" cultures, where food supplies are precarious, human survival beyond the normal years of reproduction could have an adverse impact upon the prospects of other family members. Rapid aging and early death minimize the competition between a forbear and its offspring.[195] Early death also increases population turnover, and thus could benefit a community by promoting genetic drift.[31]

The extension of survival into the postreproductive years is a unique and puzzling characteristic of humans.[241] However, a long life span could have positive adaptive value if it were linked to some other trait that conferred success in mating or rearing of children.[212] For example, large strength or aerobic power in a young male might be attractive to fertile females, and at the same time enhance survival prospects in old age. Likewise, functional capacity allowing life in an extreme environment might allow a population of fertile age to avoid dangerous predators. Prolonged survival could also have intrinsic value to the development of a community if it allowed grandparents to teach important skills to subsequent generations.[131]

Horiuchi[99] has pointed to gender differences in patterns of age-related functional losses and longevity. In women, functional losses accelerate with the distinct end point of menopause, but in men the process begins at a later age, and develops more gradually, as does the decline of fecundity.[99] Nevertheless, average longevity is less for males than for females. The adaptive value of a gender difference in longevity is difficult to explain in evolutionary terms. One suggestion has been that there is less "need" for the gender with a higher rate of reproductive activity (the male) to invest in body maintenance;[242] so men die at a younger age than women. However, the majority

TABLE 3.1

Difference in Life Expectancy at Birth between Males and Females in Various Countries, Based on Statistics for 1990, 1950, and 1990

Country	1900	1950	1990
Australia	3.5 (6.6)	5.1 (7.6)	6.3 (8.6)
Canada	4.5 (6.8)	—	6.7 (9.0)
England/Wales	3.7 (7.9)	4.9 (7.4)	5.9 (8.0)
France	3.4 (7.5)	5.7 (8.9)	8.5 (11.5)
Hungary	1.6 (4.1)	4.1 (6.9)	8.2 (12.2)
Japan	1.5 (3.5)	3.5 (5.9)	5.7 (7.5)
Spain	1.8 (5.3)	4.5 (7.5)	6.8 (9.1)
Sweden	2.5 (4.7)	2.7 (3.9)	6.0 (8.0)
Switzerland	2.8 (6.1)	4.4 (6.6)	7.4 (9.8)
United States	2.8 (5.8)	5.7 (8.6)	6.9 (9.6)
Mean	2.6 (5.7)	4.5 (7.0)[a]	6.8 (9.3)[b]
SD	0.81 (1.48)	0.93 (1.41)	0.95 (1.52)

Note: Figures show absolute advantage of the female, and in parentheses the percentage advantage.

[a] Absolute difference from 1900 statistically significant; percentage difference approaching statistical significance.

[b] Both absolute and percentage difference from 1900 and 1950 statistically significant.

of men die after their reproductive contribution has ceased; a more plausible argument might be that, in general, they make a smaller contribution to family welfare as grandparents.

Natural selection has progressively less impact on survival prospects as the age of an individual increases [257], because there is an age-related increase in the likelihood of death from acquired mutations[68] and other more direct environmental dangers (predators, disease, accidents, and starvation). Apparently, "successful" reproduction at an advanced age may have an adverse effect on the long-term prospects of a community by allowing the transmission of acquired genetic abnormalities to subsequent generations. Gavrilov et al.[67] noted that, among European aristocrats, an advanced paternal age (50 to 59 years) shortened the life span of female offspring by an average of 4.4 years. They hypothesized that, in this closed community, crucial housekeeping genes sensitive to mutational load were being transmitted through the paternal X-chromosome.

3.2.2 Gender Differences in Longevity

Official statistics show that women have had a substantially longer average survival than men in all countries of the world throughout the past century (Table 3.1). Although genetic factors may account for some of the gender differential, sex differences in traditional social roles, lifestyle, and behavior are major and possibly dominant factors. One recent modification of the traditional Gompertzian analysis concluded that the genetic influence upon age-specific mortality was essentially similar in men and women.[187]

From a biological perspective, women have an inherent advantage, since the presence of two X-chromosomes in female tissues allows some cells to compensate for the biosynthetic deficiencies of others. Moreover, cell selection in women proceeds according to which X-chromosome is active, allowing an optimal development of the organism in terms of cell viability and proliferative capacity.[220] The extent to which this in-built, constitutional difference influences aging, morbidity, and mortality seems likely to depend on the level of stress to which the individual is exposed, and thus the need for tissue repair. In other words, one should anticipate a substantial gene–environment interaction.

Sex differences in life span are shown by many animal species.[41,102,153] In general, the female lives longer, but this is not invariably the case; moreover, many animal studies have not considered the issue of survival to an advanced age.[219] Further, the common causes of death differ between animals and humans, so animal data cannot be extrapolated directly to the human situation. Relative to their male peers, human females show less vulnerability to many of the principal causes of death (Chapter 11); this advantage is seen from an early age.[120] In 1990, the gender difference in average life span at birth ranged from 5.9 to 8.2 years across various developed nations (Table 3.1).

Lifestyle and other environmental factors plainly modulate any underlying effect of constitution, since gender discrepancy increased very substantially in almost all countries during the first two thirds of the 20th century (Table 3.1). In the U.S., for example, the gender differential increased from 5.8% in 1900 to 9.6% in 1990. There are large regional differences of morbidity and mortality within many countries. In Great Britain, the largest and widening gender differentials have been observed in economically deprived areas, where both men and women die at a relatively early age.[181] Similarly, in Canada the gender gap in life span widens by 4 years from areas with the highest quintile of incomes to areas in the lowest quintile.[1] The importance of economic influences is supported by a narrowing of the sex differential in life expectancy at birth in 12 industrialized nations as average living standards have improved since the early 1970s.[124,125,232,244]

Gains in life expectancy during the present century have been much larger in women than in men.[206,236] Thus, a large fraction of the elderly population and an even larger fraction of those who are very old are now women. Part of the gender difference reflects the fact that, until recently, women in most countries were not eligible for front-line military service, with its associated high mortality. Up till now, women have also sustained fewer premature deaths from lung cancer and myocardial infarction,[250] reflecting both the protective action of estrogens against cardiovascular disease and historic differentials in cigarette consumption. Prior to menopause, the risk of sudden death during a bout of vigorous physical activity is ten times greater in men than in women.[194] On the other hand, body fat content is substantially greater in women than in men; this has several adverse consequences for health and longevity: (1) it changes the pathway of estradiol metabolism, increasing the formation of carcinogenic 16-hydroxylation products;[63] (2) it decreases estradiol binding, particularly after menopause;[119,123] and (3) it increases the potential for conversion of estrogens to more potent carcinogens.[216] Thus, women are vulnerable to premature death from breast and reproductive tract cancers.

Secular changes in mortality from specific conditions have differed between the two sexes. For instance, in the U.S., the decline in stroke mortality between 1951 and 1986 was 52% in men, but only 31% in women.[187] At least some of these secular changes reflect a decreased prevalence of cigarette smoking among men, and an increased prevalence in women (see later discussion).

Although women currently have a much longer average survival than men, many aspects of function such as aerobic power and muscular strength deteriorate at a similar absolute rate in the two sexes (Chapters 4 through 6). Thus, women face a substantially longer period than men when their level of function is insufficient to undertake instrumental and other activities of daily living[43,210,224] (see Chapter 5). Indeed, their active life expectancy[112] may be no greater than that of their male counterparts. Already, among Canadians aged 55 to 64 years, 31% of women have noted some limitation of physical activity, compared with 25% of men.[40] In those over the age of 65 years, the corresponding figures are 37% and 31%.[88] In the U.S., the total number of disabled life years averages 10.8 years for men and 14.0 years for women,[223] and in some countries the gender discrepancy in chronic disability is even larger.

3.2.3 Twin and Family Studies of Longevity and Functional Loss

Early life insurance statistics suggested the importance of family history as a determinant of longevity. Dublin et al.[52] noted a strong association between the life span of parents and that of their immediate male offspring. Likewise, Vaillant[237] found that the longevity of parents and grandparents was a strong predictor of a person's risk of chronic illness at the age of 60 years, and of mortality by the age of 68 years.

Nevertheless, a history of early death within a given family could reflect either an adverse genetic characteristic such as a familial hypertrophic cardiomyopathy[140] or hemophilia,[32] or a familial concentration of undesirable behavior patterns such as cigarette smoking, overeating, and lack of physical activity. Moreover, findings concerning the predictive value of family history are far from uniform. In a 25-year follow-up of 2370 civil servants, Vandenbroucke et al.[240] found parental survival was only a weak predictor of mortality in men (odds ratio 0.63), although it was a stronger predictor in women (odds ratio 0.36). Likewise, van Doorn and Kasl[239] found no influence of parental longevity on the 3-year mortality of 70-year-old Australians.

Comparisons between the life spans of monozygotic and dizygotic twins[36] provide more convincing evidence that genes affect survival prospects — for instance, by influencing susceptibility to sudden, premature cardiac death.[251] The classic study of Kallman and Sander[110] showed that, if identical twins died between the ages of 60 and 75 years, the average interpair difference in age at death was 47.6 months for males and 24.0 months for females. In the case of nonidentical twins, the corresponding interpair differences were 107.9 and 88.7 months. Hayakawa et al.[86] also found a closer similarity of life span in monozygous than in dizygous twins (respective discordances, 6.7 and 8.7 years).

Nevertheless, a concordance of age at death among identical twin pairs is not conclusive proof of a genetic effect. It remains arguable that identical twins are exposed to more closely comparable environmental influences than dissimilar twins, or that identical twins experience a greater grief-related mortality if their twin dies. The residual gender discordance of age at death among identical twins supports the viewpoint that environment has a substantial effect. Further, Jarvik et al.[107] found that the difference in concordance of age at death between heterozygous and homozygous twins diminished as the age at death increased. Presumably, the cumulative effects of environment relative to constitution increased as individuals became older.

McGue et al.[148] examined the longevity of 218 monozygotic and 382 dizygotic twin pairs who were born in Denmark between 1870 and 1880. The similarity of age at death was statistically significant in monozygotic but not dizygotic twins. The heritability (h^2) of life span was estimated at 0.333 ± 0.058, with no difference between genders. Herskind et al.[92] completed a 28-year follow-up of 2464 Danish twins born between 1890 and 1920. The proportions of variance due to genetic and environmental influences were analyzed by covariance matrices, using a structural equation approach. They concluded that most of the genetic component of survival was effected through a direct influence upon viability, with only a very small part being mediated through genetic influences upon other determinants of health such as smoking behavior and body mass index.

Iachine et al.[101] applied the maximum likelihood technique to determine the relative contributions of constitution and environment to frailty in 31,000 pairs of twins from Denmark, Sweden, and Finland. The narrow-sense heritability of frailty was estimated at 0.5. Hayakawa et al.[86] examined two commonly used measures of aging (hair-graying and presbyopia), finding greater similarities in monozygous than in dizygous twins. Finkel et al.[62] assessed the biological age of 140 monozygous and 97 dizygous twin pairs from three groups of measures: physiological variables, cognitive abilities, and processing speed. Their estimates of heritability varied greatly among the three components of biological age.

A number of twin studies have looked at specific risk factors for premature death. A longitudinal examination of 630 women (185 monozygotic and 130 dizygotic twin pairs) concluded that, over a 10-year interval between average ages of 41 and 51 years, genetic factors influenced the extent of increases in body-mass index.[11] A cross-sectional analysis of body-mass and body mass index based on 586 monozygotic and 447 like-sex dizygotic twin pairs concluded that the additive genetic component of variance in this aspect of body composition remained stable over the age range from 18 to 81 years, but the environmental component increased. The heritability of body mass thus decreased from 0.86 in the youngest to 0.70 in the oldest individuals examined, with corresponding figures of 0.82 and 0.63 for body-mass index [37]. A study of 322 twin pairs noted significant gender differences in the heritability of waist to hip ratio and waist circumference, with respective values of 28% and 46% in males, and 48% and 66% in females.[162] Bouchard and Després[29] estimated that, after standardizing their data for age, gender, and overall body fatness, 32% of intersubject variation in the cardiac risk from a centripetal distribution of fat was attributable to sociocultural inheritance, and 25% to genetic inheritance. Computed tomography data from 382 members of the Quebec family study suggested that an autosomal recessive gene accounted for a substantial fraction of visceral fat.[30] Heller et al.[90] compared serum lipids in 302 twin pairs, 146 of which were separated at an early age. Genetic factors had a substantial impact on total cholesterol, HDL-cholesterol, triglycerides, and apolipoproteins A-1 and B, although no single factor could be identified that influenced all components of the lipid profile. A shared home environment contributed to the phenotypic correlations of total cholesterol and apolipoprotein B, but not to other components of the lipid profile. A similarly designed study looked at the insulin resistance syndrome in 289 twin pairs aged 66 years, 140 of which were apart.[97] It was concluded that a single latent genetic factor influenced all five components of the syndrome (body-mass index, insulin resistance, triglycerides, HDL-cholesterol, and systolic blood pressure). The upper limits of heritability for systolic and diastolic pressures were 0.44 and 0.34, respectively, but shared family effects contributed 27% of the variance in resting blood pressures.[96]

McClearn and associates[146] examined lung function in 230 twin pairs of average age 65 years, some of whom had been reared apart. Allowance was made for smoking habits in terms of pack-years. Heritability estimates were 0.48 for vital capacity and 0.67 for one-second forced expiratory volume.

The genetic influence on cognitive abilities was tested in 80 same-sex twin pairs over the age of 80 years.[145] Resemblance was consistently greater for identical than for fraternal twins. Heritability estimates were 62% for cognitive ability, 55% for verbal ability, 32% for spatial ability, 62% for speed of mental processing, and 52% for memory. Locus of control was evaluated in 554 twin pairs, some of whom were reared apart. Two of the three components of locus of control (life direction and responsibility) showed a heritability of 30%;[172] likewise, genetic factors contributed to perceptions of the adequacy of social support.[20,21] Another study involving adopted twins noted substantial genetic effects on emotionality, activity level, and sociability, all of which could influence survival in later life.[179]

There is thus considerable evidence of a genetic influence on risk factors for premature death, but a linkage to the sex chromosomes is less clearly established.

3.2.4 Aging Genes

Although some authors do not like to use the term "biological clock" when describing the aging of body tissues,[184] many investigators believe that the human genome modulates a number of mechanisms regulating the rate of loss of function in key cell populations.[69] Aging seems associated with a progressive repression of growth-stimulating genes, an increased expression of growth-inhibiting genes, a failure of repair processes, and a progressive build up of metabolic errors. These changes are associated with a depletion of key enzymes such as those dealing with reactive species.[73,196,235]

Gene variants may either accelerate or slow the rate of functional loss. Variants that speed the rate of aging have, in essence, escaped the forces of natural selection,[141] presumably because their effects only become manifest late in life. Little is known about variants that favor a prolonged life span. In *Drosophila*, certain mutations can accelerate aging,[78] and, conversely, artificial selection can extend the survival of this species by as much as 50%.[6] Likewise, selection for a small body size can increase the survival of dogs,[156] and single mutations can increase the life span of laboratory mice by as much as 50%.[75] However, critics of such studies have pointed out that inbreeding is an artificial situation, and that, in such circumstances, the offspring tend to live longer than either parent, irrespective of selection criteria. Hybridization of animals increases their life span, although at the same time it reduces the influence of genes relative to environmental factors.[102] Under natural conditions, hybridization occurs, and an unusual longevity presumably reflects a high resistance to various forms of environmental stress. Conversely, it seems likely that, in our modern human society, limited exposure to environmental stressors is reducing the likelihood that resistant individuals will be selected.[169]

Some authors have argued for the existence of specific human senescence loci — for example, on chromosome I between 1q12 and 1q31, and between 1q42–43.[243] However, the major effect of genotype is probably in terms of increasing an individual's susceptibility to various causes of disability and premature death. Examples include the genes modulating obesity[29] and thus the risk of diabetes mellitus,[178] cardiovascular disease,[136] chronic chest disease,[137,197] osteoporosis,[19] various forms of cancer,[9,54,218] Parkinson's disease[226] and Alzheimer's disease.[185,225] The likelihood that a given constitutional disadvantage will impair the quality of life and/or shorten an individual's life span depends strongly on the interaction between genes and environment. For example, people with familial hypertrophic cardiomyopathy who are moderately active may survive to an advanced age, whereas others who engage in vigorous competitive sports may die as young adults.[211] Likewise,

TABLE 3.2

Genes Implicated in the Aging Process

Gene	Species	Function	Ref.
hic-5	Human fibroblasts	Cellular senescence	214
clk-1	Mouse and human	Biosynthesis of ubiquinone in heart and skeletal muscle	8
p66shc	Mouse	Increases susceptibility to ultraviolet light and oxidants	154
APP/RK transgene	Mouse	Amyloid processing; APP/RK mice die prematurely with neurodegeneration and apoptosis	158
CYP2D6, NAT-2, CYP2E1	41 nonagenarians vs. 217 healthy adults	Metabolism of xenobiotics; no differences of genotype in elderly	4
TP53 mutations	Families with Li-Fraumeni syndrome	Cell cycle control, genomic stability, susceptibility to DNA damage and cancer	33
J mtDNA hablogroup	212 centenarians vs. 275 subjects	Frequency of J hablogroup higher HG1-14	45
TGF-beta	287 postmenopausal women	Synthesis of TGF-beta and thus risk of osteoporosis	252
Presenilin genes PS1, PS2		Metabolism of amyloid beta-protein; mutations associated with premature Alzheimer's disease, apoptosis	225 249 28 248
C677T point mutation	224 healthy adults, 75 coronary disease, 63 peripheral vasc. dis.	Metabolizes homocysteine; related to longevity but not cardiovascular disease	231
APO AIV (360:His) Allele	120 Alzheimer patients, 119 healthy elderly	Presence of gene associated with longevity, but unrelated to Alzheimer's disease	152
APO A-IV (Hinf1347; Fnu4H1360; VNTR)	Centenarians vs. normal adults	Hinfl genotypes differ in centenarians; lower HDL-cholesterol	174
APO E-2	1068 non-institutionalized adults >64 years, not on lipid-lowering drugs	Reduces LDL- and Total/LDL-cholesterol; prevalence of genotype Afro-American> Hispanic>Caucasian	165
APO E-2	253 Italians	Trend to lower LDL- and total/HDL cholesterol with APO E-2 genotype; no relation to CV disease or dementia	12
APO E variation	1988 multigenerational pedigrees, ages 5–90 yr	Heritability greatest in young adults	256
APO E-4; ACE	338 centenarians vs. adults 20–70	APO E-4 less prevalent in centenarians; paradoxically ACE variant predisposing to atherosclerosis more common	204
APO E-2, APO C-1 ACE, methylenetetrahydrofolate reductase	182 F, 100 M .84 yr s., 100 F and 100 M <17 yr	Apo C-I linked to longevity in F but not in M; ACE I/I depleted in M elderly, but not F	66
APO E-4	1316 M, 246 F aged 20–108 yr	Longevity negatively related to APO E-4	108

TABLE 3.2 (continued)
Genes Implicated in the Aging Process

Gene	Species	Function	Ref.
APO E-4	5888 adults >65 yr	Association of APO E-4 with atherosclerosis or diabetes accelerates cognitive decline	80 185
ACE genotype	249 type I diabetics, 162 control	ACE genotype influences survival in diabetes, but not nephropathy	93
ACE D/D genotype	French centenarians vs. controls	Unclear; no sex difference, prevalence of D/D phenotype in centenarians unrelated to cardiovascular risk	57 2
ACE D/D genotype	210 patients with diabetes mellitus	D/D genotype linked to risk of insulin dependent diabetes	178
HLA-DRBI, HLA-DQ	Okinawan centenarians	Alleles of these genes influence MHC, and thus immune response and longevity	5
HLA-DRBI	533 centenarians vs. 163 nonagenarian siblings	DR7 frequency elevated in men DR11 increased in women, DR 13 increased in centenarians of both sexes	105
HLA-B40, HLA-DR5	964 adults >85 yr	HLA-B40 lower, HLA-DR5 higher in elderly. Differences more marked in women; unrelated to diseases	126
HLA-DR53	432 healthy subjects	HLA-DR53 negatively associated with longevity, predisposes to leukemia	49
delta F508 deletion	112 cystic fibrosis families	Influences susceptibility to cystic fibrosis	197
fas/fasL1 and bax	Isolated lymphocytes from young and older subjects	Promotion of apoptosis	3

the adverse health effects of genetic susceptibility to chronic obstructive lung disease[137] and lung cancer[54,218] are most likely to be revealed if there has been prolonged exposure to cigarette smoke or other air pollutants.

Formal analysis of critical gene combinations is complicated by the polygenic nature of the processes regulating aging.[230] Some of the relevant genes are listed in Table 3.2. In humans, there is good evidence that genes influence the synthesis of apolipoproteins and, thus, the risk of an adverse lipid profile and atherosclerosis. Specific insertion/deletion polymorphism also influences the activity of angiotensin-converting enzyme[57,66] and survival in patients with type I diabetes mellitus.[93] However, with the exception of specific cardiomyopathies, linkages between cardiovascular death and ACE or apolipoprotein genotype are less well established.[12,57,66,126,161,231]

A gene that influences the synthesis of transforming growth factor-beta affects the risk of osteoporosis.[252] Mutations of the presenilin genes PS1 and PS2 are associated with the early onset of Alzheimer's disease.[225] Other genes are known to influence susceptibility to cystic fibrosis,[197] and the formation of enzymes that can help in processing carcinogens[4] and other DNA-damaging agents,[33,154] although a specific link between genotype and susceptibility to neoplasms has been demonstrated less consistently. Finally, specific gene combinations influence the HLA/MHC component of the immune response and thus an individual's resistance to disease and neoplasia.[5,49,91,105,126]

Thus, good evidence exists that constitutional factors underlie the aging process, although the extent of interactions with gender is less clearly established. Moreover, the precise impact of genetic factors upon vulnerability to major diseases and thus prognosis remains to be clarified and, in most populations, a broad range of environmental and lifestyle factors have played an important role in modulating genetic predispositions to early morbidity and mortality.

3.3 Influences of Environment and Lifestyle upon the Aging Process

Exposure to a stressful environment or adoption of an adverse lifestyle may modify survival in its own right, and may also reveal an inherent weakness of genotype. Further, in a more long-term perspective, it may encourage the emergence of a new genotype that enhances prognosis in the face of an adverse environment. Gender differences in either exposure or susceptibility to a hostile environment or an adverse lifestyle contribute to differences in patterns of disability and mortality between men and women.

3.3.1 Effects of Environmental Stressors

The immediate environment, physical, biological, and psychological, can have either a positive or negative influence upon an individual's ability to cope with a given level of disability, thus affecting the overall quality of life.

Adaptations of the home environment and the introduction of assistive technology can do much to reduce the difficulties that elderly people experience when living independently. Such innovations have a substantial short-term cost, but there are long-term savings through a reduced need for long-term expenditures on institutional care.[139] For example, a study of 800 Finns aged 65 to 84 years showed that difficulties in getting about outdoors were more common in women than in men, but such difficulties could also be greatly reduced by simple environmental modifications.[198]

3.3.1.1 Physical Stressors

Elderly individuals react adversely to a number of potential physical stressors, including extremes of heat and cold and low oxygen pressures.

Hot weather. Hot weather increases demand for blood flow to the skin, and thus augments the cardiovascular load associated with a given intensity of physical activity. The level of stress experienced in any particular environment also depends on the fraction of maximal oxygen intake utilized and, partly for this reason, older people have poor tolerance of exercise in the heat.[114] Impaired regulation of skin blood flow and an accumulation of subcutaneous fat exacerbate the problem, as do many age-associated pathologies (for instance, hypertension, diabetes mellitus, and cardiovascular insufficiency).[113,116-118] The central drive to sweating is similar to that seen in a young adult,[103,104] but there is a reduction in sweat rate with aging.[103,104] This reflects decreased sensitivity of the glands to cholinergic stimuli and/or sluggish vasodilatation, and it may also be linked to the age-related decrease in maximal oxygen intake.[51,85]

In the southern U.S., heat waves are associated with increased death rates in the oldest members of the community.[114,117] Nevertheless, the vascular regulation of such individuals can be improved by an exercise program,[229] and it remains unclear how far a lack of physical conditioning, obesity, and cardiovascular disease are responsible for physiological and clinical problems experienced by the frail elderly under hot conditions.

Disagreement on the extent of gender differences in heat tolerance[50,51] reflects difficulties in matching subjects for body size and aerobic fitness (Chapter 1). If the environment permits heat exchange, women tend to be helped by a larger body surface/body mass ratio; on the other hand, a smaller body mass reduces their potential for heat storage in conditions where external heat loss is restricted. Lower maximal oxygen intake and a thicker layer of subcutaneous fat also increase a woman's vulnerability relative to a man's, and heat-related deaths thus tend to be more common in women than in men.

Cold weather. Very cold weather also poses a challenge to the elderly. In physiological terms, the zone of thermal comfort seems similar for young and elderly individuals, but slower perceptions of body cooling and less rapid adjustment of indoor heating systems contribute to poorer tolerance of cold conditions among older individuals.[39]

Under cold conditions, cutaneous vasoconstriction increases both preloading and afterloading of the heart. These changes increase the cardiac work rate, and thus the risk of a cardiac catastrophe. The problem is compounded because snow and ice increase the energy cost of common activities such as walking.[53] Specific winter tasks such as shoveling wet snow and pushing stalled vehicles can impose a heavy isometric load upon the heart. Most authors accept that the performance of such tasks predisposes the vulnerable older individual with coronary atherosclerosis to sudden cardiac death during periods of severe cold and heavy snowfall.[10,13,27,55,70,208] Nevertheless, some moderately sized studies have found no significant correlations between snowfall and the incidence of cardiac emergencies.[71,176]

The likelihood of sudden cardiac death under severe winter conditions is greater in men than in women, in part because tasks such as snow shoveling are usually deputed to men, and in part because men have a greater likelihood of pre-existing coronary vascular disease. Although older individuals face the apparent disadvantage of lower maximal aerobic power when shoveling snow, in fact, most people adjust their rate of shoveling so that they use between 60 and 68% of their personal maximal oxygen intake.[207]

If clothing is inadequate, cutaneous vasodilatation is induced by consumption of alcohol, or if the weather is extremely cold, death can arise from hypothermia. An age-related sarcopenia decreases both body insulation and the ability to generate heat by vigorous physical activity and shivering.[115] Elderly women are more vulnerable to loss of muscle than men and they also have a greater surface area to mass ratio; however, a greater adiposity may provide a compensating increase of thermal insulation, and exposure to cold tends to differ between men and women. Thus no convincing evidence exists of inherent, constitutional differences in the risk of hypothermia between men and women.

High altitudes. The low partial pressures of oxygen encountered at high altitudes theoretically increase the risk that physical activity will precipitate a heart attack, particularly in older individuals.[159] A study of elderly people who traveled to moderate altitudes typical of many ski resorts (2500 m) found that myocardial ischemia developed at lower work rates than at sea level.[130] Nevertheless, there is no great increase in the prevalence of electrocardiographic abnormalities at moderate altitudes,[253] and the morbidity rate remains low.[79,81] Moreover, adaptation to high altitudes quickly reduces both the risk of cardiac arrhythmias[150] and the extent of myocardial necrosis following infarction.[234]

The extent of any gender differences in cardiac risks at high altitude depends on the nature of the task to be undertaken. If body mass is to be displaced, as when walking or climbing, then men and women are likely to use rather similar fractions of their peak aerobic power, and any difference in the incidence of cardiac catastrophes reflects the greater prevalence of atherosclerosis in men. However, if a given amount of heavy external work must be performed, then the typical woman must use a larger fraction of her maximal aerobic power, which tends to offset any advantage she may have gained from a lesser likelihood of advanced atherosclerosis.

Air pollutants. Exposure to air pollutants progressively increases the accumulation of mitochondrial DNA mutations, and in those over the age of 40 years such mutations make a substantial contribution to the aging of lung tissues.[56]

Physical activity necessarily increases exposure to polluted air, both by increasing ventilation and by causing mouth or oro-nasal breathing. Women typically have a smaller respiratory minute volume than men, and thus inhale smaller quantities of pollutants even when they engage in equally intense activity. Against this apparent advantage, the inhaled pollutants act on a smaller volume of pulmonary tissue, so that no substantial gender difference in the response to air pollutants may be anticipated.

3.3.1.2 Biological Stressors

The impact of biological stressors on the prospects for health and survival depends on the likelihood of exposure to noxious agents and the resistance of the host.

Some isolated communities rarely encounter a new microorganism; in the short term, there is a corresponding decrease in the risk of infectious disease.[212] However, if a new microorganism is introduced into such a community (as, for example, with a measles epidemic that afflicted the Inuit of Arctic Canada), it can have devastating effects.[94] The likelihood of infection within a community is increased by contact with small children, thus placing women at greater inherent risk than men.

In terms of host resistance, the risks of infection are augmented by abnormalities of genotype that depress the overall immune response (discussed earlier). In the specific case of tuberculosis, the risk of developing an active disease depends also on body calcium reserves, thus augmenting the risk for pregnant and lactating women. In many conditions, the risk that disease will cause death is influenced ultimately by functional reserves of the cardiorespiratory system.

Vulnerability to many other disabling and fatal illnesses is influenced by gender. Perhaps the most obvious example is cardiovascular disease, where, in men, the adverse effects of cigarette smoking (discussed later) and a lack of estrogens[109] may be supplemented by a greater increase in blood pressure during exercise.[163] Likewise, men are more vulnerable to Parkinson's disease than women, although if women acquire this condition, it appears to reduce their life expectancy to that of their male peers.[48] Many of the conditions to which men seem more susceptible (for example, chronic bronchitis, lung cancer, and peptic ulcer) are heavily influenced by the habit of cigarette smoking.[151] Nevertheless, even after adjusting for smoking habits, myocardial ischemia and peptic ulcer still seem to be more frequent in men than in women, whereas cholecystectomy, intermittent claudication, and hypertension are more prevalent in women.[151]

3.3.1.3 Psychological Stressors

Both the quality of life of the elderly and their ultimate will to survive are strongly influenced by the level of psychological stress which they experience. This depends, in turn, on the frequency and severity of adverse life events, the extent of external support, coping skills, and the level of external resources.[14] In men, survival is adversely affected by either upward or downward social mobility, but such mobility does not seem to affect prognosis in women.[201]

Cohort differences in psychological stresses associated with aging can arise due to such factors as changing structures of religious belief.[59,247] A high level of trust is associated with greater life satisfaction, better self-rated health, and enhanced survival.[15,247] A comparison between sexagenarians and centenarians found a higher proportion of type B personalities (people who are less time conscious and less hostile) among those who survived to an advanced age; this favorable personality characteristic was more common in women than in men.[215]

In general, women have fewer material resources than men during old age.[132] They are much more likely to be living on their own,[16] and thus tend to receive less psychological support than men.[42,149,167] They are also more likely to be disabled. In general, disability increases social isolation, but car ownership and the ability to drive are also important variables; a proportion of those quite severely disabled thus manage to sustain at least daily social interactions.[217] When institutionalization occurs, it seems to have a more depressant effect on men than on women.[238]

Some gender differences are seen in cross-sectional analyses, where multiple regressions relate social status to survival.[202] In men, the risk of death before the age of 80 years is linked to being single,[100,202] and either upward or downward social mobility.[202] In contrast, marriage to a younger partner is linked to longer survival.[246] Among women, being single[100,202] or currently married is an important risk factor for early death, whereas widows and those who are divorced enjoy better prospects.[202] One author has suggested that, in women, divorce reflects a termination of shared environmental risk factors.[222]

Despite physical limitations, most old people want to continue living at home, and are happiest if they can do so.[164,183] Regular physical activity can make an important contribution to the achievement of this goal;[210] however, widowhood and increasing physical disability limit the potential of the oldest females to realize this option.

A Swedish study has argued that mental health is more important to survival than social networks, mobility, and religious attitudes.[135] In men, poor cognitive function has an adverse influence on prognosis and, because of a selective mortality, the oldest men (those aged 90 to 99 years) have a greater cognitive ability than either their younger male peers or women of the same age.[175] Growing evidence suggests that physical activity helps to maintain social contacts, enhances mental health, and sustains cognitive ability in the very old.[210]

Among many indigenous populations, the process of acculturation to a modern, industrial lifestyle has led to social alienation, with a substantial increase in the risk of suicide and other forms of violent death.[212]

3.3.2 Effects of an Adverse Lifestyle

The rate of functional aging and survival prospects are strongly influenced by an individual's personal lifestyle. Such factors as smoking, excessive consumption of alcohol, overeating, and lack of regular physical activity interact with each other and with an inherent weakness of genotype to exacerbate the changes associated with healthy aging. Problems of an adverse lifestyle commonly reflect a low socioeconomic status, and risk-taking behavior is particularly frequent among those currently adapting to modern, urban society. For instance, Campos et al.[35] compared men and women from urban and rural areas of Costa Rica. They noted that the inherent impact of APO-A-IV alleles on lipid profile was greatly exacerbated among those undergoing urbanization, apparently because those from urban areas had a higher consumption of saturated fat and were more likely to be cigarette smokers.

3.3.2.1 Cigarette Smoking

Cigarette smoking can shorten life expectancy by as much as eight years in young men and five years in young women;[17] the gender difference probably reflects in part male vulnerability to premature cardiac death, and in part gender differences in patterns of smoking. Unfortunately, heavy smokers substantially underestimate the risk to which they are exposing themselves.[205] The main effect of smoking is upon the lungs and airways; here, carcinogenic mutations accumulate more rapidly, and the normal, age-related decreases in vital capacity and forced expiratory volume are accelerated.[228] However, the aging process is also adversely affected in many other organs.

The cumulative effects of smoking upon life expectancy seem somewhat less dramatic in the elderly than in younger individuals, but this arises partly because a substantial proportion of those genetically vulnerable to smoking have already died.

Gender differences in the prevalence of cigarette smoking have in the past explained much of the shorter average life span of the male. Indeed, after allowing for a somewhat greater incidence of traumatic deaths among men, there is almost no gender difference in life expectancy among nonsmokers.[155] Now that the prevalence of smoking also shows little sex difference, a progressive equalization of average life span between men and women can be anticipated.[173]

Physical activity enhances prognosis, in both smokers and nonsmokers, although the benefits of a physically active lifestyle are probably somewhat smaller in those who smoke. In middle age, the main protection is against cardiovascular disease and, here, a larger benefit may be anticipated in men than in women.

3.3.2.2 Alcohol Consumption

Excessive consumption of alcohol has a direct influence in exacerbating the age-related deterioration in hepatic and cardiac function. Alcoholism may also serve as a marker of underlying psychological problems that influence survival prospects.

Much of the dramatic decline of male longevity in Russia during recent years seems attributable to an increase in excessive consumption of alcohol, particularly among men displaced from heavy industry; between 1986 and 1994, life expectancy dropped from 65 to 59 years in men, and from 74.8 to 73.2 years in women.[34] Likewise, high mortality rates and shortened life span seen in economically disfavored regions[26,188,221] reflect a potent combination of psychological discouragement, heavy cigarette consumption, excessive intake of alcohol, and inadequate physical activity. Typically, these factors are linked to downward social mobility, loss of home ownership, and marriage breakdown.[160] In the western world, too, the pace of change has been greatest in male-dominated "heavy" industries; in consequence many men have now lost their traditional social role as economic provider. Therefore, the adverse impact of deindustrialization has been greater in men than women.

3.3.2.3 Dietary Factors

The ability of dietary restriction to lengthen life span has long been recognized in laboratory animals.[143,199] It has been hypothesized that production of reactive species increases in proportion to total daily energy expenditure. In support of this hypothesis, restriction of the overall intake of nutrients reduces the peroxidation of hepatic mitochondria in rats.[7]

However, the implications of such observations for humans remain unclear. Women restrict their food intake much more frequently than men, but they commonly adopt a cyclic rather than a sustained reduction of food consumption. Unfortunately, a cyclic pattern of weight loss appears to have an adverse rather than favorable effect upon an individual's prognosis. One study of male veterans noted that longevity was greater in short and light individuals than in those who were tall and heavy.[200] Others have also noted a shorter life span among athletes with a muscular, mesomorphic body build than in tall, thin ectomorphs.[203] These observations seem to agree with findings in experimental animals, although they need repeating on a mixed gender population to see whether a reduction in body mass and/or a decrease in body size would enhance the survival of women.

Mortality is adversely affected by an accumulation of body fat; thus there is a marked interaction among diet, habitual physical activity, and longevity. Longevity is increased by the choice of a high fiber diet rich in omega-three unsaturated fatty acids. The health of traditional indigenous populations with a fishing economy profits from a high intake of the omega-three fatty acids. Men tend to consume more protein and animal fat than women,[133] and meat consumption also increases with "modernization." Thus, elderly Greek migrants to Australia had a greater intake of meat and beer and a lower intake of cereals, carbohydrates, and olive oil than their peers still living in rural Greece.[122] Moreover, dietary changes adopted by migrants were associated with an increased prevalence of heart disease (especially in men) and cancer (especially in women).

3.3.2.4 Habitual Physical Activity

The ability of regular physical activity to prolong survival has long been recognized from animal studies.[74] In humans, most data on longevity and habitual physical activity have been collected on men.[23,180] Regular physical activity generally augments maximal aerobic power[210] and muscle strength[60] by similar percentages in young and elderly individuals, although a poor fluid intake and a low concentration of circulating protein may limit the expansion of plasma volume and cardiac stroke volume in some older adults.[255]

A questionnaire survey of Harvard alumni suggested that the life expectancy of young adults was 1 to 2 years greater in those who engage in 8.4 MJ/week of leisure activity than in those who were sedentary.[166] However, if physical activity was not begun until old age, the gain in life span was reduced to a few months.[166] Indeed, a survey of Seventh-Day Adventist men suggested that vigorous (as opposed to moderate) physical activity could even shorten life span in the oldest age groups.[134] A study of Framingham adults over the age of 75 years found that women who pursued moderate activity had substantially lower mortality over the next ten years, whereas men and women who were vigorously active gained no advantage.[213] Furthermore, at this stage in life much of the apparent benefit of physical activity disappears after allowing for the effects of age, gender, education, marital status, ethnicity, and self-rated health.[129] Any independent benefit of activity depends mainly on current rather than former lifestyle. Thus, in the Zutphen study, recent physical activity (walking or cycling for at least 20 minutes 3 times per week) had a greater influence upon mortality than did activity undertaken 5 years previously. The risk among those who currently were most active, relative to the least active tertile, was 0.44.[24]

Particularly in the final years of life, the greatest dividend from regular physical activity may be an increase in the individual's functional capacity and thus quality of life (Chapter 5), rather than an extension of life span.[209] A progressive physical activity program can increase muscle strength and aerobic power by what is equivalent to a 10- to 20-year reversal of the aging process.[210] Because women generally have a smaller functional margin than men, they are likely to show a larger gain in quality of life as a result of participating in a regular physical activity program (Chapter 5).

3.4 Ethnic Differences in Rates of Functional Loss and Longevity

The prevalence of adverse genotypes is greater in some ethnic groups than in others.[165] Moreover, there are gender differences in the impact of specific gene combinations upon longevity (see, for instance References 66, 105, 126).

However, regional and ethnic differences in the course of aging and in total life span reflect not only constitutional factors, but also influences of environment, lifestyle, and interactions between constitution and external factors. Formal genetic studies have been conducted in populations isolated by geographic or class barriers. Other investigators have looked at the course of aging in isolated or multiracial communities.

3.4.1 Genetic Studies of Isolated Populations

Intensive intermarriage in geographically or socially isolated communities has allowed the emergence of small groups carrying disadvantageous recessive genes, resulting in a substantial shortening of average life span. Canadian examples include the Lac St. Jean region of Northern Québec, the outports of Newfoundland, and the circumpolar regions.

In the area around Lac St. Jean, an autosomal recessive gene in the 13q11 region has been associated with the development of spastic ataxia in later life.[186] The Lac St. Jean community also has an above-normal prevalence of cystic fibrosis[44] and hereditary hemochromatosis.[46] Other genetic abnormalities have been explored in the isolated fishing communities of the Newfoundland coastline. Families with a PKDI mutant gene on the short arm of chromosome 16 have a high prevalence of polycystic disease of the kidneys,[168] and those with polymorphism of the D2S123 locus on 2p15–16 have a susceptibility to hereditary nonpolyposis colon cancer.[77] The royal families of Europe are a third closed community where the adverse effect of recessive genes has become manifest; most noticeably, susceptibility to hemophilia has led to a shortening of the average male life span in this population.[32,68]

Formal genetic studies conducted under the auspices of the International Biological Programme (I.B.P.) began from the opposite premise: that life in a challenging environment such as the high Arctic might lead to the emergence of genetic traits with positive adaptive value.[212] In practice, little evidence was found for emergence of unusual genotypes that favored survival in a harsh environment. Several explanations were advanced. Firstly, although the populations concerned were small and apparently isolated, there had been a continuing admixture of genes from outside the community. Secondly, many of the indigenous populations studied by the I.B.P. lived at the junction of two or more ecosystems. Thus, an unusual characteristic contributing to successful exploitation of one type of environment could prove a disadvantage to colonization of the second environment.[212] Finally, survival in the face of a challenging natural environment depends more upon intelligence than on emergence of a high physical working capacity or unusual muscular strength.[212]

Nevertheless, the Inuit of the circumpolar regions do show minor constitutional anomalies, including lactose and sucrose malabsorption.[84] In theory, certain apolipoprotein polymorphisms might also interact with heavy physical activity[72] and high consumption of marine oils[89,193] to yield a favorable lipid profile,[47,121] thereby reducing risks of cardiovascular disease. The incidence of cardiovascular deaths is reputed to be low in the circumpolar regions, although documentation of the cause of death is often limited in these populations. Suggestions have also been made that a whale-hunting economy has favored the emergence of a robust skeleton among coastal Inuit, in both men and in women,[38] although others have found low bone calcium levels and attribute this to lack of exposure to sunlight for much of the year.[212] In American Indians, a polymorphic genetic variant of the pyrimidine pathway enzyme uridine monophosphate kinase-3 has left this population highly susceptible to *Haemophilus* influenza type b (Hib) disease,[58,177] and an interaction between constitution and environment has increased their susceptibility to various types of gall bladder disease.[245]

To the extent that these various diseases show a gender bias, the ethnic differences in susceptibility have had a differential effect on the longevity of men and women in indigenous communities.

3.4.2 Aging in Isolated Communities

Considerable excitement was aroused by early reports of unusual longevity in certain isolated, mountainous communities, including the village of Vilcabamba in the Ecuadorian Andes, the Hunza region in the Himalayas, and parts of Georgia.[128] It was hypothesized that the active lifestyle imposed by primitive agriculture in a rugged terrain had enhanced health and longevity. However, subsequent access to formal birth records disclosed that most of those who claimed to be exceptionally old had exaggerated their ages, sometimes by as much as 30 years.[127,144] In fact, the average life expectancy in these communities was below the world average.

Early death has indeed been a feature of most primitive communities. This is hardly surprising, given the risks imposed by physical dangers, starvation, and untreated disease. Traditional patterns of agriculture in rugged mountainous terrain sometimes involve very high daily energy expenditures,[53] but an exceptional level of physical fitness is not necessarily characteristic of older residents in these regions.[18] Nevertheless, people living in some of these communities appear to have shown a slower rate of functional aging than that which is usual in "developed" societies. Further, this advantage has been lost progressively with acculturation to the lifestyle of developed societies.[212] Modernization has brought a heavy toll of physical inactivity, obesity, cigarette smoking, alcoholism, substance abuse, and violent death, compounded by growing risks of diabetes mellitus and chronic respiratory disease.[138]

3.4.3 American Indians

Modernization of the indigenous Indian populations of the Americas has been associated with obesity and maturity-onset diabetes.[157,212] The prevalence of diabetes among those over the age of 20 years is still less than 1%

in the rural Mapuche Indians of Chile, but it is now more than 50% among Pima Indians living in the U.S. The better health prospects of traditional Indian populations reflect a diet which contains less animal fat, more complex carbohydrates, and a greater total energy content than that of their "modernized" peers.[182] After adjusting data for body fat content, plasma concentrations of the appetite regulator leptin were higher in Mexican Pima Indians than among their peers living in Arizona. This difference was correlated both with levels of habitual physical activity and the proportion of carbohydrate in the diet.[64]

3.4.4 Mexicans

Mexicans who have migrated to the southern U.S. show a high prevalence of diabetes as they become older. These figures show a strong inverse socioeconomic gradient, from 16% in low-income barrios to 5% in high-income suburbs.[157] Mexican Americans also seem vulnerable to gall bladder disease. By the age of 85 years, 40% of Mexican American females have undergone a cholecystectomy. The relative contributions of constitution and diet to this finding need to be clarified,[245] but the risk shows little correlation with the extent of Native American heritage.[233]

3.4.5 Pacific Islanders

The lifestyle of most Pacific Islanders has changed dramatically over the past 30 years. Modernization has brought increases in body mass, serum cholesterol, and blood pressure, with related clinical disorders.[61,170,171] The prevalence of overweight among adult females is 46% among traditional Western Samoans, but 80% in those who have migrated to Hawaii.[147] Likewise, Samoan migrants to California show a high prevalence of hypertension.[170] Changes in diet, physical activity, and levels of stress have all contributed to urban/rural differences within Samoa.[227] As a consequence of growing obesity, the maximal oxygen intake per kg of body mass has decreased at any given age, and the relative work rate has increased when undertaking heavy physical activity. This in turn has led to an increased 24-hour excretion of norepinephrine.[171] The prevalence of hypercholesterolemia and diabetes also rose dramatically between 1978 and 1991.[95] One consequence of modernization is that many Samoan women now take jobs outside the home; such an arrangement seems associated with higher blood pressure in their husbands, but not in the women themselves.[25]

As in other indigenous populations, the increase in body fat with modernization has been particularly marked in women. In men, increases in both overall and abdominal adiposity are correlated with worsening of the serum lipid profile and thus an increase in cardiovascular risk. On the other hand, the measures of body fat content in women are poorly correlated with either the serum lipid profile[65] or the risk of diabetes,[227] possibly because of statistical problems arising from the high prevalence of obesity. The risks of stroke and cardiovascular death remain lower for Samoan Americans than for other North American populations. One group of investigators has suggested that, among traditional Samoans, high social status associated with aging may serve as a buffer against overt manifestations of ischemic heart disease, despite high levels of other risk factors.[106]

3.4.6 Circumpolar Populations

Various circumpolar communities are at differing points in the process of acculturation to a modern lifestyle.[192] However, the patterns of aging observed among the Inuit of Igloolik in the Canadian Northwest Territories illustrate the impact of modernization. When measurements were first made (1969 to 1970), both men and women began adult life with a much greater maximal aerobic power than their "white" counterparts in the cities of Southern Canada.[189] This reflected a high level of habitual physical activity,[72] and very low stores of body fat compared to their white counterparts.[189] Cross-sectional data suggested that loss of function over the first half of adult life was less than in southern Canada. Despite a widespread prevalence of chronic respiratory disease, and almost universal cigarette consumption, the average loss of pulmonary function was also much as in nonsmoking adults from southern Canada.[190] However, the aging curve was convex, with rapid loss of function among those over the age of 40 years. In this particular population, changes of functional capacity in the latter part of adult life seemed attributable to a change in social roles; habitual physical activity decreased dramatically as offspring assumed responsibility for the heavy physical tasks of hunting.

By 1990, the pattern of aging in Igloolik had moved much closer to that observed in the white communities of developed societies. The young adults of the community no longer engaged in regular hunting expeditions, and, consequently, the aging of maximal aerobic power showed a concave rather than a convex curve, much as in southern Canada.[191] Further, instead of remaining very thin throughout adult life, the Inuit began adulthood with a thickness of subcutaneous fat similar to that of people in southern Canada, and (particularly in women) the thickness of subcutaneous fat increased substantially as they became older. Regional peculiarities of aging seen in 1969 to 1970 were thus due to the lifestyle of that era, rather than any genetic characteristics emerging in what was then a relatively isolated community. The functional advantage conferred by a traditional, physically active lifestyle was similar to that observed in comparisons between athletes and sedentary individuals in white society — namely, a halving of the rate of aging of maximal aerobic power. Other factors being equal, this would have extended the period of disability-free life by as much as 20 years.[210]

Studies of the bone mineral content of the tibia in Alaskan Inuit showed a 50% decrease in women between the ages of 30 and 60 years; however, male values showed no significant change over the same age range.[142] It was suggested that a continuing high level of physical activity, particularly walking, might account for maintenance of bone mineral among older male participants in this study.[142]

3.4.7 Multiracial Communities

There are often substantial ethnic differences in the prevalence of disease, functional mobility, and quality of life among the elderly members of multiracial communities. For instance, U.S. black and Native Americans not only have a shorter average life span than their white peers, but also face a longer period with chronic disability.[87] Nevertheless, such differences seem to reflect education, income, and living environment,[22] rather than the influence of inherent constitutional factors upon the aging process. Influences adversely affecting black and Native Americans include poverty, dislocation through immigration, and/or separation from their ethnic community and lack of family support.[98]

For example, the prevalence, complications, and mortality from diabetes mellitus are higher among African Americans, Hispanic Americans, and Native Americans than in the general U.S. population of similar age.[111] Paradoxically, and for reasons as yet poorly understood, the prevalence of coronary heart disease in Hispanic and Native American populations remains much lower than would be predicted from their levels of obesity, diabetes, and hypertension.[254]

3.5 Conclusions

Specific genes can now be identified that increase the risk of various chronic diseases, affecting an individual's quality of life and survival prospects. Furthermore, the frequency of occurrence of such genes in some instances differs between the two sexes. Nevertheless, various environmental challenges exert a powerful influence, both in their own right and as the reason why adverse genetic characteristics become manifest. The gender difference in survival thus seems determined almost entirely by environmental factors, with cigarette smoking playing a dominant role. Likewise, regional and ethnic differences in life span reflect mainly the impact of various environmental constraints, including (in isolated indigenous populations) the favorable influence of a high level of physical activity and an unusual diet, offset by exposure to physical dangers, lack of immunity to certain major diseases, and (particularly as modernization develops) adoption of an adverse lifestyle.

References

1. Adams, O., Life expectancy in Canada: an overview, *Health Rep.*, 2, 361–376, 1990.
2. Agerholm-Larsen, B., Nordestgaard, B.G., Steffensen, R., et al., ACE gene polymorphism: ischemic heart disease and longevity in 10,150 individuals. A case-referent and retrospective cohort study based on the Copenhagen city heart study, *Circulation*, 10, 2358–2367, 1997.
3. Aggarwal, S. and Gupta, S., Increased apoptosis of T cell subsets in aging humans: altered expression of Fas (CD 95), fas ligand, Bcl-2, and Bax, *J. Immunol.*, 160, 1627–1637, 1998.
4. Agidez, J.A., Rodriguez, I., Olivera, M., et al., CYP2D6, NAT2 and CYP2E1 genetic polymorphisms in nonagenarians, *Age Ageing*, 26, 147–151, 1997.
5. Akisaka, M., Suzuki, M., and Inoko, H., Molecular genetic studies on DNA polymorphism of the HLA class II genes associated with human longevity, *Tissue Antigens*, 50, 489–493, 1997.
6. Arking, R., Successful selection for increased longevity in *Drosophila*; analysis of the survival data and presentation of a hypothesis on the genetic regulation of longevity, *Exp. Gerontol.*, 23, 59–76, 1987.
7. Armeni, T., Tomasetti, M., Svegliati-Baroni, S., et al., Dietary restriction affects antioxidant levels in rat liver mitochondria during aging, *Mol. Aspects Med.*, 18 (Suppl.), S247–S250, 1997.
8. Asaumi, S., Kuroyanaji, H., Seki, N., et al., Orthologues of the *Caenorhabditis elegans* longevity gene clk-1 in mouse and human, *Genomics*, 58, 293–301, 1999.
9. Au, W.W., Sierra-Torres, C.H., Cajas-Salazar, N., et al., Inheritance of polymorphic metabolizing genes on environmental disease and quality of life, *Mutat. Res.*, 428, 131–140, 1999.
10. Auliciems, A. and Frost, D., Temperature and cardiovascular deaths in Montreal, *Int. J. Biometeorol.*, 33, 151–156, 1989.
11. Austin, M.A., Friedlander, Y., Newman, B., et al., Genetic influences on changes in body mass index, *Obes. Res.*, 5, 326–331, 1997.
12. Bader, G., Zuliani, G., Kostner, G.M., et al., Apolipoprotein E polymorphism is not associated with longevity or disability in a sample of Italian octo- and nonagenarians, *Gerontology*, 44, 293–299, 1998.
13. Baker-Blocker, A., Winter weather and cardiovascular mortality in Minneapolis–St. Paul, *Am. J. Publ. Health*, 72, 261–265, 1982.
14. Baltes, M.M. and Lang, F.R., Everyday functioning and successful aging: the impact of resources, *Psychol. Aging*, 12, 433–443, 1997.
15. Barefoot, J.C., Maynard, K.E., Beckham, J.C., et al., Trust, health, and longevity, *J. Behav. Med.*, 21, 517–526, 1998.
16. Barer, B.M., Men and women aging differently, *Int. J. Aging Hum. Develop.*, 38, 29–40, 1994.
17. Basavaraj, S., Smoking and loss of longevity in Canada, *Can. J. Publ. Health*, 84, 341–345, 1993.
18. Beall, C.M., Goldstein, M.C., and Feldman, E.S., Social structure and intracohort variations in physical fitness among elderly males in a traditional third world society, *J. Am. Geriatr. Soc.*, 33, 406–412, 1985.
19. Beamer, W.G., Donahue, L.R., Rosen, C.J., et al., Genetic variability in adult bone density among inbred strains of mice, *Bone*, 18, 397–403, 1996.

20. Bergeman, C.S., Plomin, R., Pedersen, N.L., et al., Genetic mediation of the relationship between social support and psychological well-being, *Psychol. Aging*, 6, 640–646, 1991.
21. Bergeman, C.S., Plomin, R., Pedersen, N.L., et al., Genetic and environmental influences on social support: the Swedish adoption/twin study of aging, *J. Gerontol.*, 45, P101–P106, 1990.
22. Berkman, C.S. and Gurland, B.J., The relationship between ethnoracial group and functional level in older persons, *Ethnic Health*, 3, 175–188, 1998.
23. Berlin, J.A. and Coldlitz, G.A., A meta-analysis of physical activity in the prevention of coronary heart disease, *Am. J. Epidemiol.*, 132, 612–628, 1990.
24. Bijnen, F.C., Feskens, E.J., Caspersen, C.J., et al., Baseline and previous physical activity in relation to mortality in elderly men: the Zutphen elderly study, *Am. J. Epidemiol.*, 150, 1289–1296, 1999.
25. Bindon, J.R., Knight, A., Dressler, W.W., et al., Social context and psychosocial influences on blood pressure among American Samoans, *Am. J. Phys. Anthropol.*, 103, 7–18, 1997.
26. Black, D., *Inequalities in Health: Report of a Research Working Group*, Department of Health and Social Services, London, 1980.
27. Blindauer, K.M., Rubin, C., Morse, D.L., et al., The 1996 New York blizzard: impact on non-injury emergency visits, *Am. J. Emerg. Med.*, 17, 23–27, 1999.
28. Borchelt, D.R., Ratovitski, T., van Lare, J., et al., Accelerated amyloid deposition in the brains of transgenic mice coexpressing mutant presenilin I and amyloid precursor proteins, *Neuron*, 19, 939–945, 1997.
29. Bouchard, C. and Després, J.-C., Variation in fat distribution with age and health implications, in *Physical Activity and Aging. The Academy Papers 22*, Spirduso, W. and Eckert, H., Ed., Human Kinetics Publishers, Champaign, IL, 1988, 78–106.
30. Bouchard, C., Rice, T., Lemieux, S., et al., Major gene for abdominal visceral fat area in the Québec Family Study, *Int. J. Obesity*, 20, 420–427, 1996.
31. Bowles, J.T., The evolution of aging: a new approach to an old problem of biology, *Med. Hypoth.*, 51, 179–221, 1998.
32. Boyd, W., *A Textbook of Pathology. Structure and Function in Diseases*, Lea & Febiger, Philadelphia, 1961.
33. Boyle, J.M., Mitchell, E.L., Greaves, M.J., et al., Chromosome instability is a predominant trait of fibroblasts from Li-Fraumeni families, *Br. J. Cancer*, 77, 2181–2192, 1998.
34. British Medical Journal, news item: Life expectancy in Russia falls, *Br. Med. J.*, 308, 553, 1994.
35. Campos, H., Lopez-Miranda, J., Rodriguez, C., et al., Urbanization elicits a more atherogenic lipoprotein profile in carriers of the apolipoprotein A-IV-2 allele than in A-IV-! homozygotes, *Arterioscler. Thromb. Vasc. Biol.*, 17, 1074–1081, 1997.
36. Carmelli, D., Intrapair comparisons of total life span in twins and pairs of sibs, *Hum. Biol.*, 54, 525–537, 1982.
37. Carmichael, C.M. and McGue, M., A cross-sectional examination of height, weight, and body mass index in adult twins, *J. Gerontol.*, 50, B237–B244, 1995.
38. Collier, S., Sexual dimorphism in relation to big-game hunting and economy in modern human populations, *Am. J. Phys. Anthropol.*, 91, 485–504, 1993.
39. Collins, K.J., Exton-Smith, A.N., and Doré, C., Urban hypothermia: preferred temperature and thermal perception in old age, *Br. Med. J.*, 282, 175–177, 1981.

40. Colvez, A. and Blanchet, M., Potential gains in life expectancy free of disability: a tool for health planning, *Int. J. Epidemiol.*, 12, 86–91, 1983.
41. Comfort, A., *The Biology of Senescence*, 3rd ed. Elsevier Science, New York, 1979.
42. Connidis, I., *Family Ties and Aging*, Butterworth, Toronto, Ontario, 1989.
43. Coroni-Huntley, J., Brock, D.B., Ostfeld, A.M., et al., Established populations for epidemiological studies of the elderly: resource data book, U.S. Public Health Service, National Institute on Aging, Washington, D.C. 1986.
44. Daigneault, J., Aubin, G., Simard, F., et al., Genetic epidemiology of cystic fibrosis in Saguenay–Lac St.Jean, *Clin. Genet.*, 40, 298–303, 1991.
45. De Benedictis, G., Rose, G., Carrieri, G., et al., Mitochondrial DNA inherited variants are associated with successful aging and longevity in humans, *FASEB J.*, 13, 1532–1536, 1999.
46. de Braekeleer, M., Vigneault, A., and Simard, H., Population genetics of hereditary hemochromatosis in Saguenay Lac St. Jean (Québec, Canada), *Ann. Genet.*, 35, 202–207, 1992.
47. de Maat, M.P., Bladbjerg, E.M., Johansen, L.G., et al., DNA polymorphisms and plasma levels of vascular disease risk factors in Greenland Inuit — is there a relation with the low risk of cardiovascular disease in the Inuit? *Thromb. Haemostas.*, 81, 547–552, 1999.
48. Diamond, S.G., Markham, C.H., Hoehn, M.M., et al., An examination of male–female differences in progression and mortality of Parkinson's disease, *Neurology,* 40, 763–766, 1990.
49. Dorak, M.T., Mills, K.I., Gaffney, D., et al., Homozygous MHC genotypes and longevity, *Hum. Hered.*, 44, 271–278, 1994.
50. Drinkwater, B., Women and exercise. Physiological aspects, *Ex. Sport Sci. Rev.*, 12, 21–52, 1984.
51. Drinkwater, B.L., Bedi, J.F., Loucks, A.B., et al., Sweating sensitivity and capacity of women in relation to age, *J. Appl. Physiol.*, 53, 671–676, 1982.
52. Dublin, L.L., Lotka, A.J., and Spiegelman, M., *Length of Life: A Study of the Life Table*, Ronald Press, New York, 1949, Chap. 6.
53. Durnin, J.V.G.A. and Passmore, R., *Energy, Work and Leisure*, Heinemann, London, 1967.
54. el-Zein, R., Zwischenberger, J.B., Wood, T.G., et al., Combined genetic polymorphism and risk for development of lung cancer, *Mutation Res.*, 381, 189–200, 1997.
55. Emmett, J.D. and Hodgson, J.L., Cardiovascular responses to snow-shoveling in a thermoneutral, cold and cold with wind environment, *J. Cardiopulm. Rehabil.*, 13, 43–50, 1993.
56. Fahn, H.J., Wang, L.S., Hsieh, R.H., et al., Age-related 4977 bp deletion in human mitochondrial DNA, *Am. J. Resp. Crit. Care Med.*, 154, 1141–1145, 1996.
57. Faure-Delanef, L., Baudin, B., Benet-Burnet, B., et al., Plasma concentration, kinetic constants, and gene polymorphism of angiotensin-I- converting enzyme in centenarians, *Clin. Chem.*, 44, 2083–2087, 1998.
58. Feeney, A.J., Atkinson, M.J., Cowan, M.J., et al., A defective Vkappa A2 allele in Navajos which may play a role in increased susceptibility to *Haemophilus* influenza type b disease, *J. Clin. Invest.*, 97, 2277–2282, 1996.
59. Felton, B.J., Cohort variation in happiness: some hypotheses and exploratory analyses, *Int. J. Aging Hum. Develop.*, 25, 27–42, 1987.
60. Fiatarone, M.A., Marks, E.C., Ryan, N.D., et al., High-intensity strength training in nonagenarians: Effects on skeletal muscle, *JAMA*, 263, 3029–3034, 1990.

61. Finau, S.A., Prior, I.A., and Evans, J.G., Aging in the South Pacific. Physical changes with urbanization, *Soc. Sci. Med.*, 16, 1539–1549, 1982.
62. Finkel, D., Whitfield, K., and McGue, M., Genetic and environmental influences on functional age: a twin study, *J. Gerontol.*, 50, P104–P113, 1995.
63. Fishman, J., Boyar, R.M., and Hellman, L., Influence of body weight on estradiol metabolism in young women, *J. Clin. Endocrinol. Metab.*, 41, 989–991, 1975.
64. Fox, C., Esparza, J., Nicolson, M., et al., Plasma leptin concentrations in Pima Indians living in drastically different environments, *Diabetes Care*, 22, 413–417, 1999.
65. Galanis, D.J., McGarvey, S.T., Sobal, J., et al., Relations of body fat and fat distribution to the serum lipid, apolipoprotein and insulin concentrations of Samoan men and women, *Int. J. Obesity*, 19, 731–738, 1995.
66. Galinsky, D., Tysoe, C., Brayne, C.E., et al., Analysis of the apo E/apo CI, angiotensin converting enzyme and methylenetetrahydrofolate reductase genes as candidates affecting human longevity, *Atherosclerosis*, 129, 177–183, 1997.
67. Gavrilov, L.A., Gavrilova, N.S., Kroutko, V.N., et al., Mutation load and human longevity, *Mutat. Res.*, 377, 61–62, 1997.
68. Gavrilova, N.S., Gavrilov, L.A., Evdokushkina, G.N., et al., Evolution, mutation and human longevity: European royal and noble families, *Hum. Biol.*, 70, 799–804, 1998.
69. Gelman, R., Watson, A., Bronson, R., et al., Murine chromosomal regions correlated with longevity, *Genetics*, 118, 693–704, 1988.
70. Glass, R.I., Wiesenthal, A.M., Zack, M.M., et al., Risk factors for myocardial infarction associated with the Chicago snowstorm of Jan 13–15, 1979, *JAMA*, 245, 164–165, 1981.
71. Gnecchi-Ruscone, T., Crosignani, P., Micheletti, T., et al., Meteorological influences on myocardial infarction in the metropolitan area of Milan, *Int. J. Cardiol.*, 9, 75–80, 1985.
72. Godin, G. and Shephard, R.J., Activity pattern of the Canadian Eskimo, in *Polar Human Biology,* Edholm, O.G. and Gunderson, E.K.E., Eds., Heinemann Medical Books, London, 1973, 193–215.
73. Goldstein, S., Replicative senescence: the human fibroblast comes of age, *Science*, 249, 1129–113, 1990.
74. Goodrick, C.L., Effects of long-term voluntary wheel exercise on male and female Wistar rats. I. Longevity, body weight, and metabolic rate, *Gerontol.*, 26, 22–33, 1980.
75. Goodrick, C.L., Ingram, D.K., Reynolds, M.A., et al., Differential effects of intermittent feeding and voluntary exercise on body weight and life span in adult rats, *J. Gerontol.*, 38, 36–45, 1983.
76. Gori, G.B., Richter, B.J., and Yu, W.K., Economics and extended longevity: a case study, *Prev. Med.*, 13, 396–410, 1984.
77. Green, R.C., Narod, S.A., Morasse, J., et al., Hereditary nonpolyposis colon cancer: analysis of linkage to 2p15–16 places the COCAI locus telomeric to D2S123 and reveals genetic heterogeneity in seven Canadian families, *Am. J. Hum. Genet.*, 54, 1067–1077, 1994.
78. Grigliatti, T.A., Programmed cell death and aging in *Drosophila melanogaster,* in *Evolution of Longevity in Animals: A Comparative Approach,* Woodhead, A.D. and Thompson, K.H., Eds., Plenum Press, New York, NY, 1987, 193–208.
79. Grover, R.F., Tucker, C.E., McGroarty, S.R., et al., The coronary stress of skiing at high altitude, *Arch. Int. Med.*, 150, 1205–1208, 1990.

80. Haan, M.N., Shemanski, L., Jagust, W.J., et al., The role of APOE epsilon4 in modulating effects of other risk factors for cognitive decline in elderly persons, *JAMA*, 282, 40–46, 1999.
81. Halhuber, M.J. and Humpeler, K.J., Does altitude cause exhaustion of the heart and circulatory system? *Med. Sci. Sports Exerc.*, 19, 192–202, 1985.
82. Harris, J.R., Pedersen, N.L., McClearn, G.E., et al., Age differences in genetic and environmental influences for health from the Swedish adoption/twin study of aging, *J. Gerontol.*, 47, P213–P220, 1992.
83. Harrison, D.E. and Roderick, T.H., Selection for maximum longevity in mice, *Exp. Gerontol.*, 32, 65–78, 1997.
84. Harvald, B., Genetic epidemiology of Greenland, *Arct. Med. Res.*, 36, 364–367, 1989.
85. Havenith, G., Inoue, Y., Luttiholt, V., et al., Age predicts cardiovascular, but not thermoregulatory, responses to humid heat stress, *Eur. J. Appl. Physiol.*, 70, 88–96, 1995.
86. Hayakawa, K., Shimizu, T., Ohba, Y., et al., Intrapair differences of physical aging and longevity in identical twins, *Acta Genet. Med. Gemellol.*, 41, 177–185, 1992.
87. Hayward, M.D. and Heron, M., Racial inequality in active life among adult Americans, *Demography*, 36, 77–91, 1999.
88. Health and Welfare Canada, The Active Health Report on Seniors. Health and Welfare Canada, Ottawa, Ontario, 1989.
89. Hegele, R.A., Young, T.K., and Connelly, P.W., Are Canadian Inuit at increased risk for coronary heart disease? *J. Mol. Med.*, 75, 364–370, 1997.
90. Heller, D.A., Pedersen, N.L., de Faire, U., et al., Genetic and environmental correlations among serum lipids and apolipoproteins in elderly twins reared together and apart, *Am. J. Hum. Genet.*, 55, 1255–1267, 1994.
91. Henon, N., Busson, M., Dehay-Martuchou, C., et al., Familial vs. sporadic longevity and MHC markers, *J. Biol. Regulat. Homeostat. Agents*, 13, 27–31, 1999.
92. Herskind, A.M., McGue, M.I., Iachine, I.A., et al., Untangling genetic influences on smoking, body mass index and longevity: a multivariate study of 2464 Danish twins followed for 28 years, *Hum. Genet.*, 98, 467–475, 1996.
93. Hibberd, M.L., Millward, B.A., and Demaine, A.G., The angiotensin-I-converting enzyme (ACE) locus is strongly associated with age and duration of diabetes in patients with type I diabetes, *J. Diabetes Complic.*, 11, 2–8, 1997.
94. Hildes, J., Health problems in the Arctic, *Can. Med. Assoc. J.*, 39, 1255–1257, 1960.
95. Hodge, A.M., Dowse, G.K., Toelupe, P., et al., The association of modernization with dyslipidaemia and changes in lipid levels in the Polynesian population of Western Samoa, *Int. J. Epidemiol.*, 26, 297–306, 1997.
96. Hong, Y., de Faire, U., Heller, D.A., et al., Genetic and environmental influences on blood pressure in elderly twins, *Hypertension*, 24, 663–670, 1994.
97. Hong, Y., Pedersen, N.L., Brismar, K., et al., Genetic and environmental architecture of the features of the insulin-resistance syndrome, *Am. J. Hum. Genet.*, 60, 143–152, 1997.
98. Hopper, S.V., The influence of ethnicity on the health of older women, *Clin. Geriatr. Med.*, 9, 231–259, 1993.
99. Horiuchi, S., Post-menopausal acceleration of age-related mortality increase, *J. Gerontol.*, 52, B78–B92, 1997.
100. Hu, Y. and Goldman, N., Mortality differentials by marital status: an international comparison, *Demography*, 27, 233–250, 1990.

101. Iachine, I.A., Holm, N.V., Harris, J.R., et al., How heritable is individual susceptibility to death? The results of an analysis of survival data on Danish, Swedish and Finnish twins, *Twin Res.*, 1, 196–205, 1998.
102. Ingram, D.K., Reynolds, M.A., and Les, E.P., The relationship of genotype, sex, body weight, and growth parameters to life span in inbred and hybrid mice, *Mech. Ageing Dev.*, 20, 253–266, 1982.
103. Inoue, Y. and Shibasaki, M., Regional differences in age-related decrements of the cutaneous vascular and sweating responses to passive heating, *Eur. J. Appl. Physiol.*, 74, 78–84, 1996.
104. Inoue, Y., Shibasaki, M., Ueda, H., et al., Mechanisms underlying the age-related decrement in the human sweating response, *Eur. J. Appl. Physiol.*, 79, 121–126, 1999.
105. Ivanova, R., Henon, N., Lepage, V., et al., HLA-DR alleles display sex-dependent effects on survival and discriminate between individual and familial longevity, *Hum. Mol. Genet.*, 7, 187–194, 1998.
106. Janes, C.R. and Pawson, I.G., Migration and biocultural adaptation: Samoans in California, *Soc. Sci. Med.*, 22, 821–834, 1986.
107. Jarvik, L., Falek, A., Kallman, F.J., et al., Survival trends in a senescent twin population, *Am. J. Hum. Genet.*, 12, 170–179, 1960.
108. Jian-Gang, Z., Yong-Xing, M., Chuan-Fu, W., et al., Apolipoprotein E and longevity among Han Chinese population, *Mech. Ageing Dev.*, 104, 159–167, 1998.
109. Johansson, S., Longevity in women, *Cardiovasc. Clin.*, 19, 3–16, 1989.
110. Kallman, F.G. and Sander, G., Twin studies on aging and longevity, *J. Hered.*, 39, 349–357, 1948.
111. Kamel, H.K., Rodriguez-Salda, J., Flaherty, J.H., et al., Diabetes mellitus among ethnic seniors: contrasts with diabetes in whites, *Clin. Geriatr. Med.*, 15, 265–278, 1999.
112. Katz, S., Branch, L.G., Branson, M.H., et al., Active life expectancy, *N. Engl. J. Med.*, 309, 1218–1824, 1983.
113. Kenney, W.L., Control of heat-induced cutaneous vasodilatation in relation to age, *Eur. J. Appl. Physiol.*, 57, 120–125, 1988.
114. Kenney, W.L., Body fluid and temperature regulation as a function of age, in *Exercise in Older Adults*, Lamb, D.R., Gisolfi, C.V., and Nadel, E.R., Eds., Cooper Publications, Carmel, IN, 1995, 305–351.
115. Kenney, W.L. and Buskirk, E.R., Functional consequences of sarcopenia: effects on thermoregulation, *J. Gerontol.*, 50, 78–85, 1995.
116. Kenney, W.L. and Ho, C.W., Age alters regional distribution of blood flow during moderate-intensity exercise, *J. Appl. Physiol.*, 79, 1112–1119, 1995.
117. Kenney, W.L. and Hodgson, J.L., Heat tolerance, thermoregulation and aging, *Sports Med.*, 4, 446–456, 1987.
118. Kenney, W.L., Morgan, A.L., Farquhar, W.B., et al., Decreased active vasodilator sensitivity in aged skin, *Am. J. Physiol.*, 272, H1609–H1614, 1997.
119. Key, T.J.A. and Pike, M.C., The role of estrogens and progestagens in the epidemiology and prevention of breast cancer, *Eur. J. Clin. Oncol.*, 24, 29–43, 1988.
120. Kinsella, H.G., Changes in life expectancy, *Am. J. Clin. Nutr.*, 55, 1196S-1202S, 1992.
121. Klausen, I.C., Hansen, P.S., Poulsen, J.V., et al., A unique pattern of apo(a) polymorphism in an isolated east Greenlandic Inuit (Eskimo) population, *Eur. J. Epidemiol.*, 11, 563–568, 1995.

122. Kouris-Blazos, A., Wahlqvist, M.L., Trichopoulou, A., et al., Health and nutritional status of elderly Greek migrants to Melbourne, Australia, *Age Ageing*, 25, 177–189, 1996.
123. Kramer, M. and Wells, C.L., Does physical activity reduce risk of estrogen-dependent cancer in women?, *Med. Sci. Sports Exerc.*, 28, 322–334, 1996.
124. Kranczer, S., Mixed life expectancy changes, *Stat. Bull. Metr. Ins. Co. N.Y.*, 77 (4), 29–36, 1996.
125. Kranczer, S., Continued United States longevity increases, *Stat. Bull. Metr. Ins. Co. N.Y.*, 80 (4), 20–27, 1999.
126. Lagaay, A.M., D'Amaro, J., Ligthart, G.J., et al., Longevity and heredity in humans. Association with human leucocyte antigen phenotype, *Ann. N.Y. Acad. Sci.*, 621, 78–89, 1991.
127. Leaf, A., Long-lived populations (extreme old age), in *Principles of Geriatric Medicine*, Andres, R., Bierman, E.L., and Hazzard, W.R., Eds., McGraw Hill, New York, 1985, 82–86.
128. Leaf, A. and Lannois, J., Search for the oldest people, *Nat. Geograph.*, 143, 93–119, 1973.
129. Lee, D.J. and Markides, K.S., Activity and mortality among aged persons over an eight-year period, *J. Gerontol.*, 45, S39–S42, 1990.
130. Levine, B.D., Zuckerman, J.H., and deFilippi, C.R., Effect of high altitude in the elderly: the tenth mountain division study, *Circulation*, 96, 1224–1232, 1997.
131. Lewis, K., Human longevity: an evolutionary approach, *Mech. Ageing Dev.*, 109, 43–51, 1999.
132. Lewis, M., Older women and health: an overview, *Women Health*, 10, 1–16, 1985.
133. Lieberman, H.R., Wurtman, J.J., and Teicher, M.H., Aging, nutrient choice, activity and behavioral responses to nutrients, *Ann. N.Y. Acad. Sci.*, 561, 196–208, 1989.
134. Linsted, K.D., Tonstad, K., and Kuzma, J., Self-report of physical activity and patterns of mortality in Seventh-Day Adventist men, *J. Clin. Epidemiol.*, 44, 355–364, 1991.
135. Ljungquist, B. and Sundström, G., Health and social networks as predictors of survival in old age, *Scand. J. Soc. Med.*, 24, 90–101, 1996.
136. Luft, F.C., Bad genes, good people, association, linkage, longevity and the prevention of cardiovascular disease, *Clin. Exp. Pharmacol. Physiol.*, 26, 576–579, 1999.
137. Luisetti, M., Gile, L.S., Bombieri, C., et al., Genetics of chronic obstructive pulmonary disease and disseminated bronchiectasis, *Monaldi Arch. Chest Dis.*, 53, 614–616, 1996.
138. MacMillan, H.L., MacMillan, A.B., Offord, D.R., et al., Aboriginal health, *Can. Med. Assoc. J.*, 155, 1569–1578, 1996.
139. Mann, W.C., Ottenbacher, K.J., Fraas, L., et al., Effectiveness of assistive technology and environmental interventions in maintaining independence and reducing home care costs for the frail elderly. A randomized controlled trial, *Arch. Fam. Med.*, 8, 210–217, 1999.
140. Marian, A.J., Kelly, D., Mares, A., et al., A missense mutation in the beta-myosin heavy chain gene is a predictor of premature sudden death in patients with hypertrophic cardiomyopathy, *J. Sports Med. Phys. Fitness*, 34, 1–10, 1994.
141. Martin, G.M., Genetics and the pathobiology of aging, *Phil. Trans. Roy. Soc. Lond., Series B (Biol. Sci.)*, 352, 1363, 1773–1780, 1997.

142. Martin, R.B., Burr, D.B., and Schaffler, M.B., Effects of age and sex on the amount and distribution of mineral in Eskimo tibiae, *Am. J. Phys. Anthropol.* 67, 371–380, 1985.
143. Masoro, E.J., Dietary restriction and aging, *J. Am. Geriatr. Soc.*, 41, 994–999, 1993.
144. Mazess, R.B. and Mathiesen, R.W., Lack of unusual longevity in Vilcabamba, Ecuador, *Hum. Biol.*, 54, 517–524, 1982.
145. McClearn, G.E., Johansson, B., Berg, S., et al., Substantial genetic influence on cognitive abilities in twins 80 or more years old, *Science*, 276, 1560–1563, 1997.
146. McClearn, G.E., Svartengren, M., Pedersen, N.L., et al., Genetic and environmental influences on pulmonary function in aging Swedish twins, *J. Gerontol.*, 49, 264–268, 1994.
147. McGarvey, S.T., Obesity in Samoans and a perspective on its etiology in Polynesians, *Am. J. Clin. Nutr.*, 53, 1586S-1594S, 1991.
148. McGue, M., Vaupel, J.W., Holm, N., et al., Longevity is moderately heritable in a sample of Danish twins born 1870–1880, *J. Gerontol.*, 48, B237–B244, 1993.
149. McPherson, B.D., *Aging as a Social Process*, Butterworth, Toronto, Ontario, 1990.
150. Meerson, F.Z., Ustinova, E.E., and Orlova, E.H., Prevention and elimination of heart arrhythmias by adaptation to intermittent high altitude hypoxia, *Clin. Cardiol.*, 10, 783–789, 1987.
151. Mellström, D. and Svanborg, A., Tobacco smoking — a major cause of sex differences in health, *Compr. Gerontol.*, 1, 34–39, 1987.
152. Merched, A., Xia, Y., Papadoulou, A., et al., Apolipoprotein AIV codon 360 mutation increases with human aging and is not associated with Alzheimer's disease, *Neurosci. Lett.*, 242, 117–119, 1998.
153. Michell, A.R., Longevity of British breeds of dog and its relationship with sex, size, cardiovascular variables and disease, *Vet. Record*, 145, 625–629, 1999.
154. Migliaccio, E., Giorgio, M., Mele, S., et al., The p66shc adaptor protein controls oxidative stress response and life span in mammals, *Nature*, 402, 309–313, 1999.
155. Miller, G.H. and Gerstein, D.R., The life expectancy of nonsmoking men and women, *Publ. Health Rep.*, 98, 343–349, 1983.
156. Miller, R.A., Kleemeier award lecture: are there genes for aging?, *J. Gerontol.*, 54, B297–B307, 1999.
157. Mitchell, B.D. and Stern, M.P., Recent developments in the epidemiology of diabetes in the Americas, *Wld. Health Stat. Quart.*, 45, 347–349, 1992.
158. Moehars, D., Lorent, K., and Van Leuven, F., Premature death in transgenic mice that overexpress a mutant amyloid precursor protein is preceded by severe neurodegeneration and apoptosis, *Neuroscience*, 91, 819–830, 1999.
159. Morgan, B., Alexander, J., Nicoli, S., et al., The patient with coronary heart disease at altitude, *J. Wilderness Med.*, 1, 147–153, 1990.
160. Moser, K.A., Goldblatt, P.O., Fox, A.J., et al., Unemployment and mortality: comparison of the 1971 and 1981 longitudinal census samples, *Br. Med. J.*, 294, 86–90, 1987.
161. Nassar, B.A., Dunn, J., Title, L.M., et al., Relation of genetic polymorphism of apolipoprotein E angiotensin converting enzyme apolipoprotein B-100, and glycoprotein IIIa and early onset coronary heart disease, *Clin. Biochem.*, 32, 275–282, 1999.
162. Nelson, T.L., Vogler, G.P., Pedersen, N.L., et al., Genetic and environmental influences on waist-to-hip ratio and waist circumference in an older Swedish twin population, *Int. J. Obesity*, 23, 449–455, 1999.

163. Nygaard, E., Madsen, A.G., and Christensen, H., Endurance capacity and longevity in women, *Health Care Wom. Int.*, 11, 1–10, 1990.
164. Oswald, F., The importance of the home for healthy and disabled elderly adults, *Z. Gerontol.*, 27, 355–365, 1994.
165. Pablos-Mendez, A., Mayeux, R., Ngai, C., et al., Association of apo E polymorphism with plasma lipid levels in a multiethnic elderly population, *Arterioscl. Thromb. Vasc. Biol.*, 17, 3534–3541, 1997.
166. Paffenbarger, R.S., Hyde, R.T., Wing, A.L., et al., Some interrelations of physical activity, physiological fitness, health and longevity, in *Physical Activity, Fitness and Health,* Bouchard, C., Shephard, R.J., and Stephens, T., Eds., Human Kinetics, Champaign, IL., 1994, 119–133.
167. Page, R.M. and Cole, G.E., Demographic predictors of self-reported loneliness in adults, *Psychol. Rep.*, 68, 939–945, 1991.
168. Parfrey, P.S., Bear, J.C., Morgan, J., et al., The diagnosis and prognosis of autosomal dominant polycystic kidney disease, *N. Engl. J. Med.*, 323, 1085–1090, 1990.
169. Parsons, P.A., The limit to human longevity: an approach through a stress theory of aging, *Mech. Ageing Dev.*, 87, 211–218, 1996.
170. Pawson, I.G. and Janes, G., Biocultural risks in longevity: Samoans in California, *Soc. Sci. Med.*, 16, 183–190, 1982.
171. Pearson, J.D., Hanna, J.M., Fitzgerald, M.H., et al., Modernization and catecholamine excretion of young Samoans, *Soc. Sci. Med.*, 31, 729–736, 1990.
172. Pedersen, N.L., Gatz, M., Plomin, R., et al., Individual differences in locus of control during the second half of the life span for identical and fraternal twins reared apart and reared together, *J. Gerontol.*, 44, P100–P105, 1989.
173. Pelletier, F., Marcil-Gratton, N., and Legare, J., A cohort approach to tobacco use and mortality: the case of Québec, *Prev. Med.*, 25, 730–740, 1996.
174. Pepe, G., Di Perna, V., Resta, F., et al., In search of a biological pattern for human longevity: impact of apo A-IV genetic polymorphisms on lipoproteins and the hyper-Lp(a) in centenarians, *Atherosclerosis*, 137, 407–417, 1998.
175. Perls, T.T., Morris, J.N., Ooi, W.L., et al., The relationship between age, gender and cognitive performance in the very old: the effect of selective survival, *J. Am. Geriatr. Soc.*, 41, 1193–1201, 1993.
176. Persinger, M.A., Ballance, S.E., and Moland, M., Snowfall and heart attacks, *J. Psychol.*, 127, 243–252, 1993.
177. Petersen, G.M., Silimperi, D.R., Scott, E.M., et al., Uridine monophosphate kinase 3: a genetic marker for susceptibility to *Haemophilus* influenza type B disease, *Lancet,* 2 (8452), 417–419, 1985.
178. Pfohl, M., Frost, D., Koch, M., et al., Lack of association between the insertion/deletion polymorphism of the angiotensin-converting gene and diabetic neuropathy in IDDM patients, *Horm. Metabol. Res.*, 30, 276–280, 1998.
179. Plomin, R., Pedersen, N.L., McClearn, G.E., et al., EAS temperaments during the last half of the life span: twins reared apart and twins reared together, *Psychol. Aging*, 3, 43–50, 1988.
180. Powell, K.E., Thompson, P.D., Caspersen, C.J., et al., Physical activity and the incidence of coronary heart disease, *Ann. Rev. Publ. Health*, 8, 253–287, 1987.
181. Raleigh, V.S. and Kiri, V.A., Life expectancy in England: variations and trends by gender, health authority, and level of deprivation, *J. Epidemiol. Comm. Health*, 51, 649–658, 1997.

182. Ravussin, E., Valencia, M.E., Esparza, J., et al., Effects of a traditional lifestyle on obesity in Pima Indians, *Diabetes Care*, 17, 1067–1074, 1994.
183. Receputo, G., Rapisarda, R., and Motta, I., Centenarians: health status and life conditions, *Ann. Ital. Med. Intern.*, 10, 41–45, 1995.
184. Refinetti, R., *Circadian Physiology,* CRC Press, Boca Raton, FL, 2000.
185. Regland, B., Blennow, K., Germgard, T., et al., The role of the polymorphic genes apolipoprotein E and methylene-tetrahydrofolate reductase in the development of dementia of the Alzheimer type, *Dementia Geriatr. Cogn. Disorders,* 10, 245–251, 1999.
186. Richter, A., Rioux, J.D., Bouchard, J.P., et al., Location score and haplotype analyses of the locus for autosomal recessive spastic ataxia of Charlevoix–Saguenay, in chromosome region 13q11, *Am. J. Hum. Genet.*, 64, 768–775, 1999.
187. Riggs, J.E., The dynamics of aging and mortality in the U.S., 1900–1988, *Mech. Ageing Dev.*, 66, 45–57, 1992.
188. Robine, J.M. and Ritchie, K., Healthy life expectancy: evaluation of global indicator of change in population health, *Br. Med. J.*, 302, 457–460, 1991.
189. Rode, A. and Shephard, R.J., Cardiorespiratory fitness of an Arctic community, *J. Appl. Physiol.*, 31, 519–526, 1971.
190. Rode, A. and Shephard, R.J., Pulmonary function of Canadian Eskimos, *Scand. J. Resp. Dis.*, 54, 191–205, 1973.
191. Rode, A. and Shephard, R.J., Physiological consequences of acculturation: a 20-year study of Canadian Inuit and Siberian nGanasan, *Eur. J. Appl. Physiol.*, 69, 516–524, 1994.
192. Rode, A. and Shephard, R.J., Comparison of physical fitness between Igloolik Inuit and Volochanka nGanasan, *Am. J. Hum. Biol.*, 7, 623–630, 1995.
193. Rode, A., Shephard, R.J., Vloshinsky, P.E., et al., Plasma fatty acid profiles of Canadian Inuit and Siberian nGanasan, *Arct. Med. Res.*, 54, 10–20, 1995.
194. Romo, M., Factors relating to sudden death in acute ischaemic heart disease: a community study in Helsinki, *Acta Med. Scand.*, 547 (Suppl.), 7–92, 1972.
195. Rossler, R., Kloeden, P.E., and Rossler, O.E., Slower aging in women: a proposed evolutionary explanation, *Biosystems*, 36, 179–185, 1995.
196. Rothstein, M., Altered proteins, error and aging, in *Protein Metabolism in Aging,* Segal, H.L., Rothstein, M., and Bergamini, E., Eds., Wiley-Liss, New York, 1990, 139–154.
197. Rozen, R., Schwartz, R.H., Hilman, B.C., et al., Cystic fibrosis mutations in North American populations of French ancestry: analysis of Quebec French Canadian and Louisiana Acadian families, *Am. J. Hum. Genet.*, 47, 606–610, 1990.
198. Sakari-Rantala, R., Heikkinen, E., and Ruoppila, I., Difficulties in mobility among elderly people and their association with socioeconomic factors, dwelling environment and use of services, *Aging (Milano)*, 7, 433–440, 1995.
199. Salmon, G.K., Leslie, G., Roe, F.J., et al., Influence of food intake and sexual segregation on longevity, organ weights and the incidence of nonneoplastic and neoplastic diseases in rats, *Food Chem. Toxicol.*, 28, 39–48, 1990.
200. Samaras, T.T. and Storms, L.H., Impact of height and weight on life span, *Bull. Wld. Hlth. Org.*, 70, 259–267, 1992.
201. Samuelsson, G. and Dehlin, O., Social class and social mobility — effects on survival. A study of an entire birth cohort during an 80-year life span, *Z. Gerontol.*, 22, 156–161, 1989.

202. Samuelsson, G. and Dehlin, O., Family network and mortality: survival chances through the life span of an entire age cohort, *Int. J. Aging Hum. Develop.*, 37, 277–295, 1993.
203. Sarna, S. and Kaprio, J., Life expectancy of former athletes, *Sports Med.*, 17, 149–151, 1994.
204. Schächter, F., Faure-Delanef, L., Guénet, F., et al., Genetic associations with human longevity at the APOE and ACE loci, *Nat. Genet.*, 6, 29–32, 1994.
205. Schoenbaum, M., Do smokers understand the mortality effects of smoking? Evidence from the health and retirement study, *Am. J. Publ. Health*, 87, 755–759, 1997.
206. Seely, S., The gender gap: why do women live longer than men?, *Int. J. Cardiol.*, 29, 113–119, 1990.
207. Sheldahl, L.M., Wilke, N.A., Dougherty, S.M., et al., Effect of age and coronary artery disease on response in snow shoveling, *J. Am. Coll. Cardiol.*, 20, 1111–1117, 1992.
208. Shephard, R.J., How cold weather affects the heart, *Perspect. Cardiol.*, 8, 35–51, 1992.
209. Shephard, R.J., Habitual physical activity and the quality of life, *Quest*, 48, 354–365, 1996.
210. Shephard, R.J., *Aging, Physical Activity and Health*, Human Kinetics Publishers, Champaign, IL., 1997.
211. Shephard, R.J., Cardiovascular risks of endurance sport, in *Endurance in Sport*, Shephard, R.J. and Åstrand, P.-O., Eds., Blackwell Scientific Publications, Oxford, U.K., 2000.
212. Shephard, R.J. and Rode, A., *The Health Consequences of "Modernization": Evidence from Circumpolar Peoples*, Cambridge University Press, London, 1996.
213. Sherman, S.E., D'Agostino, R.B., Cobb, J.L., et al., Does exercise reduce mortality rates in the elderly? Experience from the Framingham heart study, *Am. Heart J.*, 128, 965–972, 1994.
214. Shibanuma, M., Mochizuki, E., Maniwa, R., et al., Induction of senescence-like phenotypes by forced expression of hic-5, which encodes a novel LIM motif protein, in immortalized human fibroblasts, *Mol. Cell. Biol.*, 17, 1224–1235, 1997.
215. Shimonaka, Y., Nakazato, K., and Homma, A., Personality, longevity, and successful aging among Tokyo metropolitan centenarians, *Int. J. Aging Hum. Develop.*, 42, 173–187, 1996.
216. Siiteri, P.K., Adipose tissue as a source of hormones, *Am. J. Clin. Nutr.*, 45, 277–282, 1987.
217. Simonsick, E.M., Kasper, J.D., and Phillips, C.I., Physical disability and social interaction: factors associated with low social contact and home confinement in disabled older women (the women's health and aging study), *J. Gerontol.*, 53, S209–S217, 1998.
218. Sjalander, A., Birgander, R., Rannug, A., et al., Association between the p21 codon 31 A1 (arg) allele and lung cancer., *Hum. Hered.*, 46, 221–225, 1996.
219. Smith, D.W., Is greater female longevity a general finding among animals? *Biol. Rev. Camb. Philosoph. Soc.*, 64, 1–12, 1989.
220. Smith, D.W. and Warner, H.R., Does genotypic sex have a direct effect on longevity? *Ex. Gerontol.*, 24, 277–288, 1989.
221. Smith, G.D., Bartley, M., and Blane, D., The Black report on socioeconomic inequalities in health ten years on, *Br. Med. J.*, 301, 373–376, 1990.

222. Smith, K.R. and Zick, C.D., Linked lives, dependent demise? Survival analysis of husbands and wives, *Demography,* 31, 81–93, 1994.
223. Spirduso, W., *Physical Dimensions of Aging*, Human Kinetics Publishers, Champaign, IL, 1995.
224. Sports Council and Health Education Authority, *The Allied Dunbar National Fitness Survey: The Main Findings,* Sports Council and Health Education Authority, London, 1992.
225. Sudoh, S., Kawamura, Y., Sato, S., et al., Presenilin I mutations linked to familial Alzheimer's Disease increase the intracellular levels of amyloid beta-protein I-42 and its N-terminally truncated variants which are generated at distinct sites, *J. Neurochem.*, 71, 1535–1543, 1998.
226. Tanner, C.M., Chen, B., Wang, W.Z., et al., Environmental factors in the etiology of Parkinson's Disease, *Can. J. Neurol. Sci.*, 14, 419–423, 1987.
227. Taylor, R.J. and Zimmet, P.Z., Obesity and diabetes in Western Samoa, *Int. J. Obesity,* 5, 367–376, 1981.
228. Terry, P. and Tockman, M.S., Chronic airways obstruction, in *Principles of Geriatric Medicine,* Andres, R., Bierman, E.L., and Hazzard, W.R., Eds., McGraw Hill, New York, 1985, 571–578.
229. Thomas, C.M., Pierzga, J.M., and Kenney, W.L., Aerobic training and cutaneous vasodilatation in young and older men, *J. Appl. Physiol.*, 86, 1676–1686, 1999.
230. Thurmon, T.F., Genetics, aging and the heart, *J. Louisiana State Med. Soc.*, 150, 356–366, 1998.
231. Todesco, L., Angst, C., Litynski, P., et al., Methlenetetrahydrofolate reductase polymorphism, plasma homocysteine and age, *Eur. J. Clin. Invest.*, 29, 1003–1009, 1999.
232. Trovato, F. and Lalu, N.M., Narrowing sex differentials in life expectancy in the industrialized world: early 1970s to early 1990s, *Soc. Biol.*, 43, 20–37, 1996.
233. Tseng, M., Williams, R.C., Maurer, K.R., et al., Genetic admixture and gallbladder disease in Mexican Americans, *Am. J. Phys. Anthropol.*, 106, 361–371, 1998.
234. Turek, Z., Kubat, K., Rignalda, B.E., et al., Experimental myocardial infarction in rats acclimated to simulated high altitude, *Basic Res. Cardiol.*, 75, 544–554, 1980.
235. Turner, T.R. and Weiss, M.L., The genetics of longevity in humans, in *Biological Anthropology and Aging: Perspectives on Human Variation over the Lifespan,* Crews, D.E. and Garutto, R.M., Eds., Oxford University Press, New York, 1994, 76–100.
236. United Nations, Sex differentials in survivorship in the developing world: levels, regional patterns and demographic determinants, *Populat. Bull. U.N.*, 25, 51–64, 1988.
237. Vaillant, G.E., The association of ancestral longevity with successful aging, *J. Gerontol.*, 46, P292–P298, 1991.
238. Valliant, P.M. and Furac, C.J., Type of housing and emotional health of senior citizens, *Psychol. Rep.*, 73, 1347–1353, 1993.
239. van Doorn, C. and Kasl, S.V., Can parental longevity and self-related life expectancy predict mortality among older persons? Results from an Australian cohort, *J. Gerontol.*, 53, S28–S34, 1998.
240. Vandenbroucke, J.P., Matroos, A.W., van der Heide-Wessel, C., et al., Parental survival, independent predictor of longevity in middle-aged persons, *Am. J. Epidemiol.*, 119, 742–750, 1984.

241. Vaupel, J.W., Carey, J.R., Christensen, K., et al., Biodemographic trajectories of longevity, *Science*, 280, 855–860, 1998.
242. Vinogradov, A.E., Male reproductive strategy and decreased longevity, *Acta Biotheoretica*, 46, 157–160, 1998.
243. Vojta, P.J., Futreal, P.A., Annab, L.A., et al., Evidence for two senescence loci on human chromosome I, *Genes Chromosom. Cancer*, 16, 55–63, 1996.
244. Weiss, J.E. and Mushinski, M., International mortality rates and life expectancy: selected countries, *Stat. Bull. Metropol. Ins. Co. N.Y.*, 80 (1), 13–21, 1999.
245. Weiss, K.M., Ferrell, R.E., Harris, C.L., et al., Genetics and epidemiology of gallbladder disease in new world native peoples, *Am. J. Hum. Genet.*, 36, 1259–1278, 1984.
246. Williams, C.L. and Durm, M.W., Longevity in age-heterogeneous marriages, *Psychol. Rep.*, 82, 872–874, 1998.
247. Wingard, D.L., The sex differential in mortality rates: demographic and behavioral factors, *Am. J. Epidemiol.*, 115, 205–216, 1982.
248. Wisniewski, T. and Frangione, B., Molecular biology of brain aging and neurodegenerative disorders, *Acta Neurobiol. Exper.*, 56, 267–279, 1996.
249. Wolozin, B. and Alexander, P.P., J., Regulation of apoptosis by presenilin I, *Neurobiol. Aging*, 19, S23–S27, 1998.
250. World Health Organization, The uses of epidemiology in the study of the elderly. Geneva, Switzerland. 1984.
251. Wright, K., Nature, nurture and death, *Sci. Am.*, 258, 34–38, 1988.
252. Yamada, Y., Miyauchi, A., Goto, J., et al., Association of a polymorphism of the transforming growth factor-beta1 gene with genetic susceptibility to osteoporosis in postmenopausal Japanese women, *J. Bone Min. Res.*, 13, 1569–1576, 1998.
253. Yaron, M., Hultgren, H.N., and Alexander, J.K., Low risk of myocardial ischemia in the elderly visiting moderate altitude, *Wilderness Environ. Med.*, 6, 20–28, 1995.
254. Yu, P.N., Heart disease in Asians and Pacific-Islanders, Hispanics and Native Americans, *Circulation*, 83, 1475–1477, 1991.
255. Zappe, D.H., Bell, G.W., Swartzentruber, H., et al., Age and regulation of fluid and electrolyte balance during repeated exercise sessions, *Am. J. Physiol.*, 270, R71–R79, 1996.
256. Zerba, K.E., Ferrell, R.E., and Sing, C.F., Genotype-environment interaction: apolipoprotein E (ApoE) gene effects and age as an index of time and spatial context in the human, *Genetics*, 143, 463–478, 1996.
257. Zwaan, B.J., The evolutionary genetics of aging and longevity, *Heredity*, 82, 589–597, 1999.

4

Limitations to Oxygen Transport with Aging

Jack M. Goodman and Scott G. Thomas

CONTENTS

0-8493-1027-X/02/$0.00+$1.50

4.1 Introduction

It is generally agreed that a decline in maximal oxygen transport ($\dot{V}O_{2max}$) is one of the characteristics of aging. In examining the age-associated decline in $\dot{V}O_{2max}$, the Fick equation is useful in isolating the several factors that limit oxygen conductance. This equation may be expressed as:

$$\dot{V}O_{2max} = (SV_{max} \cdot HR_{max})\ (av0_2D_{max}) \tag{4.1}$$

where $av0_2D$ = the arterial-mixed venous oxygen difference, HR = heart rate, max = maximum, and SV = stroke volume. Although this arrangement allows for a description of cardiac output and peripheral oxygen extraction, cardiac output can be solved using an alternative approach:

$$\dot{V}O_{2max} = (MAP_{max}/TPR_{max})\ (av0_2D_{max}) \tag{4.2}$$

where MAP = mean arterial pressure and TPR = total peripheral resistance; and therefore,

$$(SV_{max} \cdot HR_{max})(av0_2D_{max}) = \dot{V}O_{2max} = (MAPmax/TPRmax)(av02Dmax) \tag{4.3}$$

There are age-dependent changes in each of the above variables, in addition to gender-related factors that modulate the acute response to exercise and strategies used in chronic adaptation. Mechanisms explaining the decline in $\dot{V}O_{2max}$ through the aging process are multifactoral. In addition, it is possible that resistors to oxygen delivery change throughout the aging process, uncoupling certain relationships along the way.[1]

4.2 Changes in Aerobic Power with Age

The decline in aerobic power ($\dot{V}O_{2max}$) with increased age is secondary to three primary causes: (1) reduced physical activity, (2) physiological aging, and (3) increased prevalence of pathological conditions. The decline in aerobic power with increased age is well documented,[2] but the estimated rate of decline varies widely among individuals, contingent on the magnitude of each of the primary factors mentioned earlier (see Figure 4.1). The degree of screening of a population for chronic diseases (especially coronary heart disease) is also a key factor in determining the average change in $\dot{V}O_{2max}$ observed with age, particularly when comparing data for older men and women. For example, there is typically a ten-year delay in the onset of coronary symptoms for women compared to men and, given the lower

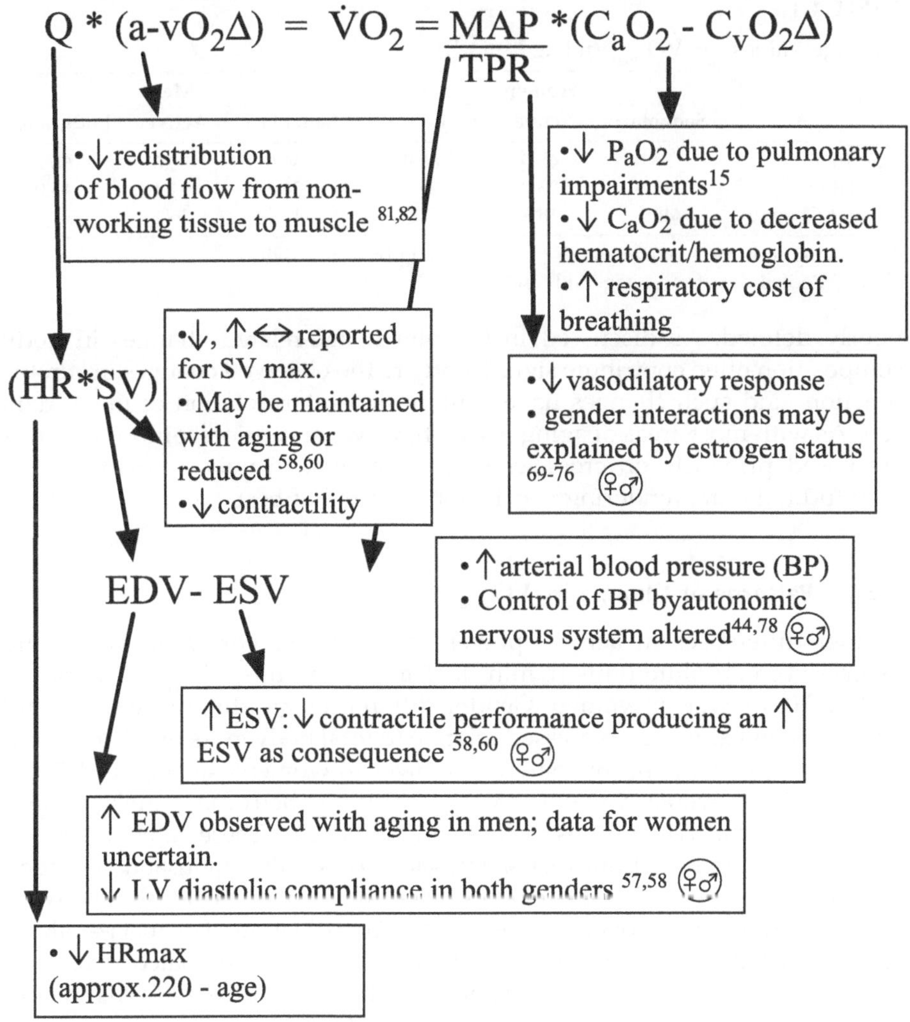

FIGURE 4.1
Age and gender interactions in the cardiorespiratory limitations to exercise. Where: $a\text{-}vO_2$ = arterio-mixed venous oxygen difference; $C_aO_2–C_vO_2$ = oxygen content of arterio-venous oxygen difference Δ; EDV = end-diastolic volume; ESV = end-systolic volume; HR_{max} = maximal heart rate; LV = left ventricle; MAP = mean arterial pressure; P_aO_2 = partial pressure arterial oxygen; $\dot{Q}$ = cardiac output; SV = stroke volume; TPR = total peripheral resistance; $\dot{V}O_2$ = oxygen intake.

diagnostic power of most screening tools for coronary heart disease in females, they are more likely to be considered free of cardiac pathology.

A recent position statement from the American College of Sports Medicine indicated a broad range of decline (5 to 15%) in $\dot{V}O_{2max}$ per decade.[3] The interactive effects of age, gender, and habitual physical activity appear to account for a considerable amount of the variance in rate of decline among apparently healthy individuals, but their relative contributions remain

TABLE 4.1

Average Values for $\dot{V}O_{2max}$ ($ml \cdot kg^{-1} \cdot min^{-1}$)*

	Women			Men		
	Sedentary	Active	Endurance	Sedentary	Active	Endurance
Age 20 yr	36.8	45.0	60.0	46.0	53.6	68.0
Age 70 yr	19.3	23.2	29.0	26.2	34.1	45.0
Percent Change	48%	48%	52%	43%	36%	34%

* Showing influences of age, gender, and habitual physical activity.
Source: Pooled data from Fitzgerald[5] and Wilson.[5,6]

poorly defined. As discussed in Chapter 1, age-related changes in body composition often contribute significantly to the observed changes in aerobic function, and such changes have confounded interpretation of many data sets. As with most areas of aging research, views of cardiorespiratory change are based primarily on cross-sectional studies with only a smattering of longitudinal data, rendering conclusions limited at best.

4.2.1 Patterns of Change in $\dot{V}O_{2max}$

Gender differences in aerobic power are most evident when values are expressed in absolute units ($L \cdot min^{-1}$). Using such units, $\dot{V}O_{2max}$ is approximately 30% lower in women. Gender differences are diminished, but still persist when values are expressed relative to total body mass or fat-free mass (the $\dot{V}O_{2max}$ is then approximately 5% lower in women;[4] see Figure 4.2).

Table 4.1 lists average values for $\dot{V}O_{2max}$ relative to body mass ($ml \cdot kg^{-1} \cdot min^{-1}$) by gender and activity groups in youth and in old age. These values are based on equations derived from meta-analyses incorporating thousands of study participants.[5,6] Notice that the equations assume a linear relationship between age and aerobic power over the age range of 20 to 70 years. The meta-analyses suggest that the effect of habitual activity on the age-associated decline in $\dot{V}O_{2max}$ is gender specific. In males aged 20 to 70 years, Wilson and colleagues[6] observed similar absolute (–4 to –4.6 $ml \cdot kg^{-1} \cdot min^{-1}$/decade) and relative (–9 to –7%/decade) rates of decline, irrespective of habitual activity level. However, the same group[5] observed a similar relative (approximately –10%/decade) but faster absolute rate of decline in endurance-trained women (–6 $ml \cdot kg^{-1} \cdot min^{-1}$/decade) compared to sedentary women (–3 $ml \cdot kg^{-1} \cdot min^{-1}$/decade; see Figure 4.2d).

These observations illustrate how the difference in aerobic power between well-trained men and women increases from youth to old age and decreases between sedentary men and women. The decreased difference between sedentary and fit older women may reflect changes in responsiveness to training of the central circulation in older women,[7] and the greater degree of training achieved at a young age.

Recent data from the Baltimore Longitudinal Study of Aging[8] suggest that the rate of decline is not in fact linear, but rather accelerates from 6% per decade between the ages of 20 and 30 to over 15% after the age of 60. Analysis further indicates more rapid declines in older men compared to women; the latter maintain a more linear decline in the later ages.

The age-associated decline in aerobic function becomes critical to independent function only in later life, when $\dot{V}O_{2max}$ becomes an important predictor of independence[9] (see also Chapter 5). In addition, low aerobic power is associated with increased risk of disability in older adults.[10] Nonlinear, allometric modeling of the influences of age, body mass, and gender for men and women aged 55 to 86 years suggests an average decline of 15% per decade.[11]

Gender differences in age-associated aerobic change are related to changes in body composition and lean body mass. In later life, the reduction in lean body mass is more pronounced in older men than in older women.

4.2.2 Responses to Submaximal Exercise

The ability to perform submaximal aerobic exercise may decline at a slower rate than maximal oxygen intake. The ventilation threshold is a noninvasive marker of the ability to perform exercise without causing a significant rise in plasma lactate levels. It is correlated with the lactate threshold, and is used to identify the anaerobic threshold. The ventilation threshold decreases at a slower rate than $\dot{V}O_{2max}$ between the ages of 20 and 65 years and 55 to 85 years.[12] As a result of its slower decline, the ventilation threshold is reached at a higher percentage of $\dot{V}O_{2max}$ in older compared to younger people (~80% vs. ~45%). The low-intensity activities of older adults may be sufficient to slow the decline in ventilation threshold. Moreover, these observations may indicate that central cardiovascular deconditioning contributes more significantly to the decline in exercise performance than do changes in peripheral metabolic factors.

4.3 Ventilatory Response to Acute Exercise

There is little evidence to support the idea that ventilatory performance limits oxygen uptake in healthy older adults. Notwithstanding, a reduced ability to ventilate the lungs and an increased demand for ventilation are hallmarks of aging in both men and women.[13] Underlying physiological changes include decreases in elastic recoil of the lungs, compliance of the chest wall, and respiratory muscle strength.[14]

Changes in lung volumes include a rise in functional residual capacity and a fall in vital capacity.[14] The $FEV_{1.0}$ declines slightly faster in older men (–42 $ml \cdot y^{-1}$) than in older women (–37 $ml \cdot y^{-1}$), although smoking greatly accelerates the rate of decline for both genders (to an average value of –48 $ml \cdot y^{-1}$).[15]

In combination with loss of elastic recoil, hyperinflation associated with aging may limit the increase in ventilation during aerobic exercise. Evidence of mechanical constraint of ventilation includes expiratory airflow limitation, and excessive expiratory pressure generation.[16] The effect of gender upon the mechanical constraints of exercise ventilation has not been explored.

These changes have direct implication for ventilatory efficiency during exercise. This is quantified as the ratio of change in ventilation to change in $\dot{V}_{CO2}$ at intensities of effort below the ventilatory threshold. Reports consistently observe smaller ratios (and thus a higher efficiency) in young adults compared to older adults.[13] Studies over an older age range (55 to 86 years) suggest that age-related declines are greater for men than women.[17]

Decreased ventilatory efficiency may also reflect an increased dead space to tidal volume ratio and a small increase in ventilation/perfusion ($\dot{V}_A / \dot{Q}$) inequalities.[18] Those changes may contribute to the small age-associated decline in arterial oxygen partial pressures observed in studies contrasting young (20 years) and older adults (from a Pa_{O2} of approximately 100 to 85 mmHg).[14]

The increased load consequent upon increased work of breathing and decreased ventilatory efficiency must be met by decreased respiratory muscle strength. Average values for maximum inspiratory and expiratory pressures fall below clinical thresholds for respiratory muscle dysfunction at age 65 for women and 75 for men.[14] Given a reduced $\dot{V}O_{2max}$ with age, the oxygen cost of breathing accounts for a significant portion of oxygen delivery when elderly individuals exercise.

In summary, ventilatory function declines with age; it also requires more work and may be mechanically constrained; however, current evidence does not support the hypothesis that it limits $\dot{V}O_{2max}$ per se. Gender differences in lung function persist across age groups, but the overall differences are smaller in the elderly because of the slower declines observed in women. The decline observed in apparently healthy older women may be accelerated if osteoporosis-related vertebral fractures lead to kyphosis, increased work of breathing, and decreased force-generating ability.[14]

4.4 Acute Cardiovascular Responses to Exercise

4.4.1 Maximal Cardiac Output

There is overwhelming evidence that maximal cardiac output ($\dot{Q}max$) is slightly reduced with age.[19-23] Only two studies have reported maintenance of $\dot{Q}max$ with age.[24,25] Rodeheffer's group[26] later cited abstracted data from the Baltimore Longitudinal Study of Aging reporting a decline in cardiac output with increased age.[1]

4.4.2 Submaximal Cardiac Output

The submaximal $\dot{Q}$ response to exercise is well maintained with age,[27-29] although there is some evidence of a minor reduction in the elderly.[30] Consequently, the slope of the $\dot{Q}/\dot{V}O_2$ relationship remains reasonably constant with increasing age, regardless of gender or state of training.[24,28] With advancing age, strategies used to augment cardiac output during exercise shift from codependence on catecholamine-mediated inotropic, chronotropic, and volumetric means, to greater dependence on changes in ventricular end-diastolic volume via the Frank–Starling mechanism. Possible factors underlying this shift are outlined later, including the manner in which cardiac output is supported throughout the course of aging (in particular when considering adaptive responses to endurance training), together with any gender differences.

Given close matching of $\dot{Q}$ to $\dot{V}O_2$ throughout aging (a consistent slope of 5–6 l/l), it seems dubious to ascribe the reduction in $\dot{V}O_{2max}$ exclusively to a decrease in $\dot{Q}max$.[23] A combination of small changes in ventilatory function, muscle mass, and hematological factors together may account for diminished work capacity, not to mention the influence of age-related changes in distribution of cardiac output during exercise.[28,31] These various factors are considered next.

4.4.3 Heart Rate

Maximal heart rate (HR) declines with age, regardless of gender or state of training.[20-25,32-35] A sedentary lifestyle and increased likelihood of disease with the aging process do not seem to be contributing factors.[1] The popular equation for prediction of maximal HR (220 – the individual's age, in years) provides a reasonably accurate guide to age-related change in HR, although many authors have observed higher maximal heart rates than this equation would predict in elderly individuals. The quality of the exercise test also contributes significantly to the heart rate achieved.[36]

A lower adrenergic responsiveness with increasing age is the leading explanation of diminished heart rate response to exercise.[1,37-39] Myocardial tissue sensitivity to catecholamines decreases with increasing age across a large number of animal species.[40] Because catecholamines are key stimulatory agonists during exercise and are the first stimulatory extra-sarcolemmic signals within the myocyte,[41] their modulating effect on cardiac function is critical to a normal chronotropic (and inotropic) response. Catecholamine secretion seems to be maintained with advanced age,[1,38] and older endurance-trained individuals have higher levels of catecholamines than those who are untrained, except when data are expressed at a similar relative workrate.

A number of factors lead to diminished sensitivity. Alterations in postreceptor adrenergic signaling,[41] rather than a change in absolute receptor number,[38] are seen as the primary cause. The key signaling proteins involved in both the amplification and integration of extracellular signals in the myocyte (from the sarcoplasmic reticulum to the intracellular effectors) include β-adrenergic receptors, G proteins, and adenyl cyclase. Aging is associated with significant reductions in all of these mediators. As animal studies indicate, the older sedentary heart displays a 30 to 40% reduction in G-protein- and receptor-dependent adrenergic responsiveness.[40,41] Almost all of this decline can be reversed with aerobic training, yet the age-related reduction in adenyl cyclase-dependent production of cAMP does not respond to training.[41]

It is highly unlikely that reduction in maximal heart rate is related to changes in vagal tone. Although some rat studies show a lower vagal nerve stimulus threshold with increased age, atropine blockade in older dogs failed to alter the age-dependent maximal heart rate.[1] Variability in the R-R interval, used as an index of parasympathetic tone, is augmented with aerobic training, and has been associated with a lower risk of coronary heart disease.[42] A similar age-related decrease in heart rate variability and cardiac baroreflex sensitivity (another measure of vagal tone) has been observed at rest[43] and has been seen in sedentary and physically active men and women.[42,44-48] However, despite the decline with age, physically active men and women continue to demonstrate higher levels of heart rate variability and cardiac baroreflex sensitivity than their sedentary peers.[42,43,45] These responses argue against changes in parasympathetic tone contributing to the changes in left ventricular chronotropic function observed during exercise.

4.4.4 Left Ventricular Contractility

There has been limited investigation of inotropic state in the intact human because an interaction of loading conditions affects left ventricular function at rest and, in particular, during exercise. Although various noninvasive indices of myocardial contractility have been used to characterize left ventricular function at rest and during exercise, analysis of the inotropic state remains problematic. Consequently, it is not surprising to find conflicting data describing differences in inotropic state with age and gender. For example, at rest, the peak systolic blood pressure/end-systolic volume ratio (PVR) and other echocardiographic (fiber shortening) measures of contractility are unchanged[1,49] or only minimally affected[50] by age, regardless of gender. However, there is convincing evidence for a lower resting inotropic reserve from animal models, when rate of tension development, velocity of cell shortening, sarcoplasmic Ca^{2+} release rates, and troponin I phosphorylation are measured.[1,51] Undoubtedly, the mechanisms for many of these changes relate to alterations in β-adrenergic sensitivity as described earlier.[37-41,51] Recent data also indicate that changes in myocyte shortening rates may relate to an age-induced shift towards a slower myosin, heavy-chain isoform.[52]

Augmented inotropic function during exercise is a significant response to dynamic exercise in young adults, particularly as exercise reaches higher intensities.[53] Studies in older men using a combination of β-blockade have demonstrated an impairment of inotropic reserve with age.[54,55] Ventricular loading conditions may contribute significantly to these observations, as acute afterload reduction can reverse age-related changes in the ejection fraction and peripheral vascular resistance.[56] Unfortunately, no data examining gender differences during exercise are available. Data from training studies suggest that older women fail to increase their inotropic state as much as men, and in older women the left ventricular ejection fraction does not increase significantly during supine exercise.[57] Turner and colleagues[58,59] have observed both age and gender differences in the cardiovascular response to phenylephrine and isoproterenol. Older women had a more pronounced increase in systolic blood pressure with phenylephrine (α-agonist) and less age-related decline in inotropic and chronotopic response to isoproterenol (β-agonist).

4.4.5 Stroke Volume, End-Diastolic, and End-Systolic Volume Responses to Exercise

Studies examining age-related changes in left ventricular volume responses to exercise have produced disparate results because of sampling bias, differences in methodology, and apparent gender differences. As mentioned earlier, both $\dot{V}O_{2max}$ and $\dot{Q}$ are reportedly lower in older adults. The changes in stroke volume at peak exercise remain equivocal. Early work by Rodeheffer's group suggested that stroke volume increased[25] or showed no change[25,60] with advancing age. However, others have reported a decrease of stroke volume in untrained[19] and trained[22] individuals. Interstudy differences in the time when stroke volume was measured, or the relative intensity of exercise, may contribute to these disparate findings, since changes in stroke volume over a range of exercise intensities are not uniform.[53,60-62] Older women may not increase stroke volume significantly during an acute bout of exercise,[57] although conflicting data suggest a significant rise in stroke volume to maximum effort.[23] However, data on healthy older females are lacking, limiting conclusions concerning gender differences.

4.4.6 Left Ventricular Volume Changes during Exercise

The changes in left ventricular filling (end-diastolic volume) and emptying (end-systolic volume), and their relative contributions to the stroke volume response during exercise remain unclear. Aging appears to be associated with greater reliance on the Frank–Starling mechanism to augment stroke volume, in part as a countermeasure to the decline in myocardial contractility.[25,63] Data from the Baltimore Longitudinal Study of Aging indicated that ejection fraction, heart rate, and cardiac index were all reduced with age; the end-diastolic volume index increased 35% with age in men, but changes in end-diastolic volume index were unrelated to age in women.[60]

The age-associated dependence on an increase of left ventricular filling to compensate for diminished inotropic reserve is interesting, given observations of an age-related impairment in left ventricular filling during both rest and exercise. Numerous studies have demonstrated an impairment of left ventricular filling characteristics with increasing age.[64-68] Despite these observations, a less compliant ventricle appears capable of compensating partially for the decline in adrenergic-dependent inotropic reserve. Nevertheless, there are few studies of diastolic filling characteristics during exercise, due to limited temporal resolution of the early rapid filling phase associated with high heart rates. Mechanisms contributing to early diastolic filling during exercise include the so-called "diastolic suction" effect (a downward shift of the left ventricular pressure-volume loop) secondary to enhanced sympathetic stimulation, and increases in left atrial pressure.[67] There are no data describing changes in these characteristics in the older population. Although data support a training-induced improvement in lusitrophic function (relaxation) in an aged rat model,[69] there are no parallel findings in older men or women exposed to volume loading following training.

4.5 Peripheral Vascular Function during Exercise

4.5.1 Vasodilatory Capacity and Age

The direct relationship between maximal oxygen intake and peak vascular blood flow[70] is maintained in both health and disease.[71] Information is limited concerning the older population, but the relationship appears to be preserved with increasing age[72] provided there is no peripheral vascular disease. Nevertheless, when considering the relationship between muscle blood flow and exercise performance, the cardiac output response to exercise may not reflect the local perfusion of skeletal muscle accurately because of reduced shunting ability in the elderly. Thus, peak vasodilatory capacity is diminished with age,[31,72-77] and even if submaximal cardiac output is well maintained, the regional blood flow to the exercising muscle may be reduced. The flow-mediated impairment in vasodilatory capacity is seen in both genders. Older women may demonstrate a disproportionately greater increase in peripheral vascular resistance, both at rest and during exercise, when compared to age-matched men.[28] Women receiving estrogen therapy do not show an elevated peripheral vascular resistance relative to men,[72] but they still experience a reduction in peak blood flow with increasing age. Estrogen status seems important to gender differences in blood flow and conductance because estrogen increases endothelial-dependent vasodilatation, specifically through its ability to upregulate nitric oxide production.[51,78-81] Both endothelial-dependent vasodilatation and estrogen levels decline after menopause;[82] however, impairment can be attenuated and possibly arrested by estrogen replacement therapy.[78-80,82] Preliminary data from our laboratory[83] indicate that, in postmenopausal women, opposed estrogen replacement therapy (with progesterone) increased reactive hyperemic blood flow after 16 weeks, although it failed to increase exercise performance.

4.5.2 Regional Blood Flow Changes with Age

Changes in regional blood flow may explain why exercise performance diminishes with aging, despite a well-maintained submaximal $\dot{Q}$. Renal and splanchnic vasoconstriction during exercise are attenuated in older men and women,[84] and training may not reverse these changes.[85] The age-related impairment of exercise capacity may be exacerbated in hot environments, since older individuals also show a smaller increase in skin blood flow under such conditions.[85]

4.5.3 Changes in Vascular Function and Structure

Age-related changes in vascular function develop throughout the vascular tree; these changes include a loss of compliance in the large arteries of the thorax.[86] This increased stiffness may explain the increase in left ventricular wall mass,[65] and the matched left ventricular systolic stiffening[87] seen with aging. Considerable changes develop in vessels that regulate vascular resistance. An impairment of endothelial-dependent vasodilatation in the elderly[88] involves reduced functioning of the L-arginine nitric oxide pathway, considered to be active in augmenting local blood flow during exercise. Improvements in endothelial-dependent vasodilatation following training[89] indicate the potential for training-induced upregulation of nitric oxide production.[74,75] Age-related changes in microcirculation are less clearly established; modest reductions have been reported in the elderly,[90] but if data are expressed per muscle fiber, capillarization does not seem to be affected significantly by age.[91] The direct relationship between oxygen kinetics and capillarization appears to become uncoupled in older subjects,[91] suggesting that other muscular factors may control oxygen kinetics, for instance mitochondrial oxidative capacity (known to diminish by as much as 50% in aging human skeletal muscle;[92] see further discussion in Chapter 7).

4.6 Adaptation to Increased Physical Activity

4.6.1 Maximal Oxygen Intake

Debate continues about the relative importance of physical activity and physical fitness, yet higher levels of both are associated with better health and function in older adults (see Chapter 5). The relative (percentage) increase in aerobic power observed with physical training is comparable across a wide age range. Although the absolute magnitude of $\dot{V}O_{2max}$ increase varies widely between individuals,[93] the mean increases are similar in young and old if similar training stimuli are employed. An effective aerobic training program will increase $\dot{V}O_{2max}$ by 10 to 30%. The magnitude of the change in $\dot{V}O_{2max}$ depends on the magnitude of the training stimulus in both men[93] and women.[94]

Aerobic training is equally effective in young men and women.[4] The absolute increase of $\dot{V}O_{2max}$ is larger in men, but the percentage increase of aerobic power is similar in men and women. In contrast, some studies suggest that the training-induced gain in $\dot{V}O_{2max}$ is smaller in older women than in older men.[4,95] Reasons for these differences are now being explored.

4.6.2 Responses to Submaximal Exercise

In addition to training-induced increases in $\dot{V}O_{2max}$, responses to submaximal exercise are modified. The ventilation threshold is increased with training in young[96] and older[97] men and women.[98] Exercise training which increases $\dot{V}O_{2max}$ and augments the ventilation threshold by 10 to 15% may increase the time to fatigue by as much as 180% when exercising at a fixed intensity. Improvement in submaximal aerobic exercise performance is believed to result in part from change in skeletal muscle metabolism. These changes in submaximal performance have a profound effect on the ability of older people to function in daily life.[99]

4.7 Strategies for Adaptation: Central and Peripheral Factors

4.7.1 General Considerations

Although both men and women appear to have similar adaptive potential with respect to $\dot{V}O_{2max}$, there seem to be gender differences in how this is achieved. Whereas older men increase $\dot{V}O_{2max}$ through a combination of increased arterio-mixed venous oxygen content difference and increased maximal cardiac output, older women seem to rely exclusively on increased oxygen extraction.[61] However, cross-sectional comparisons have also documented high maximal cardiac outputs in well-trained older women.[23]

4.7.2 Cardiac Adaptations

Whether inherent gender differences exist in growth factors specific to the adaptive potential of the left ventricle (i.e., eccentric or eccentric hypertrophic adaptation) is unknown. Women seem to demonstrate a lower capacity for left ventricular hypertrophy than men, secondary to either estrogen-mediated signaling that attenuates the hypertrophic response[100] or the absence of an androgenic growth factor found in males.[101] The presence of physiological levels of estrogen in premenopausal women or the use of hormone replacement therapy by postmenopausal women may be key factors in interpreting changes in their central and peripheral adaptation relative to men, given the systemic effects of estrogen.[102]

Cross-sectional data suggest that trained postmenopausal women have a 38% greater $\dot{Q}$ than young sedentary women,[103] reflecting almost entirely a larger stroke volume. These data are contrary to the findings of Spina et al.,[95,103,104] who suggested that older women do not increase their stroke volumes with training. More recent data indicate that older women fail to increase their stroke volumes at high intensities of exercise, and demonstrate a drop in stroke volume between 70 and 90% of $\dot{V}O_{2max}$,[28,95,103,104] or sometimes as early as 40 to 50% $\dot{V}O_{2max}$.[105] However, the study by McCole et al.[105] confirmed that a high degree of training was associated with higher stroke volumes in postmenopausal women.

Contrary to cross-sectional data, longitudinal training studies do not support the concept of training-induced cardiac adaptations in older women, as they do for men. Prolonged training (9 months or more) failed to improve the stroke volume in older women compared to age-matched men.[95]. Recent data confirm earlier laboratory work demonstrating that 11 months of training failed to change either left ventricular systolic function or left ventricular dimensions in postmenopausal women.[106] The failure of women to increase their exercise-end-diastolic volume after training may reflect a limited ability to improve the parameters of diastolic filling.[7] Both animal[69] and human[7,67,69] studies indicate that older males have the capacity to improve their diastolic filling. Part of the adaptive response may relate to favorable changes in cardiac connective tissue content, as rats exposed to endurance training demonstrate lower collagen gene mRNA activity.[107]

4.7.3 Peripheral Vascular Adaptations

Few data describe peripheral vascular changes with training in the older population. Cross-sectional studies support a relationship between calf muscle vasodilatory reserve and $\dot{V}O_{2max}$,[72] and regular physical activity has been associated with enhanced availability of nitric oxide and greater endothelial-dependent vasodilatation in the elderly.[74,75] Training studies support these observations, showing significant improvements in peak leg blood flow after 3 months of aerobic training[77] and an enhanced capillary/perimeter ratio following resistance training in men.[108] The improved blood flow appears to arise from more effective distribution of cardiac output;[77] it may reflect an overall improvement in vascular control, since aerobic training can also enhance selectively the skin blood flow response of older men to exercise and heat stress.[73]

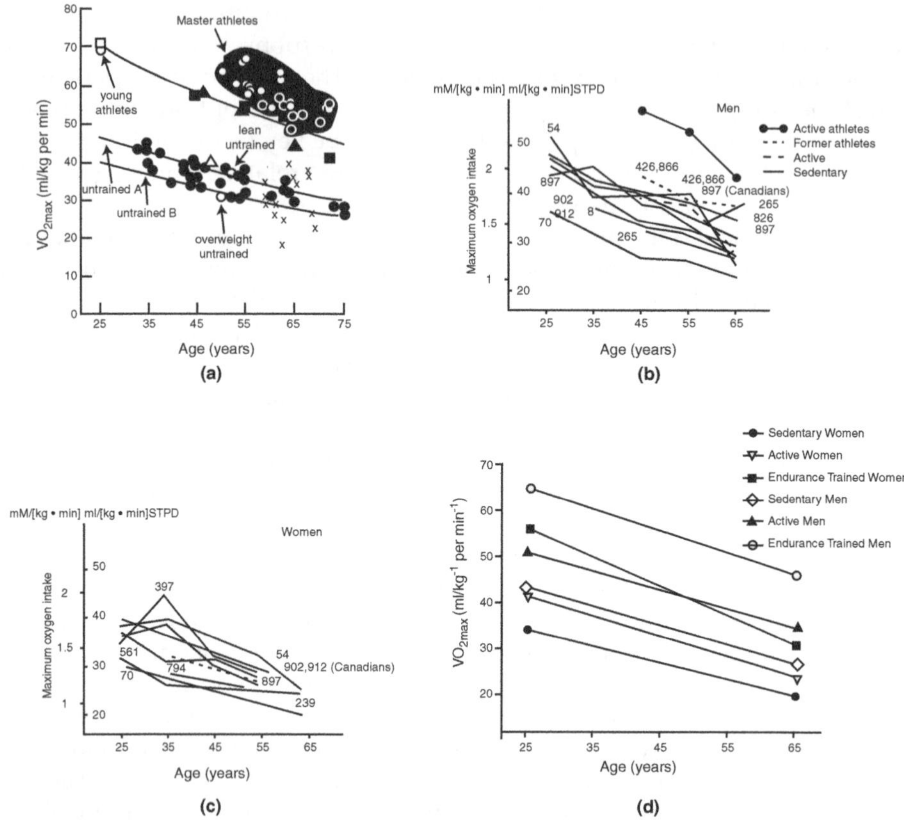

FIGURE 4.2
Patterns of change in maximal oxygen intake ($\dot{V}O_{2max}$) with age. (a) pooled data from Lakatta,[1] with permision; (b) and (c) pooled data from Shephard,[36] with permission; (d) regression lines for $\dot{V}O_{2max}$ derived from data of meta-analyses.[5,6] Note: For panels a, b, and c, see original publication for sources of individual data sets.

These training-induced changes in blood flow indicate that older individuals can adapt peripheral vascular function both at the molecular level (through enhanced production of nitric oxide) and systemically (through redistribution of available flow).

4.8 Conclusions

Aging of the cardiorespiratory system is not due to breakdown in a single step of oxygen conductance from the atmosphere to exercising muscles. Rather, there are physiological changes in each of the series of resistors. Analysis is complicated by methodological differences between and inherent limitations of cross-sectional and longitudinal studies, changes in female hormonal status through the aging process, and the need to distinguish physiological aging from pathological change. In returning to Equation 4.3, it is apparent that aging affects each step in the delivery of oxygen, often with differing effects across genders. Many of these changes are slowed or reversed by exercise training (Figure 4.1). Further research is required to identify the mechanisms responsible for gender differences in the effects of aging on various systems contributing to cardiorespiratory function and on adaptive responses to exercise training.

References

1. Lakatta, E. G., Cardiovascular regulatory mechanisms in advanced age, *Physiol. Rev.*, 73, 413–467, 1993.
2. Åstrand, I., Aerobic work capacity in men and women with special reference to age., *Acta Physiol. Scand.*, 49, 1–92, 1960.
3. American College of Sports Medicine, Exercise and physical activity for older adults, *Med. Sci. Sports Exerc.*, 30, 992–1008, 1998.
4. Shephard, R. J., Exercise and training in women, Part I: Influence of gender on exercise and training responses, *Can. J. Appl. Physiol.*, 25, 19–34, 2000.
5. Fitzgerald, M. D., Tanaka, H., Tran, Z. V., et al., Age-related declines in maximal aerobic capacity in regularly exercising vs. sedentary women: a meta-analysis, *J. Appl. Physiol.*, 83, 160–165, 1997.
6. Wilson, T. M. and Tanaka, H., Meta-analysis of the age-associated decline in maximal aerobic capacity in men: relation to training status, *Am. J Physiol. (Heart Circ. Physiol.)*, 278, H829–H834, 2000.
7. Spina, R. J., Miller, T. R., Bogenhagen, W. H., et al., Gender-related differences in left ventricular filling dynamics in older subjects after endurance exercise training, *J. Geront. Biol. Sci. Med. Sci.*, 51, B232–B237, 1996.
8. Fleg, J. L., Bos, A. G., Brant, L. H., et al., Longitudinal decline of aerobic capacity accelerates with age, *Circulation*, 102 (suppl. II), 602, 2000.
9. Cunningham, D., Paterson, D., Himann, J., et al., Determinants of independence in the elderly., *Can. J. Appl. Physiol.*, 18, 243–254, 1993.
10. Morey, M. C., Pieper, C., and Cornoni-Huntley, J., Physical fitness and functional limitations in community-dwelling older adults, *Med. Sci. Sports Exerc.*, 30, 715–723, 1998.
11. Johnson, P. J., Winter, E. M., Paterson, D. H., et al., Modelling the influence of age, body size and sex on maximum oxygen uptake in older humans, *Exp. Physiol.*, 85, 219–225, 2000.
12. Cunningham, D. A., Paterson, D. H., Koval, J. J., et al., A model of oxygen transport capacity changes for independently living older men and women, *Can. J. Appl. Physiol.*, 22, 439–453, 1997.
13. Habedank, D., Reindl, I., Vietzke, G., et al., Ventilatory efficiency and exercise tolerance in 101 healthy volunteers., *Eur. J. Appl. Physiol.*, 77, 421–426, 1998.
14. Janssens, J. P., Pache, J. C., and Nicod, L. P., Physiological changes in respiratory function associated with aging, *Eur. Resp. J.*, 13, 197–205, 1999.

15. Griffith, K. A., Sherrill, D. L., Siegel, E. M., et al., Predictors of loss of lung function in the elderly: the cardiovascular health study, *Am. J. Resp. Crit. Care*, 163, 61–68, 2001.
16. Johnson, B. D., Reddan, W. G., Seow, K. C., et al., Mechanical constraints on exercise hyperpnea in a fit aging population, *Am. Rev. Resp. Dis.*, 143, 966–977, 1991.
17. Poulin, M. J., Cunningham, D. A., Paterson, D. H., et al., Ventilatory response to exercise in men and women 55 to 86 years of age, *Am. J. Resp. Crit. Care Med.*, 149, 408–415, 1994.
18. Cardus, J., F., B., Orlando, D., et al., Increase in pulmonary ventilation–perfusion inequality with age in healthy individuals, *Am. J. Resp. Crit. Care Med.*, 156, 648–653, 1997.
19. Bogaard, H. J., Woltjer, H. H., Dekker, B. M., et al., Haemodynamic response to exercise in healthy young and elderly subjects, *Eur. J. Appl. Physiol.*, 75, 435–442, 1997.
20. Hagberg, J. M., Allen, W. K., Seals, D. R., et al., A hemodynamic comparison of young and older endurance athletes during exercise, *J. Appl. Physiol.*, 58, 2041–2046, 1985.
21. Heath, G. W., Hagberg, J. M., Ahsani, A. A., et al., A physiological comparison of young and older endurance athletes, *J. Appl. Physiol.*, 51, 634–640, 1981.
22. Ogawa, T., Spina, R. J., Martin, W. H., et al., Effects of aging, sex and physical training on cardiovascular responses to exercise, *Circulation*, 86, 494–503, 1992.
23. Weibe, C. G., Gledhill, N., Jamnik, V. K., et al., Exercise cardiac function in young through elderly endurance trained women, *Med. Sci. Sports Exerc.*, 31, 684–691, 1999.
24. Becklake, M. R., Frank, H., Dagenais, G. R., et al., Influence of age and sex on exercise cardiac output, *J. Appl. Physiol.*, 20, 938–947, 1965.
25. Rodeheffer, R. J., Gerstenblith, G., Becker, L. C., et al., Exercise cardiac output is maintained with advancing age in healthy human subjects: cardiac dilatation and increased stroke volume compensate for a diminished heart rate, *Circulation*, 69, 203–213, 1984.
26. Rodeheffer, R. J., Gerstenblith, G., Beard, E., et al., Postural changes in cardiac volumes in men in relation to adult age, *Exp. Gerontol.*, 21, 367–378, 1986.
27. Faulkner, J. A., Heigenhauser, G. F., and Schork, M. A., The cardiac output–oxygen uptake relationship of men during graded bicycle ergometry, *Med. Sci. Sports Exerc.*, 9, 148–154, 1977.
28. Proctor, D. N., Beck, K. C., Shen, P. H., et al., Influence of age and gender on cardiac output–VO2 relationships during submaximal cycle ergometry, *J. Appl. Physiol.*, 84, 599–605, 1998.
29. McElvaney, G. N., Backie, S. P., Morrison, N. J., et al., Cardiac output at rest and in exercise in elderly subjects, *Med. Sci. Sports Exerc.*, 21, 293–298, 1989.
30. Thomas, S. G., Paterson, D. H., Cunningham, D. A., et al., Cardiac output and left ventricular function in response to exercise in older men, *Can. J. Physiol. Pharm.*, 71, 136–144, 1993.
31. Proctor, D. N., Shen, P. H., Dietz, N. M., et al., Reduced leg blood flow during dynamic exercise in older endurance-trained men, *J. Appl. Physiol.*, 85, 68–75, 1998.
32. Proctor, D. N. and Joyner, M. J., Skeletal muscle mass and the reduction of $\dot{V}O_{2max}$ in trained older subjects, *J. Appl. Physiol.*, 82, 1411–1415, 1997.

33. Douglas, P. S. and O'Toole, M., Aging and physical activity determine cardiac structure and function in the older athlete, *J. Appl. Physiol.*, 72, 1969–1973, 1992.
34. Ehsani, A. A., Ogawa, T., Miller, T. R., et al., Exercise training improves left ventricular systolic function in older men, *Circulation*, 83, 96–103, 1991.
35. Jackson, A. S., Wier, L. T., Ayers, G. W., et al., Changes in aerobic power of women, ages 20–64 years, *Med. Sci. Sports Exerc.*, 28, 884–891, 1996.
36. Shephard, R. J., *Aging, Physical Activity and Health*, Human Kinetics, Champaign, IL, 1997, 114.
37. Miyamoto, A. and Ohshika, H., Cellular and molecular mechanisms of cardiovascular aging. Molecular pharmacological implications, *Ann. N.Y. Acad. Sci.*, 786, 283–293, 1996.
38. Lakatta, E. G., Deficient neuroendocrine regulation of the cardiovascular system with advancing age in healthy humans, *Circulation*, 87, 631–636, 1993.
39. Lakatta, E. G., Catecholamines and cardiovascular function in aging, *Endocr. Metab. Clin. N. Am.*, 16, 877–891, 1987.
40. White, M., Roden, R., Minobe, W., et al., Age-related changes in β-adrenergic neuroeffector systems in the human heart, *Circulation*, 90, 1225–1238, 1994.
41. Roth, D. A., White, C. D., Podolin, D. A., et al., Alterations in myocardial signal transduction due to aging and chronic dynamic exercise, *J. Appl. Physiol.*, 84, 177–184, 1998.
42. Davy, K. P., DeSouza, C. A., Jones, P. P., et al., Elevated heart rate variability in physically active young and older adult women, *Clin. Sci.*, 94, 579–584, 1998.
43. Stein, P. K., Ehsani, A. A., Domitrovich, P. P., et al., Effect of exercise training on heart rate variability in healthy older adults, *Am. Heart J.*, 138, 567–576, 1999.
44. Tulppo, M. P., Makikallio, T. H., Seppanen, T., et al., Vagal modulation of heart rate during exercise: effects of age and physical fitness, *Am. J. Physiol.*, 274, H424–H429, 1998.
45. Schuit, A. J., van Amelsvoort, L. G., Verheij, T. C., et al., Exercise training and heart rate variability in older people, *Med. Sci. Sports Exerc.*, 31, 816–821, 1999.
46. Perini, R., Milesi, S., Fisher, N. M., et al., Heart rate variability during dynamic exercise in elderly males and females, *Eur. J. Appl. Physiol.*, 82, 8–15, 2000.
47. Levy, W. C., Cerqueira, M. D., Harp, G. D., et al., Effect of endurance exercise training on heart rate variability at rest in healthy young and older men, *Am. J. Cardiol.*, 82, 1236–1241, 1998.
48. Ferrari, A. U., Age-related modifications in neural cardiovascular control, *Aging (Milano)*, 4, 183–195, 1992.
49. Gerstenblith, G., Lakatta, E. G., and Weisfeldt, M. L., Age changes in myocardial function and exercise response, *Prog. Cardiov. Dis.*, 19, 1–21, 1976.
50. Slotwiner, D. J., Devereux, R. B., Schwartz, J. E., et al., Relation of age to left ventricular function in clinically normal adults, *Am. J. Cardiol.*, 82, 621–626, 1998.
51. Lakatta, E. G., Gerstenblith, G., Angell, C. S., et al., Diminished inotropic response of aged myocardium to catecholamines, *Circ. Res.*, 36, 262–269, 1975.
52. Wahr, P. A., Michele, D. E., and Metzger, J. M., Effects of aging on single cardiac myocyte function in Fischer 344× Brown Norway rats, *Am. J. Physiol.*, 279, H559–H565, 2000.
53. Goodman, J. M., Plyley, M. J., Lefkowitz, C. A., et al., Left ventricular functional response to moderate and intense exercise [see comments], *Can. J. Sport. Sci.*, 16, 204–209, 1991.

54. Fleg, J. L., Schulman, S., O'Connor, F., et al., Effects of acute beta-adrenergic receptor blockade on age-associated changes in cardiovascular performance during dynamic exercise, *Circulation*, 90, 2333–2341, 1994.
55. Yin, F. C. P., Raizes, G. S., Guarnieri, H. A., et al., Age-associated decrease in ventricular response to haemodynamic stress during β-adrenergic blockade, *Br. Heart J.*, 40, 1349–1355, 1978.
56. Nussbacher, A., Gerstenblith, G., O'Connor, F. C., et al., Hemodynamic effects of unloading the old heart, *Am. J. Physiol.*, 277, H1863–H1871, 1999.
57. Hanley, P., Zinsmeister, A., Clements, I., et al., Gender-related differences in cardiac response to supine exercise assessed by radionuclide angiography., *J. Am. Coll. Cardiol.*, 13, 624–629, 1989.
58. Turner, M. J., Mier, C. M., Spina, R. J., et al., Effects of age and gender on the cardiovascular responses to isoproterenol, *J. Gerontol. Biol. Sci.*, 54A, B393–B400, 1999.
59. Turner, M. J., Mier, C. M., Spina, R. J., et al., Effects of age and gender on cardiovascular responses to phenylephrine, *J. Gerontol. Biol. Sci. Med. Sci.*, 54, M17–M24, 1999.
60. Fleg, J. L., O'Connor, F., Gerstenblith, G., et al., Impact of age on the cardiovascular response to dynamic upright exercise in healthy men and women, *J. Appl. Physiol.*, 78, 890–900, 1995.
61. Spina, R. J., Cardiovascular adaptations to endurance exercise training in older men and women, *Exerc. Sport Sci. Rev.*, 27, 317–332, 1999.
62. Plotnick, G. D., Becker, L. C., Fisher, M. L., et al., Use of the Frank–Starling mechanism during submaximal vs. maximal upright exercise, *Am. J. Physiol.*, 251, H1101–H1105, 1986.
63. Gerstenblith, G., Renlund, D. G., and Lakatta, E. G., Cardiovascular response to exercise in younger and older men, *Fed. Proc.*, 46, 1834–1839, 1987.
64. Iskandrian, A. S. and Hakki, A. H., Age-related changes in left ventricular diastolic performance, *Am. Heart J.*, 112, 75–78, 1986.
65. Gerstenblith, G., Frederiksen, J., Yin, F. C., et al., Echocardiographic assessment of a normal adult aging population, *Circulation*, 56, 273–278, 1977.
66. Jungblut, P. R., Osborne, J. A., Quigg, R. J., et al., Echocardiographic Doppler evaluation of left ventricular diastolic filling in older, highly trained male endurance athletes, *Echocardiography*, 17, 7–16, 2000.
67. Levy, W. C., Cerqueira, M. D., Abrass, I. B., et al., Endurance exercise training augments diastolic filling at rest and during exercise in healthy young and old men, *Circulation*, 88, 116–126, 1993.
68. Schulman, S. P., Lakatta, E. G., Fleg, J. L., et al., Age-related decline in left ventricular filling at rest and exercise, *Am. J. Physiol.*, 263, H1932–H1938, 1992.
69. Taffet, G. E., Michael, L. A., and Tate, C. A., Exercise training improves lusitrophy by isoproterenol in papillary muscles from aged rats, *J. Appl. Physiol.*, 81, 1488–1494, 1996.
70. Snell, P. G., Martin, W. H., Buckey, J. C., et al., Maximal vascular leg conductance in trained and untrained men, *J. Appl. Physiol.*, 62, 606–610, 1987.
71. Reading, J. L., Goodman, J. M., Plyley, M. J., et al., Vascular conductance and aerobic power in sedentary and active subjects and heart failure patients, *J. Appl. Physiol.*, 74, 567–573, 1993.
72. Martin, W. H. D., Ogawa, T., Kohrt, W. M., et al., Effects of aging, gender, and physical training on peripheral vascular function, *Circulation*, 84, 654–664, 1991.

73. Thomas, C. M., Pierzga, J. M., and Kenney, W. L., Aerobic training and cutaneous vasodilation in young and older men, *J. Appl. Physiol.*, 86, 1676–1686, 1999.
74. Taddei, S., Galetta, F., Virdis, A., et al., Physical activity prevents age-related impairment in nitric oxide availability in elderly athletes, *Circulation*, 101, 2896–2901, 2000.
75. DeSouza, C. A., Shapiro, L. F., Clevenger, C. M., et al., Regular aerobic exercise prevents and restores age-related declines in endothelium-dependent vasodilation in healthy men, *Circulation (Online)*, 102, 1351–1357, 2000.
76. Degens, H., Age-related changes in the microcirculation of skeletal muscle, *Adv. Exp. Med. Biol.*, 454, 343–348, 1998.
77. Beere, P. A., Russell, S. D., Morey, M. C., et al., Aerobic exercise training can reverse age-related peripheral circulatory changes in healthy older men, *Circulation*, 100, 1085–1094, 1999.
78. Gilligan, D. M., Badar, D. M., Panza, J. A., et al., Effects of estrogen replacement therapy on peripheral vasomotor function in postmenopausal women, *Am. J. Cardiol.*, 75, 264–268, 1995.
79. Gilligan, D. M., Badar, D. M., Panza, J. A., et al., Acute vascular effects of estrogen in postmenopausal women, *Circulation*, 90, 786–791, 1994.
80. McGrath, B. P., Liang, Y. L., Teede, H., et al., Age-related deterioration in arterial structure and function in postmenopausal women: impact of hormone replacement therapy, *Arterio. Thromb. Vasc. Biol.*, 18, 1149–1156, 1998.
81. Hunt, B. E., Davy, K. P., Jones, P. P., et al., Systemic hemodynamic determinants of blood pressure in women: age, physical activity, and hormone replacement, *Am. J. Physiol.*, 273, H777–H785, 1997.
82. Taddei, S., Virdis, A., Ghiadoni, L., et al., Menopause is associated with endothelial dysfunction in women, *Hypertension*, 28, 576–582, 1997.
83. Kirwan, L., MacLusky, N., Shapiro, H., et al., Effects of short and long-term estrogen replacement therapy on cardiovascular hemodynamics during exercise in postmenopausal women., *Circulation*, 102 (suppl II), 712, 2000.
84. Kenny, W. L. and Ho, C. W., Age alters regional distribution of blood flow during moderate-intensity exercise, *J. Appl. Physiol.*, 79, 1112–1119, 1995.
85. Ho, C. W., Beard, J. L., Farrell, P. A., et al., Age, fitness, and regional blood flow during exercise in the heat, *J. Appl. Physiol.*, 82, 1126–1135, 1997.
86. O'Rourke, M. O., Arterial stiffness, systolic blood pressure, and logical treatment of arterial hypertension, *Hypertension*, 15, 339–347, 1990.
87. Chen, C. H., Nakayama, M., Nevo, E., et al., Coupled systolic-ventricular and vascular stiffening with age: implications for pressure regulation and cardiac reserve in the elderly, *J. Am. Coll. Cardiol.*, 32, 1221–1227, 1998.
88. Taddei, S. A., Virdis, A., Mattei, P., et al., Aging and endothelial function in normotensive subjects and patients with essential hypertension, *Circulation*, 91, 1981–1995, 1995.
89. Clarkson, P. H., Montgomery, A., and Mullen, M. J., Exercise training enhances endothelial function in young men, *J. Am. Coll. Cardiol.*, 33, 1379–1385, 1999.
90. Coggan, A. R., Spina, R. J., King, D. S., et al., Histochemical and enzymatic comparison of the gastrocnemius muscle of young and elderly men and women, *J. Gerontol.*, 47, B71–B76, 1992.
91. Chilbeck, P. D., Paterson, D. H., Cunningham, D. A., et al., Muscle capillarization, O2 diffusion distance, and VO2 kinetics in old and young individuals, *J. Appl. Physiol.*, 82, 63–69, 1997.

92. Conley, K. E., Jubrias, S. A., and Esselman, P. C., Oxidative capacity and aging in human muscle, *J. Physiol.*, 526, 203–210, 2000.
93. Thomas, S. G., Cunningham, D. A., Rechnitzer, P. A., et al., Determinants of the training response in elderly men., *Med. Sci. Sports Exerc.*, 17, 667–672, 1985.
94. Seals, D. R., Hagberg, J. M., Hurley, B. F., et al., Endurance training in older men and women. I. Cardiovascular responses to exercise., *J. Appl. Physiol.*, 57, 1024–1029, 1984.
95. Spina, R. J., Ogawa, T., Kohrt, W. M., et al., Differences in cardiovascular adaptations to endurance exercise training between older men and women, *J. Appl. Physiol.*, 75, 849–855, 1993.
96. Londeree, B., Effect of training on lactate/ventilatory thresholds: a meta-analysis, *Med. Sci. Sports Exerc.*, 29, 837–843, 1997.
97. Thomas, S. G., Cunningham, D. A., Thompson, J. A., et al., Exercise training and "ventilation threshold" in elderly, *J. Appl. Physiol.*, 59, 1472–1476, 1987.
98. Blumenthal, J. A., Emery, C. F., Madden, D. J., et al., Effects of exercise training on cardiorespiratory function in men and women >60 years of age, *Am. J. Cardiol.*, 67, 633–639, 1991.
99. Paterson, D. H. and Cunningham, D. A., The gas transporting systems: limits and modifications with age and training, *Can. J. Appl. Physiol.*, 24, 28–40, 1999.
100. Weinberg, E. O., Thienelt, C. D., Katz, S. E., et al., Gender differences in molecular remodeling in pressure overload hypertrophy, *J. Am. Coll. Cardiol.*, 34, 264–273, 1999.
101. Marsh, J. D., Lehmann, M. H., Ritchie, R. H., et al., Androgen receptors mediate hypertrophy in cardiac myocytes, *Circulation*, 98, 256–261, 1998.
102. Mendelsohn, M. E. and Karas, R. H., The protective effects of estrogen on the cardiovascular system, *N. Eng. J. Med.*, 340, 1801–1811, 1999.
103. McCole, S. D., Brown, M. D., Moore, G. E., et al., Enhanced cardiovascular hemodynamics in endurance-trained postmenopausal women athletes, *Med. Sci. Sports Exerc.*, 32, 1073–1079, 2000.
104. Spina, R. J., Ogawa, T., Miller, T. R., et al., Effect of exercise training on left ventricular performance in older women free of cardiopulmonary disease, *Am. J. Cardiol.*, 71, 99–104, 1993.
105. McCole, S. D., Brown, M. D., Moore, G. E., et al., Cardiovascular hemodynamics with increasing exercise intensities in postmenopausal women, *J. Appl. Physiol.*, 87, 2334–2340, 1999.
106. Spina, R. J., Rashid, S., Davila-Roman, V. G., et al., Adaptations in β-adrenergic cardiovascular responses to training in older women, *J. Appl. Physiol.*, 89, 2300–2305, 2000.
107. Thomas, D. P., Zimmerman, S. D., Hansen, T. R., et al., Collagen gene expression in rat left ventricle: interactive effect of age and exercise training, *J. Appl. Physiol.*, 89, 1462–1468, 2000.
108. Hepple, R. T., Mackinnon, S. L. M., Thomas, S. G., et al., Quantitating the capillary supply and the response to resistance training in older men, *Pflügers Arch. Eur. J. Physiol.*, 433, 238–244, 1997.

5

Physical Activity, Fitness, and Gender in Relation to Morbidity, Survival, Quality of Life, and Independence in Older Age

Donald H. Paterson and Liza Stathokostas

CONTENTS

0-8493-1027-X/02/$0.00+$1.50

5.1 Introduction

The purpose of this chapter is to review the research literature, examining and analyzing gender differences with respect to the amounts and types of physical activity needed to decrease morbidity and to promote health and independence in older adults. In epidemiological studies, the dose of physical activity required for beneficial effects has been assessed in terms of the total energy expenditure, the duration or energy expenditure of physical activities termed *exercise*, or the fitness levels achieved. The terms *physical activity*, *exercise*, and *physical fitness* have distinct definitions, and their differences may have distinct effects on outcome measures as well. Physical activity is defined as any bodily movement produced by skeletal muscle that results in energy expenditure. Exercise, a type of physical activity, is planned, structured, and repetitive bodily movement undertaken to improve or maintain one or more components of physical fitness. Physical fitness is a set of attributes that people have or achieve relating to their ability to perform physical activity. The majority of the literature has focused on physical activity measurements (using questionnaires to accommodate large surveys) and the amounts and types of physical activity needed to prevent disease and promote health. Whether the physical activity is classified as exercise is determined by the quantity or intensity of physical activity, or is reflected in the measurement of physical fitness levels.

There are gender differences in life expectancy, prevalence of chronic disease among older age groups, and quality of life in later years. Gender differences in the relationship among physical activity, exercise, or fitness and morbidity, mortality, and quality of life have not been studied systematically. This chapter attempts to discern the potentially differential effects of physical activity and physical fitness on all-cause mortality, cardiovascular disease (CVD), and quality of life in older women compared with men.

5.2 Physical Activity, Fitness, and Gender in Relation to Morbidity and Mortality in Older Age

5.2.1 Physical Activity and All-Cause Mortality

Physical activity has been cited as an important intervention in altering population health or population attributable risk. One such aspect of public health is the contribution of physical activity in altering all-cause mortality or death rates at a given age. It has been widely demonstrated that greater physical activity is associated with a reduced all-cause mortality in men. However, this relationship has been studied less frequently in women.

Physical activity and longevity were investigated by Paffenbarger et al.[1] in 17,000 male Harvard alumni aged 35 to 74 years. With physical activity assessed by questionnaire in the follow up, it was estimated that those expending greater than 8.4 megajoules per week in exercise (walking, stair climbing, sports play) had a 25 to 30% lower mortality rate than those with lower weekly energy expenditures. Paffenbarger and colleagues[2,3] also showed that physical activity participation (in the form of moderately vigorous sports play) initiated in middle-age was independently associated with a 23% lower all-cause death rate. Lee et al.[4] analyzed the Harvard alumni data further to assess the relative merits of vigorous and nonvigorous exercise. Vigorous activities, at an intensity greater than 6 METS (where 1 MET is the resting metabolic rate of 3.5 ml/[kg·min]), were compared with nonvigorous, light, and moderate activities of less than 6 METS. There was no reduction in risk for those who did not report vigorous activities at any weekly energy expenditure, whereas vigorous activities were significantly and inversely related to mortality at any total weekly energy expenditure. The authors concluded that the improved cardiorespiratory fitness induced by a sufficient intensity of physical activity might be responsible for the inverse association between physical activity and mortality, rather than the amount of exercise itself.

There is a relative lack of investigations for female samples. In addition, studies of females have generally had small sample sizes and included fewer older women.[5] In a prospective study of 1405 Swedish women, Lissner et al.[5] found that a low initial level of leisure time physical activity was a strong risk factor for mortality. Furthermore, there was an increase in mortality risk among those who decreased their leisure time activity. Kushi et al.[6] investigated the relationship between physical activity and mortality in 2260 women aged 55 to 69 years who participated in a seven-year follow-up of the Iowa Women's Health Study. An increasing frequency of moderate and vigorous physical activity, from "never" to "at least four times per week," was associated with a reduced risk of death. Another finding was that the effects of physical activity were not age dependent; that is, both younger and older postmenopausal women showed an inverse association between physical activity and mortality.

Thus, greater physical activity has, in general, been associated with reduced all-cause mortality. However, there is also a strong suggestion that the physical activity must be of or include moderately vigorous intensities. The effect appears to apply to women as well as to men, although to date there is insufficient information to state whether the reduction of risk for all-cause mortality with moderate intensity physical activity is affected by gender.

5.2.2 Physical Fitness and All-Cause Mortality

A low level of physical fitness is a health risk factor comparable to or greater than other established risk factors such as cigarette smoking, elevated blood cholesterol, blood pressure, fasting blood glucose, high BMI, and history of premature coronary heart disease death in a parent.[7] Blair et al.[7] investigated the association between physical fitness and all-cause mortality in the Aerobics Center Longitudinal Study, a large sample of high-socioeconomic-status men and women. Subjects were grouped into five fitness categories, based on their endurance as observed during progressive treadmill testing. Age and risk factor-adjusted results showed a strong, graded, and consistently inverse relationship between this index of physical fitness and mortality in both men and women. Comparison of least vs. most fit groups showed a 3.5 times greater risk of mortality for the least fit group in males, and a 4.5 times greater risk in females. These data imply a 22% greater risk for unfit females vs. unfit males. A low level of fitness was a more pronounced risk factor (in terms of greater mortality rates in older age) for all-cause mortality for men aged 50+ years and for women aged 60+ years. In 1996, Blair et al.[8] reported similar findings from the Aerobics Center Longitudinal Study, with an inverse gradient of risk across fitness groups shown within strata of other predictors or risk factors. A low cardiorespiratory fitness was shown to be an independent precursor of all-cause mortality, with those in the least fit group demonstrating a relative risk of 1.52 in men and 2.10 in women. The fitness effect suggested the risk was 58% greater in women. The data also indicated that moderate fitness was associated with some reduction of risk. Adjusted all-cause death rates were 17 to 39% lower in moderately fit men compared with low-fit men with other risk factors. Women in the moderately fit category showed 48 to 67% lower risk than their less fit counterparts with other risk factors. These data emphasized the protective effect of cardiorespiratory fitness, even in the presence of other predictors of mortality. Highly fit men with two or three other risk predictors had a 15% lower death rate than the least fit men with none of the other risk predictors. Highly fit women showed an almost 50% lower death rate in the same comparison. Thus, it appears from these data that women have a greater relative risk from the inverse relationship between physical fitness and all-cause mortality, and that being in a higher fitness category has a somewhat greater protective effect in women than in men.

The association between change in physical fitness and all-cause mortality has also been examined, but only in men. Blair et al.[9] studied the changes in physical fitness in men over a 5-year period. A reduction in all-cause mortality of 44% was observed for men whose condition had improved from unfit to fit. The benefits were particularly pronounced for the 50- to 59-year olds, with a 70% lower death rate for those who increased their fitness compared to those who remained unfit. A similar result was seen in the older adult groups, with a 50% lower death rate in those aged 60+ years who increased their fitness. Erikssen et al.[10] also observed a change in mortality risk when physical fitness changed between repeated measures. In a sample of healthy men initially aged 40 to 60 years, physical fitness was a strong predictor of mortality over a 7-year follow-up.

The epidemiological data thus show a reduced risk of all-cause mortality in those of greater fitness, and in those who improve their fitness. Moreover, data comparing men and women suggest the protective effects of greater fitness in women are as strong as or stronger than those in men.

5.3 Physical Activity, Fitness, and Gender in Relation to Cardiovascular Disease in Older Age

5.3.1 Physical Activity and Cardiovascular Disease

Examination of the cause-specific contributors to all-cause mortality indicates that cardiovascular disease (CVD) is a major contributor. Furthermore, the contribution of physical activity to the reduction of all-cause mortality rates is largely related to the beneficial effects of physical activity in reducing the risk of CVD.[1] Cardiovascular disease is the leading cause of morbidity and mortality among Canadians and particularly among older adults.[11] In fact, CVD is so prevalent among the older adult population, it is often difficult to separate cardiovascular changes that occur with increasing age from effects of the disease process.[12] The coronary heart disease mortality rate for male Canadians is 288 per 100,000 persons, whereas for female Canadians the rate is 179 per 100,000 persons.[13]

Cardiovascular disease results in a reduction of cardiorespiratory fitness and may thus jeopardize function and independence, especially in an older population. Age-related changes in the cardiovascular system can be considered risk factors for the development of CVD, but in the absence of disease, cardiovascular function can remain normal into older age.[12]

In addition to age-related disease processes, another factor contributing to the prevalence of CVD is the increasingly sedentary lifestyle of older adults. As discussed later, physical activity has an independently beneficial effect, decreasing the risk of CHD (coronary heart disease) in men,[14,15] but not in women.[15] Physical activity is thought to exert this effect both by influencing the level of major cardiovascular risk factors and by affecting the cardiovascular system directly.[16] Early investigations focused on the association between occupational physical activity and CVD in studies of men, but as physical activity at work decreased, leisure physical activity became a target of investigation.

Physical activity emerged as a standard intervention to reduce the risk of CVD and for its management. An inverse association between physical activity and CVD risk is supported for men,[2,3,17-22] but the association in women remains unclear. Before menopause, women are at a decreased risk of CVD compared to men; however, the risk in women increases to a level similar to that seen in men within ten years after menopause. Furthermore, men and women share the same risk factors for CVD. Despite similar risks and rates of risks among males and females, the current literature lacks the same unequivocal evidence regarding a beneficial effect of physical activity on CVD risk factors for women as there is for men.

5.3.2 Physical Activity and Cardiovascular Disease Risk

The relative incidence of CVD in active and sedentary men is well documented. An early study relating occupational physical activity to cardiovascular events[16] compared the incidence of CVD in sedentary bus drivers with that in the conductors, who were physically more active; the conductors had 30% lower incidence of and 50% fewer deaths from CVD, although initial differences of physique contributed to this advantage. Subsequently, Paffenbarger and Hale[17] reported longitudinal observations on longshoremen; they found that the more active dockworkers were three times less likely to experience a fatal heart attack than were the inactive foremen. Morris et al.[18-20] showed that men who participated in vigorous sports or fast walking more than twice per week had strikingly low rates of coronary heart disease. Paffenbarger et al.[2,3,21] also reported on the association between physical inactivity and CHD in their group of Harvard alumni. These studies showed that moderately vigorous sports play was associated with a 30% lower risk, whereas light sport participation or activities at intensity less than 4.5 METS (including walking, golf, and gardening) did not reduce risk.

A review of early investigations[22] identified five studies that presented separate results for women. Only two found an association between physical activity and CHD,[23,24] and one found an association for angina but not for MI (myocardial infarction) or CHD death.[25] Variability among findings for women may reflect a weaker association between physical activity and CVD, or a genuine lack of effect.[26] However, other factors identified in this gender discrepancy include measurement error in the assessment of physical activity,[27] insufficient outcome measures, and compromised statistical power.

Investigations of females alone have yielded inconclusive results. No associations between activity levels and CVD morbidity or mortality were observed in a large sample of women aged 50 to 74 years.[27] Sesso et al.[25] found no association between total physical activity and CVD risk in women. However, a greater amount of walking was related to a decreased CVD risk. Lemaitre et al.[28] reported a 50% decrease in the risk of MI with modest leisure time energy expenditure in women.

In a 4- to 7-year follow-up, Folsom et al.[29] examined the association between physical activity and coronary heart disease in both men and women. Irrespective of gender, those who developed CHD showed lower indices for leisure physical activity and sports activity. However, this did not translate into a significant inverse association between the risk of CHD and either leisure physical activity or sports participation in this group of middle-aged women. Haapanen et al.[15] found that the total energy expended on leisure time physical activity in a Finnish population bore an inverse and independent association to the risk of CHD among middle-aged men, but not among women. O'Connor et al.[30] observed an insignificant association between nonfatal MI and physical activity in women and men. The relative risk of nonfatal MI tended to be greater among women in the highest quartile of moderate to vigorous sports activity compared to those in the lowest quartile, but the difference was insignificant due to wide confidence intervals.

The association between physical activity and cardiovascular risk factors has also been examined. Mensink et al.[31] reported findings on a large German sample. Men undertook more leisure time physical activity and conditioning activity than women. Highly active men and women had more favorable risk factor levels than inactive men and women; however, no significant inverse relationship with cardiovascular mortality was observed in women, largely because they sustained few fatal cardiovascular events.

Thus, whereas moderately vigorous physical activity is associated with reduced all-cause mortality in both men and women, studies to date suggest that physical activity bears little relationship to CVD in women, in contrast to the strong association observed in men.

5.3.3 Physical Fitness and Cardiovascular Disease Risk

Middle-aged and elderly Norwegian cross-country skiers were examined in a 7-year follow-up by Lie et al.[32] and a 16-year follow-up by Sandvik et al.[33] An inverse relationship between physical fitness (as assessed by cycle ergometer testing) and the risk of death from CHD was observed in this group of healthy men. The Lipid Research Clinics Mortality Study[34] followed a large sample of males aged 30 to 69 years for an average of 8.5 years. Physical fitness quartiles, as assessed by the submaximal heart rate and exercise time during a treadmill test, showed 8.5 and 6.5 times higher death rates from CVD and CHD, respectively, in the lowest level of fitness vs. the other fitness categories. In addition to observing that moderate-to-high intensity leisure-time physical activity (mean intensity of 6 METS) was associated with a reduced risk of acute MI, Lakka et al.[14] found similar results for cardiorespiratory fitness (benefit seen with a maximal oxygen intake of at least 34 ml/[kg·min]). Farrell et al.[35] showed that, among a large sample of asymptomatic males, those in moderate and high fitness categories (an aerobic power of at least 33 to 40 ml/[kg·min]) had significantly fewer CVD deaths than similar men in low fitness categories. This finding persisted even in the presence of established CVD risk predictors.

Blair et al.[8] assessed the influence of cardiorespiratory fitness on CVD in a follow-up of a large male and female sample. A low level of fitness emerged as an independent risk factor significantly associated with CVD mortality in men and of borderline significance in women ($p = 0.05$); the relative risks of CVD in the low fitness groups were 1.70 and 2.42 for men and women, respectively. As with previous investigations of CVD mortality, the authors attributed the failure to observe a greater significance in women to the small numbers of CVD deaths among the females. Haddock et al.[36] reported cardiorespiratory fitness to be an independent determinant of CVD risk factors (total cholesterol, HDL cholesterol, total/HDL ratio, triglycerides, fibrinogens) in postmenopausal women. Treadmill time to exhaustion was compared between the highest fitness quintile and four other grouped quintiles in a sample of nonsmoking women aged 53.0 ± 7.1 years; cardiorespiratory fitness was significantly associated with CVD risk factors, irrespective of whether the women were receiving hormone replacement therapy.

In order to address the issue of whether a high level of cardiorespiratory fitness (as assessed by a graded treadmill test) or high levels of physical activity (as assessed by doubly labeled water and indirect calorimetry) are needed to affect CVD risk factors, Dvorak et al.[37] studied a healthy sample of older men (68 ± 9 years) and women (67 ± 7 years). Results indicated that the level of cardiorespiratory fitness was a stronger correlate of a more favorable CVD risk profile irrespective of whether an individual had high or low physical activity. This was evident when individuals with high levels of cardiorespiratory fitness but low physical activity were compared with individuals with high levels of physical activity but low levels of cardiorespiratory fitness. Analysis by gender did not affect these conclusions.

Thus, just as cardiorespiratory fitness is inversely related to all-cause mortality in both men and women, it appears that physical fitness is related to a favorable CVD risk factor profile and a reduced risk of CVD in both women and men. The fact that fitness, but not physical activity per se, is related to reduced CVD in women speaks to the dose of physical activity required for benefit. Even more than in men, the protective effect in women is mediated through fitness and an exercise intensity that enhances cardiorespiratory fitness.

5.3.4 Gender Differences in the Effects of Physical Activity on CVD Morbidity and Mortality: Differences in Physiological Responses to Exercise

In this section, one line of physiological research from the laboratory of Dr. Earl Noble is cited that suggests that exercise may be more effective in protecting against CHD in men than in women.

Gender is a risk factor for cardiovascular disease, as the incidence of coronary heart disease is lower in women than in men. The protection against heart pathology afforded to premenopausal women is generally considered to be conferred by the ovarian hormone estrogen, as in postmenopausal women the morbidity and mortality from cardiac disease increase to levels similar to those found in age-matched men.[38–40] Estrogen is believed to attenuate the incidence of adverse cardiac events[41] through its antiatherogenic, vasorelaxant, and antioxidant properties.[42–44] Despite these results from observational and experimental studies, clinical trials investigating the efficacy of hormone replacement therapy have found no overall reduction in the incidence of coronary heart disease.[45,46]

One factor that may influence gender differences in morbidity and survival is gender-based hormonal interaction with intracellular protective systems.

For example, heat shock proteins (Hsps) are a class of rapidly inducible products of highly conserved transcriptional units. Genetically engineered animals that express high levels of the major inducible Hsp70 protein demonstrate increased resistance to myocardial trauma.[47-51] Exercise is a physiological inducer of Hsp70; this induction improves cardiac function following ischemia–reperfusion.[52,53] There are gender differences in postexercise cardiac Hsp70 expression, males exhibiting twofold greater levels than females.[54] Furthermore, estrogen-treated males demonstrate an attenuated, female-like stress response to exercise indicating the importance of the ovarian hormone to this sexual dimorphism.[55] Removal of the major endogenous source of estrogen production by ovariectomy abolished gender differences in myocardial Hsp70 levels, but physiological estrogen replacement in ovariectomized rodents reversed this effect (Paroo and Noble, manuscript in preparation). Thus, the gender-specific Hsp response to exercise is mediated in large part by the female-specific steroid hormone estrogen.

To examine the functional consequences of this gender-specific, hormone-mediated phenomenon, hearts from control and exercised groups of male and intact and ovariectomized female animals were subjected to an experimental model of myocardial infarction. In males, exercise improved postischemic cardiac function, augmenting left ventricular developed pressure, reducing end diastolic pressure, and increasing maximal rates of contraction and relaxation, whereas no beneficial effects of exercise were observed in females. Moreover, ovariectomized rodents demonstrated an exercise-conferred tolerance to myocardial ischemia–reperfusion similar to that observed in males (Paroo, Karmazyn, and Noble, manuscript in preparation). Thus, the gender-specific, hormone-mediated Hsp response to exercise results in exercise-conferred resistance to cardiac trauma in males but not in females, suggesting that males can reduce the gender gap in susceptibility to cardiovascular disease by exercising.

In these studies, animals were subjected to relatively intense exercise. This may be important in the exercise protection afforded to males. When rats were engaged in either voluntary free wheel or forced treadmill running for similar distances, only those animals who completed the more intense treadmill running program exhibited a significant increase in cardiac Hsp72 levels.[56] Others, also, have noted that the cardioprotective effect of exercise is influenced more by exercise intensity than by the total amount of physical activity.[19,20]

5.4 Physical Activity, Fitness, and Gender in Relation to Quality of Life and Independence in Older Age

5.4.1 Physical Activity and Quality of Life

The aging process, or "primary aging" should be distinguished from "secondary aging" (the age-related deterioration in functional capacity that results from diseases).[57] The natural life span appears to have biological limits, with interindividual differences in longevity genetically determined (see Chapter 3). Shephard[58] suggests that, although life expectancy (the average life span of a large population) has increased in recent years, the fundamental aging process has apparently remained unchanged. Although disease modification associated with the adoption of physical activity can retard premature death by one or two years,[1] a long-term physically active lifestyle or any other type of lifestyle intervention will not alter primary aging or the maximum life span.

There is no apparent gender difference in maximum life span, but there is a gender difference in average life expectancy. The 1999 Statistical Report on the Health of Canadians[13] noted that a person aged 65 years could expect to live an average of another 18.4 years, to 83.4 years. However, females of all ages had a greater total life expectancy than males. The difference diminished with age, but at 65 years, females could expect to live another 20.2 years, whereas males lived only an average of another 16.3 years. This may appear to be a female advantage, but in terms of "active life expectancy," it becomes a female disadvantage. Katz et al.[59] analyzed population data with respect to functional or active life expectancy. At that time, the average 65-year-old could expect to live 16.5 more years, but only 10 of those years would be characterized by independent living; moreover, the longer life expectancy of women was associated with a longer period of dependency (Figure 5.1). Loss of independence is a major concern of older adults; as suggested by Fries,[60] the idealized population mortality curve would allow people to live to old age and then to die abruptly or after a short period of illness.

Whereas the maximal achievable life span seems fixed, an increase in life expectancy has occurred throughout the previous century. The number of early deaths was greatly reduced by control of infectious diseases and, more recently, mortality in middle-age has been reduced by improved prevention and treatment, particularly for cardiovascular disease. Thus, as a greater proportion of older adults approach their maximum life span, research initiatives need, and have begun, to refocus from maximizing the quantity of life to augmenting the quality of life in older adults. This is particularly important for older individuals, since they are more likely than younger members of the population to suffer from chronic conditions, to have activity limitations, and to be dependent on others for assistance when undertaking the activities of daily living (ADL). A reduced quality of life has a strong influence not only on the present quality of life, but also on future health and survival.[61] If the quality of life with aging is associated with a loss of functional capacity, then the determinants of quality of life become the determinants of loss in functional capacity (Figure 5.2).

The progressive relationship of functional limitations and disease to the development of disability poses a further challenge to quality of life. Both age and physical activity are modifiers along this developmental pathway.[62] Morey et al.[63] summarized the models of disability in older adults, identifying the emergence of functional limitations in the performance of basic tasks

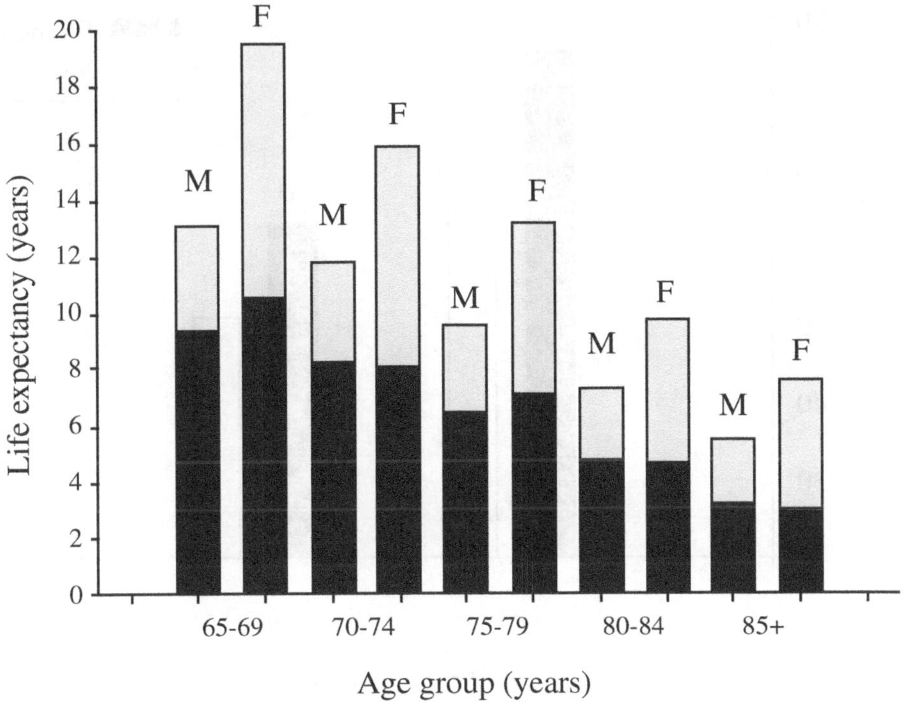

FIGURE 5.1
Life expectancy and active life expectancy for men and women. Data from Katz et al.[59] show, for each 5-year interval, total life expectancy divided into active life expectancy (shown by the darkened portion of the bar) and dependent living (shown by the lightly shaded portion of the bar).

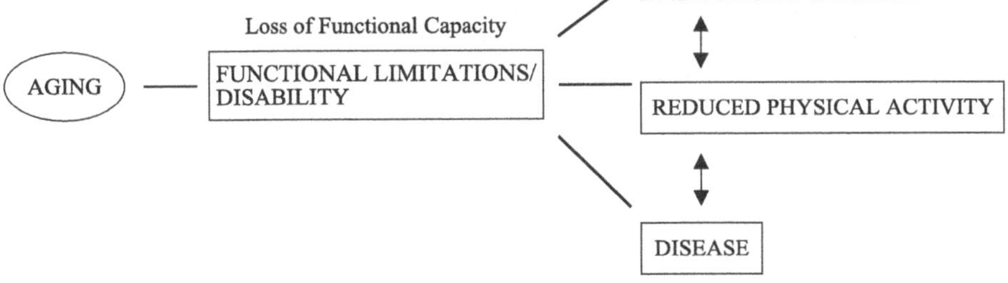

FIGURE 5.2
Interacting effects of aging, disease, and lack of physical activity upon loss of functional capacity.

as a primary consideration mediating the causal pathway from disease to disability. Based on the model by Verbrugge and Jette,[64] disability is a concept that includes difficulty in carrying out ADL. Functional limitations are restrictions in basic mental and physical actions and are influenced by physical conditions (e.g., disease) preventing persons from carrying out ADL.

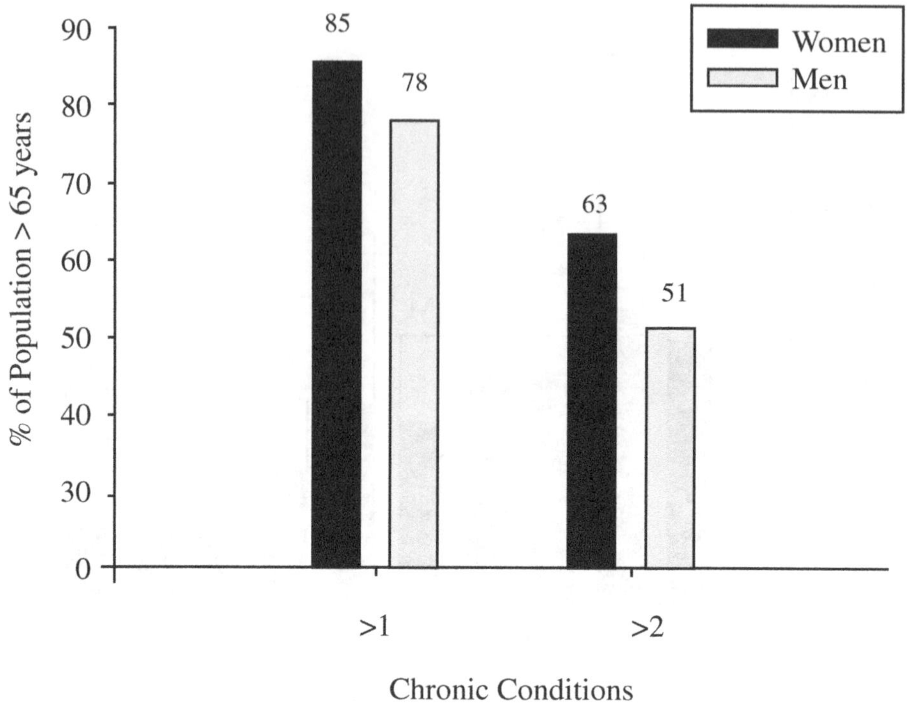

FIGURE 5.3
Incidence of chronic conditions in an older adult population (from the Health Statistics Division, Statistics Canada).[13]

TABLE 5.1

Primary Conditions Responsible for Activity Limitation in Those 65+, by Gender (Canada, 1996 to 1997)[11]

	Nervous System (%)	Back Problem (%)	Limb Problem (%)	Respiratory Problem (%)	Arthritis (%)	Heart Problem (%)
Male	13	10	10	9	11	18
Female	11	7	10	6	27	13

Reports of functional limitations are increased among older adults with age-related chronic diseases; the type of disability is dependent on the nature of the underlying disease.[65] Women tend to report more chronic conditions than men, particularly allergies, migraine headaches, and arthritis/rheumatism, whereas the prevalence of heart disease and diabetes is significantly higher among men than among women. Women also tend to report more multiple chronic conditions than men (Figure 5.3). Nevertheless, as summarized in Table 5.1, there is a broad distribution across various chronic conditions reported as primary conditions responsible for activity limitation in those aged >65 years.

TABLE 5.2
Physical Activity Levels of Canadians 65+ (1997 Physical Activity Monitor)[11]

	Active (>13 $kJ \cdot kg^{-1} \cdot d^{-1}$) %	Somewhat Active (2–13 $kJ \cdot kg^{-1} \cdot d^{-1}$) %	Sedentary (<2 $kJ \cdot kg^{-1} \cdot d^{-1}$) %
Women	20	45	35
Men	24	47	29

$kJ \cdot kg^{-1} \cdot d^{-1}$ = KiloJoules/kilogram of body mass per day; (13 $kJ \cdot kg^{-1} \cdot d^{-1}$ is equivalent to walking 1 hour every day).

As with all-cause mortality and CVD, the functional and disability status of older adults has been examined in relation to both physical activity and physical fitness.

5.4.2 Physical Activity, Fitness, and Functional Capacity

Aging is characterized by a loss of functional capacity. The 1997 Physical Activity Monitor[11] noted that 35% of Canadians over the age of 65 years reported difficulty from at least one area of functional limitation; for women alone, the figure was 42%. Huang et al.[66] reported that the prevalence of functional limitations was almost twice as high in women as in men in each of their age groupings (40 to 49, 50 to 59, and 60+ years). In a large Finnish sample of independently living men and women, Hirvensalo et al.[67] found that individuals with impaired mobility were older and had more chronic conditions than those with intact mobility. This has important implications not only for quality of life, but also for risk of death; Hirvensalo et al.[67] found that individuals with impaired mobility were at an increased risk of death. Male gender was associated with a greater risk of mortality, whereas female gender was predictive of dependency in an unadjusted analysis. It has been suggested that declines in functional capacity with age reflect age-related reductions in physical activity. Inactivity has been estimated to account for 50% of the age-related loss in function. According to the 1997 Physical Activity Monitor,[11] 79% of Canadians over the age of 65 years were inactive. Physical inactivity levels were 82% for women and 74% for men. The differences between men and women appear small (Table 5.2), although a greater percentage of women were "sedentary." Furthermore, aging was associated with a decline in vigorous activities and more time was spent in lower-intensity activities.[68]

As mentioned earlier, physical activity modifies the disease-functional limitation–disability relationship. Cardiorespiratory fitness, muscular fitness, and morphologic status are all components of physical fitness, the result of habitual and sufficient physical activity. Age-related changes in the functional capacities of the cardiorespiratory and musculoskeletal systems and in morphologic status are reviewed in other chapters of this book. Disability is presented by the International Classification of Impairments, Disability, and Handicaps[69] as a precursor to loss of independence. However, disability and functional limitation can often be defined narrowly and may not then provide a valid indication of loss of independence.

Morey et al.[63] found the cardiorespiratory, musculoskeletal, and morphologic fitness components of older men and women (mean age 72 years) to be associated directly with functional limitations independently of any existing pathologies. Huang et al.[66] showed an inverse gradient relating functional limitation with physical fitness and physical activity in a follow-up study of men and women aged 40 and older. Men and women of high and moderately high fitness had a lower prevalence of functional limitations than the unfit group after controlling for age, length of follow-up, body mass index, smoking, alcohol consumption, and presence of chronic disease (test for linear trend $p < 0.05$). The association with physical activity was also observed in the males alone ($p < 0.05$), but was insignificant for women ($p > 0.05$). Brill et al.[70] studied 3000 men and 600 women; over a 5-year follow-up, 7% of men and 12% of women reported a functional limitation. The odds of reporting a functional limitation during follow-up were almost halved for those in the high strength group. A low level of cardiorespiratory fitness (as estimated from treadmill time) was also associated with functional limitations at follow-up. In the Longitudinal Study of Aging (LSOA), Miller et al.[71] sought to determine how physical activity influences lower body functional limitations and the transition to disability in a 6-year follow-up. With gender selected as one of the covariates, subjects who reported walking 1.6 km at least once per week had a greater probability than sedentary subjects of enhancing or sustaining current function. The authors suggested that walking was of sufficient relative intensity to alter fitness in older adults and, through its influence on functional limitations, might slow the progression of disabilities affecting ADL in both men and women.

5.4.3 Physical Activity, Fitness, and Disability

In the NHANES I follow-up study, female gender was a major characteristic contributing to greater disability in an aging cohort.[72] The authors suggested that potentially greater under-representation of men with disabilities, due to selective mortality, as well as the general observation that women are more likely than men to report signs and symptoms of health-related problems, could account for some of the observed gender differences.

Physical activity has been identified as a behavioral risk factor influencing the development of disability. In the NHANES I follow-up study,[72] lower recreational and nonrecreational physical activity was found to be a common predictor of the development of physical disability in both men and women. Wu et al.[73] collected data from a survey of community-living older adults over a three-year period in order to estimate the incidence of and factors predicting the development of chronic ADL disability. The men ($n = 676$)

had a moderately greater relative risk than the women ($n = 645$), but gender had no statistically significant effect on the risk of chronic ADL disability. Leisure-time physical activity had an insignificant influence on the relative risk of chronic ADL disability ($p = 0.575$), whereas exercise had a significant effect ($p = 0.016$). Guralnik et al.[74] studied over 1000 men and women of mean age 71 years; over a 4-year follow-up, physical function was strongly associated with subsequent disability (a lower initial performance score augmenting the odds of disabilities by a factor of 2 to 4). Cunningham et al.[75] reported that objective measurements of physical fitness/capacity were associated with functional incapacities, independence, and quality of life. Posner et al.[76] studied 61 women of mean age 69 years; $\dot{V}O_{2peak}$ and calf strength predicted their ability to perform ADL needed for functional independence.

5.4.4 Determinants of Independence/Dependence: Importance of Fitness

As indicated in other chapters of this book, there are considerable age-related losses of physiological capacity and function, including losses of cardiorespiratory fitness, muscle mass, oxidative capacity and strength, shoulder flexibility, and self-selected speed of walking. Overall, a 50% loss across the life span is usual. Recognizing the loss of function with age, a *Lancet* editorial[77] stated, "A large and rapidly increasing number of people live perilously close to functional thresholds of physical ability, needing only a minor illness to render them dependent." It also noted that, "If crossing of [such] thresholds for independence could be prevented or postponed, the quality of many lives would be improved and the social and economic costs of supporting an infirm aged population would be reduced." Paterson, Cunningham, and Koval have recently examined the determinants of independence/dependence in a cohort of older adults. D. Govindasamy is analyzing the data as part of a Ph.D. thesis; however, the general findings to date are summarized here. The sample initially comprised 441 men and women aged 55 to 85 years.[78] All were living independently and were able to walk an 80-m course (a self-paced walking test). Other measurements included demographic data, anthropometric variables (skinfold thickness, body-mass index), cardiorespiratory fitness (a treadmill determination of aerobic power in $n = 373$), muscle strength (grip and plantar flexion), the flexibility of hip and shoulder joints, a leisure-time physical activity questionnaire, a medical/health assessment including history of chronic disease (cardiovascular disease, cancer, and arthritis), medications and smoking history, and a questionnaire on attitudes towards life (including a depression score).

In an 8-year follow-up, it was possible to track 189 individuals still living independently, 43 (28 women and 15 men) now categorized as dependent (30 of whom were living in long-term care or nursing home environments), and 66 who had died. A host of precursor variables was then examined to determine which might explain the subsequent transition from independence to dependent living. Among older adults the desire to remain independent is paramount. Much of the literature to date has analyzed the influence of physical activity and/or fitness, taking as its "end point" or dependent variable cardiovascular disease or all-cause mortality. Much of the literature related to quality of life has used functional limitations or disability as the dependent variable in determining whether physical inactivity and a low fitness level were related to an increase in functional limitations with age. Many of these studies have used a cross-sectional design, with subjects lying on a continuum from independent to dependent living. This design allows inferences to be drawn regarding what variables are associated with functional limitations, but cannot determine whether these variables are determinants of the impaired function (or rather are secondary to the functional limitations). Thus, the longitudinal design of the present study offered a relatively unique opportunity to explore the outcome or dependent variable of becoming "dependent" and to control for covariates or confounding variables.

Age, as would be expected, was significantly related to becoming dependent. Those in the dependent group were approximately 8 years older, and the logistic regression analysis showed that being 5 years older doubled the odds of becoming dependent in the next 8 years. The presence of disease at initial testing increased the odds of subsequent dependence three- to fourfold, even though all in the study had initially completed a fatigue-limited treadmill test. Often used health indicators such as body-mass index and resting systolic blood pressure did not differentiate between those who became dependent and those who did not, and they were not significantly related to dependence in a logistic analysis. Gender was not a significant explanatory variable of subsequent dependence, although, as noted earlier, the occurrence of dependence was nearly doubled in the women (with nearly double the all-cause mortality for the men).

The gender variable may emerge as important, with further follow-up, when greater subject numbers have passed into the dependent category, although it is also quite possible that the other explanatory variables override gender in their importance. The principal findings are that, after age adjustment, cardiorespiratory fitness ($\dot{V}O_{2max}$) and grip and plantar flexion strength were initially 10% higher in those who remained independent than in those who became dependent. In logistic regression analysis, the initial cardiorespiratory fitness was a significant explanatory variable of dependence at 8 years. After controlling for age, gender, and the presence of disease, there were 14% greater odds of dependence for each ml/[kg·min] reduction in initial $\dot{V}O_{2max}$. Daily activities of independent living require a $\dot{V}O_{2max}$ of approximately 15 ml/[kg·min],[79] and the mean $\dot{V}O_{2max}$ in those aged 70 years was approximately 22 and 20 ml/[kg·min] in men and women, respectively. When daily activities demand 75% or more of $\dot{V}O_{2max}$ it is not surprising that these activities are fatiguing and, with cessation of such activities and consequent further loss of cardiorespiratory fitness, many activities of daily living become too vigorous. Strength was not statistically significant in the logistic regression, but it may become so as the number of dependent subjects increases. The leisure-time physical activity scores did not differ between those who remained independent and those who did not; the amount of leisure-time physical activity was not a significant explanatory variable, or modifier, of the logistic regression model. Clearly, cardiorespiratory fitness was critical in maintaining independence, and participation in considerable daily physical activity per se (unless involving the type and intensity of physical activity needed to enhance cardiorespiratory fitness) was not associated with remaining independent. Similarly, Mor et al.[80] found that the regular exercise of walking at least 1.6 km once per week, but not the general level of physical activity, protected against functional decline. Miller et al.[71] reported that older adults who walked at least 1.6 km at least once per week had a reduced probability of functional decline. A recent Finnish study found that, in mobile independent elderly people, the level of physical activity did not alter the risk of becoming dependent 8 years later.[67] Systematic exercise training programs based on "brisk" walking for 30 to 45 min 3 times per week have proven effective[81,82] in raising the $\dot{V}O_{2max}$ of older adults by 3 to 4 ml/[kg·min]. The findings of the study suggest that this would decrease the odds of dependence by approximately 50%, or postpone dependence by 2 to 3 years. In support, Wu et al.[73] showed that the risk of disability was reduced by 50% in those who participated regularly (>2 times per week) in routine exercise, whereas participation in general recreational activities had no effect. As noted by Fries et al.,[60] "Insofar as frailty and dependence may be the result of loss of physical function, physical activity (or improved "fitness") is one intervention which may reduce the years of dependent living, and improve the quality of life of older adults." It appears that cardiorespiratory fitness and perhaps leg strength are critical to maintaining physical function at a level compatible with independent living in older adults.

5.5 Conclusions

Unequivocally, physical activity and/or cardiorespiratory fitness are associated with a decreased risk of heart disease and all-cause mortality. Physical inactivity (and/or a low level of physical fitness) are major risk factors, and increasing physical activity (or fitness) appears to be the most important intervention to alter population health or population attributable risk. Physical inactivity or a low level of cardiorespiratory fitness and muscle strength are associated with loss of functional capacity, disability, and loss of independence. There is strong evidence that fitness is engendered not by the amount physical activity performed, but rather by the types of physical activity undertaken, and that such fitness is critical in reducing the odds of cardiovascular disease, decreasing all-cause mortality, and maintaining the quality of life in older age. The epidemiological evidence is based in large part on studies of middle-aged men. Those studies which have included or focused on women often face the limitations that the incidence of cardiovascular disease is lower in women (with estrogen playing a role), and that women live longer than men. Thus, the number of "end-point" or outcome observations is small in studies of women, and the statistical power of relationships between activity/fitness data and cardiovascular disease and/or all-cause mortality is correspondingly reduced. Nevertheless, some gender differences in these relationships have emerged. The role of physical activity in altering the odds of cardiovascular disease appears weak in women, although the relationship between physical activity level and all-cause mortality seems similar to that in men. The "failure" of physical activity to prevent heart disease in women may be explained in part by gender differences in the response to exercise; in men, a stress protein response may "protect" the heart with moderately vigorous exercise, whereas this response is muted in the presence of estrogen. Nevertheless, epidemiological studies show that cardiorespiratory fitness level does have a strong influence on cardiovascular disease, CVD risk factors, and all-cause mortality in women, apparently at least analogous to the relationship observed in men. In regard to quality of life, women are at greater risk because they live longer, and there are gender differences in the prevalence and types of chronic disease conditions. More women live to an older age, and thus greater numbers of women have functional limitations and a dependent lifestyle. Further, insofar as cardiorespiratory fitness and muscle strength are related to loss of functional capacity, disability, and loss of independence, low fitness and strength levels would appear to put older women at risk. Nevertheless, after controlling for age, gender does not appear to be a critical variable; rather, cardiorespiratory fitness appears critical to the maintenance of an independent lifestyle in older age in both men and women. Muscle strength, particularly of the lower limbs (walking), is also important in this regard.

References

1. Paffenbarger, R.S., Hyde, R.T., Wing, A.L., et al., Physical activity, all-cause mortality, and longevity of college alumni, *N. Engl. J. Med.*, 314, 605–613, 1986.
2. Paffenbarger, R.S., Hyde, R.T., Wing, A.L., et al., The association of changes in physical-activity level and other lifestyle characteristics with mortality among men, *N. Engl. J. Med.*, 328, 538–545, 1993.
3. Paffenbarger, R.S., Kampert, J.B., Lee, I.M., et al., Changes in physical activity and other lifeway patterns influencing longevity, *Med. Sci. Sports Exerc.*, 26, 857–865, 1994.
4. Lee, I.M., Hsieh, C.C., and Paffenbarger, R.S., Exercise intensity and longevity in men: the Harvard alumni health study, *JAMA*, 273, 1179–1184, 1995.
5. Lissner, L., Bengtsson, C., Björkelund, C., et al., Physical activity levels and changes in relation to longevity, *Am. J. Epidemiol.*, 143, 54–62, 1996.
6. Kushi, L.H., Fee, R.M., Folsom, A.R., et al., Physical activity and mortality in postmenopausal women, *JAMA*, 277, 1287–1292, 1997.

7. Blair, S.N., Kohl, H.W. III, Paffenbarger, R.S., et al., Physical fitness and all-cause mortality, *JAMA*, 262, 2395–2401, 1989.
8. Blair, S.N., Kampert, J.B., Kohl, H.W. III, et al., Influences of cardiorespiratory fitness and other precursors on cardiovascular disease and all-cause mortality in men and women, *JAMA*, 276, 205–210, 1996.
9. Blair, S.N., Kohl, H.W. III, Barlow, C.E., et al., Changes in physical fitness and all-cause mortality: a prospective study of healthy and unhealthy men, *JAMA*, 273, 1093–1098, 1995.
10. Erikssen, G., Liestøl, K., Bjørnholt, J., et al., Changes in physical fitness and changes in mortality, *Lancet*, 352, 759–762, 1998.
11. 1997 Physical Activity Monitor, Canadian Fitness and Lifestyle Research Institute, Ottawa, Ontario.
12. Shulman, S.P., Cardiovascular consequences of the aging process, *Cardiol. Clin.*, 17, 35–49, 1999.
13. Statistics Canada, Health Statistics Division, Health Indicators, 1999 (Statistics Canada Catalogue No. 82-221-XCB).
14. Lakka, T.M., Venäläinen, J.M., Rauramaa, R., et al., Relation of leisure-time physical activity and cardiorespiratory fitness to the risk of acute myocardial infarction in men, *N. Engl. J. Med.*, 330, 1549–1554, 1994.
15. Haapanen, N., Miilunpalo, S., Vuori, I., et al., Association of leisure time physical activity with the risk of coronary heart disease, hypertension and diabetes in middle-aged men and women, *Int. J. Epidemiol.*, 26, 739–747, 1997.
16. Morris, J.N., Heady, J.A., Raffle, P.A.B., et al., Coronary heart disease and physical activity of work, *Lancet*, ii, 1053, 1111–1120, 1953.
17. Paffenbarger, R.S. and Hale, W.E., Work activity and coronary heart mortality, *N. Engl. J. Med.*, 292, 545–550, 1975.
18. Morris, J.N., Chave, S.P.W., Adam, C., et al., Vigorous exercise in leisure-time and the incidence of coronary heart-disease, *Lancet*, i, 333–339, 1973.
19. Morris, J.N., Everitt, M.G., Pollard, R., et al., Vigorous exercise in leisure-time: protection against coronary heart disease, *Lancet*, ii, 1207–1210, 1980.
20. Morris, J.N., Clayton, D.G., Everitt, M.G., et al., Exercise in leisure time: coronary attack and death rates, *Br. Heart J.*, 63, 325–334, 1990.
21. Paffenbarger, R.S., Wing, A.L., and Hyde, R.T., Physical activity as an index of heart attack risk in college alumni, *Am. J. Epidemiol.*, 108, 161–175, 1978.
22. Powell, K.E., Thompsom, P.D., Caspersen, C.J., et al., Physical activity and the incidence of coronary heart disease, *Ann. Rev. Publ. Health*, 8, 253–287, 1987.
23. Magnus, K., Matroos, S., and Strackee, J., Walking, cycling, or gardening, with or without seasonal interruption, in relation to acute coronary events, *Am. J. Epidemiol.*, 110, 724–733, 1979.
24. Brunner, D., Manelis, G., Modan, M., et al., Physical activity at work and the incidence of myocardial infarction, angina pectoris and death due to ischemic heart disease: an epidemiological study in Israeli collective settlements (kibbutzim), *J. Chron. Dis.*, 27, 217–233, 1974.
25. Sesso, H.D., Paffenbarger, R.S., Ha, T., et al., Physical activity and cardiovascular disease risk in middle-aged and older women, *Am. J. Epidemiol.*, 150, 408–416, 1999.
26. Blair, S.N., Kohl, H.W., and Barlow, C.E., Physical activity, physical fitness, and all-cause mortality in women: do women need to be active? *J. Am. Coll. Nutr.*, 12, 368–371, 1993.

27. Sherman, S.E., D'Agostino, R.B., Cobb, J.L., et al., Physical activity and mortality in women in the Framingham Heart Study, *Am. Heart J.*, 128, 879–884, 1994.
28. Lemaitre, R.N., Heckbert, S.R., Psaty, B.M., et al., Leisure-time physical activity and the risk of nonfatal myocardial infarction in postmenopausal women, *Arch. Intern. Med.*, 155, 2302–2308, 1995.
29. Folsom, A.R., Arnett, D.K., Hutchinson, R.G., et al., Physical activity and incidence of coronary heart disease in middle-aged women and men, *Med. Sci. Sports Exerc.*, 29, 901–909, 1997.
30. O'Connor, G.T., Hennekens, C.H., Willett, W.C, et al., Physical exercise and reduced risk of nonfatal myocardial infarction, *Am. J. Epidemiol.*, 142, 1147–1156, 1995.
31. Mensink, G.B., Deketh, M., Mul, M.D.M., et al., Physical activity and its association with cardiovascular risk factors and mortality, *Epidemiology*, 7, 391–397, 1996.
32. Lie, H., Mundal, R., and Erikssen, J., Coronary risk factors and incidence of coronary death in relation to physical fitness: seven-year follow-up study of middle-aged and elderly men, *Eur. Heart J.*, 6, 147–157, 1985.
33. Sandvik, L., Erikssen, J., Thaulow, E., et al., Physical fitness as a predictor of mortality among healthy, middle-aged Norwegian men, *N. Engl. J. Med.*, 328, 533–537, 1993.
34. Ekelund, L.G., Haskell, W.L., Johnson, J.L., et al., Physical fitness as a predictor of cardiovascular mortality in asymptomatic North American men, *N. Engl. J. Med.*, 319, 1379–1384, 1988.
35. Farrell, S.W., Kampert, J.B., Kohl, H.W., et al., Influences of cardiorespiratory fitness levels and other predictors on cardiovascular disease mortality in men, *Med. Sci. Sports Exerc.*, 30, 899–905, 1988.
36. Haddock, B.L., Hopp, H.P., Mason, J.J., et al., Cardiorespiratory fitness and cardiovascular disease risk factors in postmenopausal women, *Med. Sci. Sports Exerc.*, 30, 893–898, 1998.
37. Dvorak, R.V., Tchnernof, A., Starling, R.D., et al., Respiratory fitness, free living physical activity, and cardiovascular disease risk in older individuals: a doubly labeled water study, *J. Clin. Endocrinol. Metab.*, 85, 957–963, 2000.
38. Godsland, I.R., Wynn, V., Crook, D., et al., Sex, plasma lipoproteins, and atherosclerosis: prevailing assumptions and outstanding questions, *Am. Heart J.*, 114, 1467–1503, 1987.
39. Isles, C.G., Hole, D.J., Hawthorne, V.M., et al., Relation between coronary risk and coronary mortality in women of the Renfrew and Paisley survey: comparison with men, *Lancet*, 339, 702–706, 1992.
40. Kostis, J.B., Wilson, A.C., O'Dowd, K., et al., Sex differences in the management and long-term outcome of acute myocardial infarction. A statewide study. MIDAS Study Group. myocardial infarction data acquisition system. *Circulation*, 90, 1715–1730, 1994.
41. Grady, D.S, Rubin, S.M., Petitti, D.B., et al., Hormone therapy to prevent disease and prolong life in postmenopausal women, *Ann. Intern. Med.*, 117, 1016–1037, 1992.
42. Delyani, J.A., Murohara, T., Nossuli, T.O., et al., Protection from myocardial reperfusion injury by acute administration of 17 beta-estradiol, *J. Mol. Cell Cardiol.*, 28, 1001–1008, 1996
43. Williams, J.K., Adams, M.R., and Klopfenstein, H.S., Estrogen modulates responses of atherosclerotic coronary arteries, *Circulation*, 81, 1680–1687, 1990.

44. Kim, Y.D., Chen, B., Beauregard, J., et al., 17 beta-Estradiol prevents dysfunction of canine coronary endothelium and myocardium and reperfusion arrhythmias after brief ischemia/reperfusion, *Circulation*, 94, 2901–2908, 1996.
45. Herrington, D.M., Reboussin, D.M., Brosnihan, K.B., et al., Effects of estrogen replacement on the progression of coronary-artery atherosclerosis, *N. Engl. J. Med.*, 343, 522–529, 2000.
46. Hulley, S.D., Grady, D., Bush, T., et al., Randomized trial of estrogen plus progestin for secondary prevention of coronary heart disease in postmenopausal women. Heart and estrogen/progestin replacement study (HERS) research group, *JAMA*, 280, 605–613, 1998.
47. Gray, C.C., Amrani, M., and Yacoub, M.H., Heat stress proteins and myocardial protection: experimental model or potential clinical tool? *Int. J. Biochem. Cell. Biol.*, 31, 559–573, 1999.
48. Marber, M.S., Mestril, R., Chi, S.H., et al., Overexpression of the rat inducible 70-kD heat stress protein in a transgenic mouse increases the resistance of the heart to ischemic injury. *J. Clin. Invest.*, 95, 1446–1456, 1995.
49. Plumier, J.-C.L., Ross, B.M., Currie, R.W., et al., Transgenic mice expressing the human heat shock protein 70 have improved post-ischemic myocardial recovery. *J. Clin. Invest.*, 95, 1854–1860, 1995.
50. Radford, N.B., Fina, M., Benjamin, I.J., et al., Cardioprotective effects of 70-kDa heat shock protein in transgenic mice, *Proc. Natl. Acad. Sci. USA*, 93, 2339–2342, 1996.
51. Trost, S.U., Omens, J.H., Karlon, W.J., et al., Protection against myocardial dysfunction after a brief ischemic period in transgenic mice expressing inducible heat shock protein, *J. Clin. Invest.*, 101, 855–862, 1998.
52. Locke, M.E., Noble, E.G., Tanguay, R.M., et al., Activation of heat-shock transcription factor in rat heart after heat shock and exercise, *Am. J. Physiol.*, 268, C1387–1394, 1995.
53. Locke, M.E., Tangua, R.M., Klabunde, R.E., et al., Enhanced postischemic myocardial recovery following exercise induction of HSP 72, *Am. J. Physiol.*, 269, H320–325, 1995.
54. Paroo, Z., Tiidus, P.M., and Noble, E.G., Estrogen attenuates HSP 72 expression in acutely exercised male rodents, *Eur. J. Appl. Physiol.*, 80, 180–184, 1999.
55. Noble, E.G., Moraska, A., Mazzeo, R.S., et al., Fleshner, M., Differential expression of stress proteins in rat myocardium after free wheel or treadmill run training. *J. Appl. Physiol.*, 86, 1696–1701, 1999.
56. Williams, P.T., Relationships of heart disease risk factors to exercise quantity and intensity, *Arch. Intern. Med.*, 158, 237–245, 1998.
57. Holloszy, J.O., Mini-review: exercise and longevity: studies on rats, *J. Gerontol,*. 43, 149–151, 1988.
58. Shephard, R.J., Effects of exercise on biological features of aging, in *Biological Effects of Physical Activity*, Williams, R.S. and Wallace, A.G., Eds., Human Kinetics, Champaign, IL, 1989, 55–70.
59. Katz, S., Branch, L.G., Branson, M.H., et al., Active life expectancy, *N. Engl. J. Med.*, 309, 1218–1224, 1983.
60. Fries, J.F., Aging, natural death, and the compression of morbidity, *N. Engl. J. Med.*, 303, 130–135, 1980.
61. Svaardsudd, K., and Tiblin, G., Is quality of life affecting survival?, *Scand. J. Prim. Health Care*, Suppl 1, 55–60, 1990.
62. Lawrence, R.H., and Jette, A.M., Disentangling the disablement process, *J. Geron. Soc. Sci.*, 51B, S173–182, 1996.

63. Morey, M.C., Pieper, C.F., and Cononi-Huntley, J., Physical fitness and functional limitations in community-dwelling older adults, *Med. Sci. Sports Exer.*, 30, 715–723, 1998.
64. Verbrugge, L. and Jette, A.M., The disablement process, *Soc. Sci. Med.*, 38, 1–14, 1994.
65. Ettinger, W.H., Fried, L.P., Harris, T., et al., Self-reported causes of physical disability in older people: the cardiovascular health study, *J. Am. Geriatr. Soc.*, 42, 1035–1044, 1994.
66. Huang, Y., Macera, C.A., Blair, S.N., et al., Physical fitness, physical activity, and functional limitation in adults aged 40 and older, *Med. Sci. Sports Exerc.*, 30, 1430–1435, 1998.
67. Hirvensalo, M., Rantanen, T., and Heikkinen, E., Mobility difficulty and physical activity as predictors of mortality and loss of independence in the community-living older population, *J. Am. Ger. Soc.*, 48, 493–498, 2000.
68. Talbot, L.A., Metter, E.J., and Fleg, J.L., Leisure-time physical activities and their relationship to cardiorespiratory fitness in healthy men and women 18–95 years old, *Med. Sci. Sports Exerc.*, 32, 417–425, 2000.
69. World Health Organization, International Classification of Impairments, Disabilities and Handicaps, Geneva, 1980.
70. Brill, P.A., Macera, C.A., Davis, D.R., et al., Muscular strength and physical function, *Med. Sci. Sports Exerc.*, 32, 412–416, 2000.
71. Miller, M.E., Rejeski, W.J., Reboussin, B.A., et al., Physical activity, functional limitations, and disability in older adults, *J. Am. Geriatr. Soc.*, 48, 1264–1272, 2000.
72. Hubert, H.B., Bloch, D.A., and Fries, J.A., Risk factors for physical disability in an aging cohort: the NHANES I epidemiological follow-up study, *J. Rheumatol.*, 20, 480–488, 1993.
73. Wu Chong, S., Leu, S-Y., and Li, C-Y., Incidence of and predictors for chronic disability in activities of daily living among older people in Taiwan, *J. Am. Geriatr. Soc.*, 47, 1082–1086, 1999.
74. Guralnik, J.M., Ferrucci, L., Simonsick, E.M., et al., Lower-extremity function in persons over the age of 70 years as a predictor of subsequent disability, *N. Engl. J. Med.*, 332, 556–561, 1995.
75. Cunningham, D.A., Paterson, D.H., Himann, J.E., et al., Determinants of independence in the elderly, *Can. J. Appl. Physiol.*, 18, 243–254, 1993.
76. Posner, J.D., McCully, K.K., Landsberg, L.A., et al., Physical determinants of independence in mature women, *Arch. Phys. Med. Rehabil.*, 76, 373–380, 1995.
77. Lancet Editorial, Physical activity in old age, *Lancet*, ii, 1431, 1986.
78. Koval, J.J., Ecclestone, N.A., Paterson, D.H., et al., Response rates in a survey of physical capacity among older persons, *J. Gerontol.*, 47, S140–147, 1992.
79. Paterson, D.H., Cunningham, D.A., Koval, J.J., et al., Aerobic fitness in a population of independently living men and women aged 55–65 years, *Med. Sci. Sports Exerc.*, 31, 1813–1820, 1999.
80. Mor, V., Murphy, J., Masterson-Allen, S., et al., Risk of functional decline among well elders, *J. Clin. Epidemiol.*, 42, 895–904, 1989.
81. Cunningham, D.A., Rechnitzer, P.A., and Donner, A.P., Exercise training of men at retirement: a clinical trial, *J. Gerontol.*, 42, 17–23, 1987.
82. Blumenthal, J.A., Enery, C.F., Madden, D.J., et al., Cardiovascular and behavioral effects of aerobic exercise in healthy older men and women, *J. Gerontol.*, M147–157, 1989.

6

Aging of the Neuromuscular System: Influences of Gender and Physical Activity

Charles L. Rice and David A. Cunningham

CONTENTS

6.1 Introduction

The ability to move with purpose and to remain independent with increasing age depends to a large degree on retaining an adequate functional capacity in the neuromuscular system. This system, which governs the generation and control of muscle force, typically undergoes a substantial decline in functional capacity with age, but retains a great degree of its remarkable adaptive capabilities. Beginning at approximately 30 years of age, human muscular strength declines at a rate of 10 to 15% per decade[1] (Figure 6.1).

0-8493-1027-X/02/$0.00+$1.50

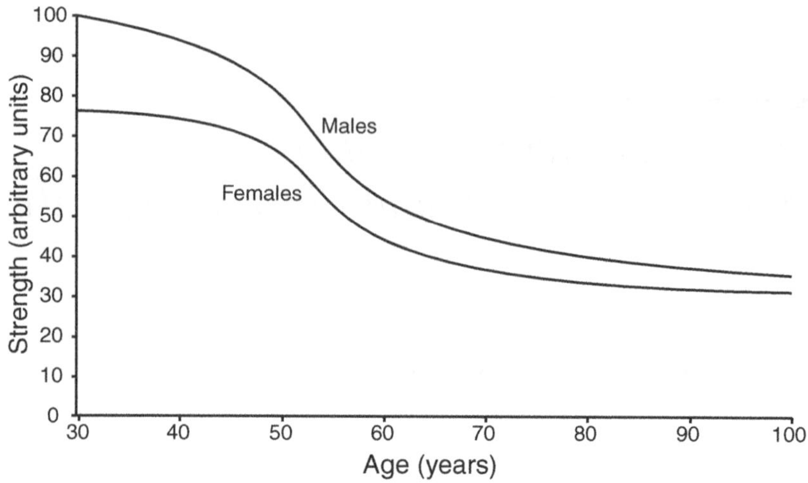

FIGURE 6.1
Hypothetical curves of changes in voluntary strength with increasing age for both males and females. The curves are based on a compilation of findings from many studies, both cross-sectional and longitudinal, that have measured voluntary strength in isometric and dynamic contractions from several limb muscles. The curves suggest that the age-related change in the strength profiles is slightly different between men and women. Strength is fairly well preserved until approximately 50 years of age, although perhaps better in females than males, with an accelerated decline during the next 20 to 25 years. Overall, males are stronger than females, but the gender difference is minimal by 80 years of age and beyond. It is suggested that the rate of strength decline in the very old is small and that, at least for ambulatory people, strength may be preserved at a minimal level required for basic activities of daily living. Further studies, especially longitudinal studies, are needed to substantiate these proposed strength curves and to identify unique curves for different muscle groups during different tasks and for each gender.

Because the activities of daily living usually do not require maximal muscular efforts, the gradual loss of strength for most individuals does not become functionally significant until after 55 to 60 years of age. Beyond ~50 years of age, the rate of loss of force may accelerate,[1,2] but eventually a minimum level of strength seems to be preserved, at least in moderately healthy and ambulatory individuals, so that the rate of decline in force approaches an asymptote in the eighth decade and beyond.[3] Thus, healthy people in the seventh and eighth decades of life may have only 50% of the strength of young adults, but the further loss over the ensuing decades may be no more than ~10% (Figure 6.1). Retention of minimum muscle strength may be related to the effort required to perform the basic tasks of daily living. More importantly, since not only strength but also speed of movement is reduced in aged adults, the power generating capacity of the neuromuscular system is affected. Indeed, the loss of power may be twice as great as the loss of strength after 65 years of age,[4] and loss of power may be most closely related to difficulties with activities of daily living and loss of independence.

There have recently been many reviews of neuromuscular aging and its effects on strength, functional capacity, and the response to exercise training.

Most reviews have centered on measurement of isometric strength, and gender has not been identified as a significant factor. The present chapter is not a comprehensive summary of the earlier literature, but rather highlights and sensitizes the reader to the influences of task and gender on changes in strength, power, and functional capacity in aged humans, relating these findings to the influence of exercise resistance training. To place these themes in context, the chapter begins with a brief overview of the major factors responsible for sarcopenia, followed by a summary of changes in voluntary strength of different types of muscle contractions with age. Problems encountered in comparing results from differently designed studies are indicated. Subsequently, the effects of age on the integrative functional neuromuscular properties of power, fatigue, and force are reviewed. The chapter concludes with a brief summary of the effects of resistance exercise training on neuromuscular function. Wherever possible, gender differences are identified, and the effects of age-related changes in the neuromuscular system on the activities of daily living are outlined. Most of the work discussed centers on results from the most recent primary and review papers of human studies, but relevant work from animal and other reduced preparations is cited to substantiate and explain certain observations.

6.2 Possible Factors Contributing to Sarcopenia

Sarcopenia is defined as a decline in skeletal muscle mass due to aging, with a concomitant loss of voluntary strength.[5] The age-associated loss in muscle mass reflects a combination of reductions in muscle fiber numbers and decreases in individual muscle fiber sizes[6] (see also Chapter 7). To a great extent, sarcopenia and its dependent changes in contractile function can be explained by morphological alterations in skeletal muscle tissue. However, depending on the muscle studied, age-related weakness cannot be explained solely by gross structural adaptations.[7,8] For example, there are age-related changes in excitation–contraction coupling mechanisms and in the contractile proteins[9-16] which reduce contractile function; also, changes in neurological factors affect voluntary force production and control.[8,10,17,18] The details of these mechanisms will not be discussed, but some key functional outcomes will be summarized briefly.

6.2.1 Central Drive

Age-related weakness may be caused to some degree by a decreased central drive, and thus a decreased ability to activate a muscle voluntarily. The threshold of excitability of the corticospinal tract, as determined by transcranial magnetic stimulation, increases progressively with age.[19] There is an accompanying increase in the electrical resistance of the cell membrane,[20] and a progressive decrease in motoneuron conduction velocities.[21] A decrease in the safety factor and a reduction of the effectiveness of synaptic transmission across the neuromuscular junction could also occur,[21] although it is uncertain to what extent such changes would be functionally significant.[22]

Using the twitch interpolation technique to assess the ability of the central nervous system (CNS) to activate a muscle, investigators have frequently reported that, in healthy aged adults, essentially all of the muscle mass in various limb muscles can be fully activated by brief isometric maximal voluntary contractions (MVCs),[8,23-27] although others have challenged this concept.[28-30] Further complete studies using refinements of this and other techniques[31,32] seem to demonstrate differences in activation abilities between older and younger subjects. However, the results to date suggest that any age-related deficits in activation ability are unlikely to be large[33] or functionally significant when compared with the substantial voluntary weakness that develops with aging. Twitch interpolation methods during controlled dynamic (isokinetic) contractions have been used in a few studies,[34,35] but no difference has been found in activation abilities between young and elderly (70 years) men for triceps surae contractions at velocities of up to 230°/s.[36] Nevertheless, some loss of activation was noted at higher contraction velocities (up to ~300°/s).[36] Thus, further studies are required to determine whether or not central activation significantly limits dynamic exercise and induces fatigue in aged humans, and whether gender and exercise training are additional factors to be considered.

6.2.2 Motor Unit Remodeling

A natural turnover of synaptic connections occurs at the neuromuscular junction by a process of denervation, axonal sprouting, and reinnervation of the muscle; this is termed motor unit remodeling.[37] The fundamental age-related change in the motor unit is a decrease in overall numbers of motor units.[8,38,39] Motor unit loss has been estimated at approximately 1% of the total number per annum, beginning in the third decade of life, and increasing in rate beyond the age of 60.[40] The reduction in the number of human lumbosacral spinal cord motoneurons evident after 60 years of age[18,40] appears to reflect losses of the largest motoneurons and their axons,[38] with a preservation of smaller motoneurons. It seems that the normal remodeling process is altered with aging; type II fibers become selectively denervated and they are reinnervated by collateral sprouting of axons from fibers of type I motor units. The reinnervated type II fibers become (or approximate) type I fibers, with respect to their physiological and biochemical properties.[37,41,42] The surviving motoneurons increase in branching complexity and exhibit collateral growth,[43] perhaps to compensate for the loss of motoneurons and an increased "load" due to increased innervation ratios. These changes may explain an apparent reduction in motoneuron excitability leading to lower motor unit discharge rates with age (see later discussion). Age-related remodeling can account for many of the observed functional changes in skeletal muscle; however, the reasons underlying the altered remodeling remain unclear.

Remodeling does not seem to affect all muscles equally.[44,45] Physiological evidence includes the generation of a greater force per action potential,[21,38,46,47] histochemical evidence is provided by fiber type grouping in various skeletal muscles in contrast to the usual heterogeneous mixture of fiber types observed in human muscle from younger adults.[48] Biochemical evidence supporting age-related fiber type transformations has been adduced from quantitative and qualitative changes in myosin heavy chain (MHC) expression.[11,49,50] The muscle fibers of very old humans show an abundant coexpression of two MHC isoforms (I and IIA) in the majority of fibers sampled.[9] Although an intriguing topic for further study, the functional significance of these biochemical changes has not yet been evaluated. It is also unknown whether remodeling is related to gender, or if exercise can affect the process.

6.2.3 Motor Unit Recruitment and Firing Rates

Muscle force is graded by recruiting an appropriate number of motor units and altering the pattern and frequency of unit discharges. From the few reports available (see later discussion), it seems that the recruitment threshold decreases with age, presumably in association with a shift towards fewer numbers of motor units and a preponderance of type I fibers.[51] Furthermore, the relationship between recruitment level and firing rate in individual motor units differs between young and old adults.[51] Although evidence is still rather limited,[8,52,53] more work has focused on age-related changes in firing rates than on recruitment during isometric contractions. In most of the muscles studied to date, motor unit firing rates are significantly lower in old than in young subjects, although there is some disagreement as to whether changes occur only at high force levels, or whether they are observed throughout the normal range of forces.[53] Differences may be muscle-specific, since some muscles seem to show a greater age-related reduction in firing rates than do others.[8,51,53] In one study, laryngeal muscle firing rates were lower and discharge variability was greater in older than in young men, but female subjects showed no change in either parameter with age.[54] Although the issue has not been studied systematically, other investigators have not noted gender differences in the firing rate properties of limb muscles; the differences seen in the laryngeal muscles likely reflect gender-specific voice characterizations.

Based on the current understanding of a matching between neural and contractile components of the motor unit for effective force generation,[55] and the common observation of slowed contractile properties with age, it is reasonable to expect an age-related reduction in firing rates. Thus, reductions may occur simply because larger motor units in the elderly are innervated primarily by slow motoneurons (see previous discussion). Alternatively, motor unit firing rates may be affected by age-related limitations in the excitability of the corticospinal tract[19] and motoneurons,[20] or a reduction in central drive.[33] However, a proportion of fast motoneurons do survive in the elderly,[56] since some motor units are capable of achieving firing rates as high as those of younger subjects.[23,24,51,57-59] Thus, it seems that changes in motor drive are not directly responsible for the substantial age-related muscle weakness found in many muscles.

Variability in motor unit firing rate is another parameter that potentially could affect optimal force production. Due to intrinsic axonal factors such as synaptic noise at low rates of discharge (see Roos et al.[8]), it appears that motor units have a specific tonic threshold tension level at which the firing rate becomes regular.[60] A few studies have measured the variability of firing rates in aged humans; observations have been made at low force levels, with equivocal results.[46,61-63] If, as has been proposed,[61-63] older humans exhibit a greater variability in their motor unit discharge pattern, it is possible that these units have not reached the rate threshold for discharge stability. This concept is compatible with the finding that firing rates are slowed with age. Functionally, this enhanced variability may adversely affect the production and control of force in aged humans (see later discussion).

Since differences in firing rate and variability in both young[64,65] and older[66] subjects have been related to habitual usage, and there is a variable response to exercise training,[58,66-68] the disparate firing rate changes observed among muscles in response to aging could be related to patterns of habitual physical activity. Alternatively, since a wide variety of firing rates have been reported for several human muscles, depending in part on the task,[52] changes in neuromodulation in relation to force could be related to anatomic or physiologic properties. How these properties and the resultant response to various tasks are affected by aging, exercise and, possibly, gender requires that appropriate experimentation be completed.

6.2.4 Contractile Properties

Besides the muscle weakness recorded from both voluntary and electrically induced contractions, another hallmark of a neuromuscular system in aged animals is a change in contractile quality, usually recorded as a slowed contractile response. During voluntary contractions there are age-related reductions in the rate of force development,[46,61-63] as well as the ability to accelerate the limb.[69] Electrically evoked isometric contractions of various whole limb muscles usually exhibit reductions in maximal twitch and tetanic tensions, and longer twitch contraction times are seen in most whole muscles[53] and individual motor units.[70] These contractile changes can be summarized functionally by an age-related leftward shift in the force–frequency relationship.[23,71-73] Although the extent to which weaker and slower muscle properties directly reflect changes in muscle composition is debatable,[74] it is reasonable to conclude, on the basis of both morphological data and slow twitch contractile properties, that type I fibers contribute proportionally more to force generation in elderly than in younger adults.[8] The shift in force–frequency relationship suggests the possibility of attenuating the age-related force loss by more effective summation within a slower contracting muscle in response to a given rate of excitation. Furthermore, older men and women show significantly less twitch potentiation than younger subjects.[75] One study of human single fiber properties indicates that aged fibers have gender-dependent differences in contractile function, reflecting fiber type rather than fiber size.[76] Given the limited data, it is unclear why female fibers would be affected differently by age, but hormonal, genetic, and immunologic factors need to be considered. Thus, not all muscles are similarly affected by age, either qualitatively or quantitatively, and the influence of gender needs to be evaluated.

6.2.5 Specific Force

One possible reason for age-related muscle weakness is a change in specific tension (force). Although not a universal finding,[26,76,77] evidence exists that, during whole muscle contractions, older humans show a reduction in the amount of force generated per unit of cross-sectional area of 20% or more.[21,78-81] Direct measurements on whole rodent muscle,[37,82] single fiber preparations,[15,83] and human muscle[76] have yielded similar findings. The mechanisms leading to a reduced specific tension in older animals remain unknown. It has been suggested that there are morphological changes in the organization of the actin and myosin contractile proteins,[49,84,85] that some substance in the cytosol of fibers in the muscles of old animals inhibits the force development of cross bridges, or that the cross bridges in intact fibers are not fully activated by calcium.[37,82,86]

Discrepancies between results from whole muscle studies in humans are related to differences in the muscle studied, and in the techniques of measurement of both the strength task (isometric, dynamic) and the method used to estimate active muscle mass and architecture.[76,204] Because of these technical problems, it is unclear if age affects specific tension, and if the effect is gender dependent. A few recent studies indicate that the muscles of old women develop a lower specific force than those of old men,[76,87] but reasons for this difference are unclear and, indeed, other studies do not find a gender difference.[26] To assess whether specific force affects whole muscle functional measures in humans, more studies making accurate measurements of muscle volume (physiologic cross-sectional area) *in vivo* from a variety of muscle groups while performing differing tasks are required. To resolve the gender issue, future studies should treat males and females separately.

TABLE 6.1

Muscle Strength Changes with Age

Muscle Group	Study	Age	Gender	MVC	Isokinetic
Knee extensors	Frontera et al.[76*]	77 ± 4	M		73%–Con
	Hortobagyi et al.[198]	60–80	M	60%	49%–Con
		60–74	F	44%	62%–Con
		60–80	M		88%–Ecc
		60–74	F		98%–Ecc
	Hunter et al.[108]	80–89	F	43%	
	Ivey et al.[177]	65–75	M	76%	
		65–75	F	75%	
	Murray et al.[109]	70–86	F	67%	68%–Con
	Poulin et al.[199]	60–75	M		68%–Con
		60–75	M		90%–Ecc
	Roos et al.[23]	73–91	M	52%	
	Vandervoort et al.[200]	66–89	F		50%–Con
		66–89	F		64%–Ecc
	Young et al.[105]	71–81	F	65%	
	Young et al.[106]	70–79	M	61%	
Knee flexors	Frontera et al.[76*]	77 ± 4	M		72%–Con
	Murray et al.[109]	70–86	F	65%	62%–Con
	Vandervoort et al.[200]	66–89	F		55%–Con
		66–89	F		73%–Ecc
Dorsiflexors	Connelly et al.[24]	80–85	M	74%	
	Kent-Braun and Ng[26]	65–83	M	92%	
		65–83	F	75%	
	Patten and Kamen[58]	66–76	M	68%	
		66–76	F	92%	
	Porter et al.[7]	60–74	F		73%–Con
		60–74	F		97%–Ecc
	Vandervoort and	80–100	M	54%	
	McComas[27]	80–100	F	63%	
Plantar flexors	Amara et al. [3]	80–86	M	61%	
		80–86	F	59%	
	Cunningham et al.[201]	63 ± 3	M		70%–Con
	Hunter et al.[108]	80–89	F	48%	
	Klein et al.[202]	64–69	M	69%	
	Porter et al.[203]	60–74	F		89%–Con
					99%–Ecc
	Vandervoort and	80–100	M	54%	
	McComas[27]	80–100	F	47%	
Elbow extensors	Frontera et al.[76*]	77 ± 4	M		86%–Con
	Klein et al.[204]	81 ± 6	M	66%	
	Poulin et al.[199]	60–75	M		69%–Con
		60–75	M		79%–Ecc
Elbow flexors	Allman and Rice[140]	80–87	M	64%	
	Bilodeau et al.[136]	65–86	M	81%	
		65–86	F	79%	
	Doherty et al.[38]	60–81	M	67%	
	Frontera et al.[76*]	77 ± 4	M		79%–Con
	Jakobi et al.[45]	79–89	M	62%	

TABLE 6.1 (continued)

Muscle Strength Changes with Age

Muscle Group	Study	Age	Gender	MVC	Isokinetic
Handgrip	Amara et al.[3]	80–86	M	64%	
		80–86	F	66%	
	Hunter et al.[108]	80–89	F	62%	
First dorsal interosseus	Kamen et al.[57]	67–85	Not stated	79%	
	Laidlaw et al.[148]	64–83	M	70%	
			F	68%	
	Semmler et al.[153]	63–81	M	66%	
		63–81	F	96%	
Adductor pollicis	Ditor and Hicks[134]	72 ± 5	M	66%	
		70 ± 5	F	84%	
	Bemben et al.[92]	70–74	M	76%	

Note: Results from several cross-sectional studies in various limb muscle groups that have measured isometric (MVC, maximum voluntary isometric contraction) force, or isokinetic torque in young and old males and females. Age is provided as a range or ± S.D. Values are expressed as a percentage of young adult strength. Concentric (Con) and eccentric (Ecc) strength are expressed as an average of the velocities tested in each study.

* Longitudinal study in which the percentage change is relative to values obtained 12 years previous (~65 years of age).

6.3 Voluntary Strength

The reduction in voluntary muscle strength due to sarcopenia is well documented (see reviews by Porter et al. and Roos et al.[7,8]). As indicated earlier, in comparison to young adults, strength can be reduced by 50% or more in 80-year-olds. Initial studies suggested that the loss of strength was stratified by anatomic location, with distal and lower limb muscles affected more than proximal and upper limb muscles,[53,88-91] but when results from many, mainly cross-sectional studies are tabulated (Table 6.1), differences in the percentage force loss cannot be categorized so simply. Longitudinal studies support the concept that no muscle group or anatomic region has a consistent and substantial preferential susceptibility to age-related loss of voluntary strength.[76,92]

For simplicity of measurement and standardization, especially in studies on larger groups of individuals, the great majority of observers have tested isometric strength. However, some studies have measured isokinetic concentric contractions in the knee, ankle, and elbow muscles; these results indicate a similar pattern of loss for peak torque and isometric force, although a trend for total loss of concentric torque to be greater by 10 to 15% than for isometric force may exist (see Vandervoort and Symons[91] and Table 6.1). There is some discrepancy among reports (see Rice[53]), but most pointed to a greater loss of peak concentric torque at high than at low test velocities.[91] Fewer studies have assessed eccentric rather than concentric isokinetic contraction strength, but in a few muscle groups eccentric contraction torque is least affected by age (Table 6.1). Compared with approximately 50% loss of isometric and concentric strength, subjects in their eighth to tenth decades of life may show decrements in eccentric strength of a few percent up to 25% for the same muscle group.[91] Reasons for the relative preservation of eccentric strength are not known; they may be related simply to changes in connective tissue properties, which enhance the force developed in this task.[93] Alternatively, or concomitantly, because eccentric strength requires less neural drive for a given force level than either concentric or isometric contractions,[52] this type of task may be less susceptible to age-related changes in various neuromuscular parameters (outlined earlier). There is much recent interest in understanding eccentric contractions and aging because aged humans may benefit from this type of training.[91] Clearly, the movement task, as reflected by the testing modality, is an important variable when considering age-related strength loss and its impact on the activities of daily living.

In addition to the possibility of the measurement task demonstrating varying degrees of strength loss with age, and the caveat of the need to compare results from the young elderly with those from the very old, other variables confounding the understanding of sarcopenia in humans include the effects of physical fitness or habitual physical activity levels, and gender. Since the neuromuscular system is very responsive to habitual activity levels even in very old humans, studies of age-related changes must be cognizant of this parameter and its effect on neuromuscular function. This is especially critical for physiological studies that often recruit fewer than 10 to 15 subjects in a given age group; for example, an active 85-year-old could have 25% greater strength than a less active 85-year-old. It seems likely from our present understanding that the physiology of two such individuals is not directly comparable, and they should not be considered as representative of the same group despite their chronological age. Current studies are increasing efforts to describe and control for the habitual activity profiles of aged subjects (e.g., References 94 through 97). In so doing, the effects of physical activity can be evaluated separately from age-related changes per se.

There is a strong relationship between limb muscle strength and muscle mass.[98,99] Even in old age and despite reductions in circulating levels of testosterone and other anabolic hormones,[16,100] males are reported to retain more absolute muscle strength than females. Gender differences in the strength of specific limb muscles have been described in some studies;[3,26,27,76,101-106] a smaller number of reports are exclusive to females.[107-109] Nevertheless, it is difficult to conclude whether females are equally or differently susceptible to age-related declines in strength compared to males. It has been suggested tentatively that, because males are initially stronger than females, they lose strength more rapidly as they age.[2,26,102,105] However, one recent study reported that from the age of 20 to 80 years, decreases in handgrip and knee extensor strength were at a consistent but greater rate for men than for women; women showed an accelerated rate of strength loss after 55 years of age.[110]

One provocative suggestion emerging from these limited studies is that perhaps the very old (>80 years) approach similar absolute strength levels, regardless of gender (Figure 6.1), and this level is related to their relative activity status.[3] Besides the few studies directed at the issue of gender, solid conclusions remain tenuous; comparisons among studies are confounded by the usual problems of differences between the muscle groups tested and the testing task, limitations of the greater number of cross-sectional studies vs. very few longitudinal studies, inclusion of individuals whose ages span several decades after the fifth decade, and the varying activity and dependency status of the subjects. Furthermore, the influence of hormone replacement therapy on the muscle strength of postmenopausal women has received minimal study; results disagree as to whether estrogen replacement therapy protects muscle function[16] (see Chapter 7). Clearly, it is imprudent to combine genders when examining changes in strength and assessing other related age-related functions such as fatigue. Results from studies in which genders have been combined need careful reconsideration. Further research must be directed at identifying possible gender differences in strength and exploring age-related alterations in levels of testosterone and estrogen.

6.4 Power

Power is a function of both strength and speed of movement. It provides a measure of the functional capacity of muscle closely related to dynamic activities of daily living. Since both force and speed of contraction are reduced in the aged, it follows that power is substantially less when compared with muscles from young adults.[111] Recent studies have focused on age-related changes in the power of the lower limb knee extensors,[112,113] the upper limb muscles,[114,115] or both.[116] In general, the loss of power is 25% greater than the loss of isometric or isokinetic strength, and is especially pronounced at high contractile velocities.[4] Muscle size and fiber type are the main determinants of maximal power. Thus sarcopenia and, specifically, the relative loss of type II fibers likely explain most of the loss of power in aged muscle.[113] Other factors affecting power and possibly related directly or indirectly to the amount of muscle and fiber type characteristics include reductions in specific tension, oxidative capacity, optimal velocity of movement,[111,117] muscle compliance,[118] and increased body fatness.[119]

Power is related to muscle mass and contractile characteristics, but it is not known whether any one muscle, or muscle group, is more susceptible to power loss with old age, since very few studies have compared power measurements between different muscle groups in the same subjects. Although the tasks are not directly comparable between these studies, the loss of power in dynamic exercise has been reported as either greater for the lower limb[115] muscles, or comparable for lower and upper limb muscles.[116] Aged women develop as little as 50% of the power of aged men;[114,120,121] despite gender differences in muscle mass, this may reflect lower levels of anabolic hormones in females.[121] Given the limited data available, it is uncertain whether there is a gender difference in the rate of power loss with age; young women also produce less power than young men.[112] As noted for strength measurements, the effects of the testing task and the activity profiles of the subjects need to be evaluated before meaningful comparisons can be made between either muscle groups or genders.

Since age affects power more than strength and most activities of daily living require an adequate combination of force and speed of movement — or a minimum power generating capacity — the preservation of muscle power with advancing age is important in reducing the risk of disability and dependency. This concept has been assessed mainly by measuring knee extensor power as related to the power required to rise from a chair, walk, or climb stairs.[120] Deterioration in these abilities may be especially critical for females, since initially they have substantially less power than males. The ability to negotiate stairs, in particular, is strongly related to other measures of functional disability in the elderly[122] and lower limb power is the strongest predictor of functional status in elderly women.[123] The minimum power required for these activities is lost at a relatively younger age in women, and a greater proportion of the population are affected. For example, the knee extensor power required to ascend a 0.5 m step may be lacking in an average 60-year-old woman, whereas the average man may retain adequate power to perform that task until almost 75 years of age.[4] The differential power loss may explain why very old women (80 to 100 years) are less able to maintain the activities of daily living than are very old men.[124] Overall, loss of power can impair efficient movement, leading to excessive muscle fatigue, reliance on accessory muscles,[91] and, conceivably, overuse injuries and falls.

6.5 Fatigability

Fatigue is defined in human neuromuscular research as any reduction in force or power during voluntary effort, regardless of whether or not the task can still be performed successfully.[125] However, in studies of aging, fatigue is usually described as fatigability, or its reciprocal, endurance capacity. Since aging is associated with substantial alterations in both the structure and function of many aspects of the neuromuscular system related to the integrative function of force generation, it is reasonable to expect that the mechanisms determining endurance capacity and muscle fatigue will be affected. Although quantitative data are limited, a reduced ability to sustain and recover from bouts of exercise is a common feature of old age.[111] Surprisingly few studies have been devoted to this topic, but it is perhaps less surprising that results are variable,[89,126] depending to a great degree on gender and the task to be undertaken.[125,127]

Because of sarcopenia and other age-related changes in the neuromuscular system, the ability to perform any task that requires an absolute workload is problematic. Further, the susceptibility to fatigue is increased because any given task represents a greater proportion of the maximal strength or power of the muscle.[111] In animal studies, the maximal sustained and normalized power is 50% less in old than in young mice, and power is further compromised as the rate of repetition of contractions is increased.[111] Studies in humans have found similar results.[128,129] Conversely, when fatigue protocols compare young and old adults in terms of force normalized to a percentage of the individual's maximum, results are inconsistent. Several studies using intermittent maximal isometric or isokinetic contractions in a variety of muscles have found no difference in the fatigability of young and old individuals;[75,130-133] however, one recent paper reported that the adductor pollicis muscle was less fatigable in old than in young subjects[134] during maximal isometric contractions. Two studies using sustained maximal contractions showed a trend towards greater endurance in small hand muscles,[135] or greater endurance of the elbow flexors in aged compared with young subjects.[136] Conversely, in studies that have tested fatigue at submaximal intensities, the only trends found suggest greater fatigue resistance in old compared with young adults.[16,137-139] In a recent study using intermittent isometric submaximal contractions of the elbow flexors in men over 80 years of age, fatigue did not differ from that seen in young men.[140] Animal studies are equally inconclusive in determining whether muscles from aged animals are more,[141] or less[142] resistant to fatigue. Clearly, findings are substantially influenced by the nature of the task.

Besides task differences per se, certain age-related factors could influence fatigue. One factor, not easy to quantify but potentially important, especially during maximal contractile intensities in aged humans, is the extent of central drive during voluntary efforts.[136] The inability to assess central drive is a major limitation when animals are used to investigate fatigue. Central drive, or activation, could influence the efficacy and mode of neural drive in the CNS, and it is important in determining whether fatigue is due to central or peripheral (muscle) factors. The enhanced endurance of the neuromuscular system observed in some situations, especially at lower contractile intensities, (and despite sarcopenia) might be explained by a remodeling of the motor unit pool, with a greater relative proportion of fatigue-resistant type I fibers. However, the oxidative potential of the muscle does not necessarily increase, since significant changes in the activity of oxidative enzymes and a decline in mitochondrial function may occur as a result of aging.[117,143] These factors, and others such as local blood flow and contractile energetics, are strongly related to the nature of the task, and they need to be evaluated critically, whether comparing results from existing fatigue studies or designing future studies. Potential sites of failure or compensation in the neuromuscular system during fatigue will respond differently, depending on whether the task is sustained or intermittent, high or low intensity, and short or long duration. Considering the age-related alterations in the neuromuscular system, the nature of the task may be a significant factor influencing fatigue in aged subjects. The few studies addressing the effects of gender and age on fatigability have added another important variable to the task-specific concept of fatigue: because of probable gender differences in the overall structure and function of muscles and possible differential age-related changes between genders, it is reasonable to expect that the effects of fatigue will be gender dependent. The limited studies currently available are inconclusive, but do suggest that in addition to the influence of task there could be gender differences to consider. Two studies that utilized intermittent maximal isokinetic knee extensor contractions found no gender differences in fatigue in subjects 65 to 75 years of age.[132,133] Women experienced less voluntary fatigue than men during intermittent isometric MVCs of the ankle dorsiflexors and the elbow flexors in subjects aged 60 to 80 years,[144] but, using an identical protocol in the adductor pollicis muscle of ~70-year-old subjects, Ditor and Hicks[134] found no gender effect on fatigue. Women aged 65 to 86 years of age had greater endurance for maximal sustained MVCs of the elbow flexors than their male peers, although in this study the number of subjects of either gender was small.[136]

Speculations about differences in fatigability focus on a combination of age-related and gender-specific factors. The possible effects of estrogen levels on fatigue are controversial.[134,145] Blood flow may not be as easily occluded in females, since they have a lower vascular reactivity to norepinephrine than males.[146] The length and mass of muscle can also affect local blood flow, and thus the smaller and shorter muscles of females generate less intramuscular pressure to impede flow and affect metabolism, and they also use less energy.[134,144] On the basis of limited data, some authors have suggested that females may have fewer type II fibers[136,144] than males, and thus have less fatigable muscles. Further studies directed specifically at understanding the effects of gender on age-related changes in fatigue, and assessing or controlling these gender factors are required. Studies on aging, especially those directed at fatigue, should take into account the task used when interpreting results, and male and female data should not be combined in analyses. Finally, the ability to recover from fatigue is an important concept to consider, especially in aged subjects, but as yet it has not been evaluated. Older people use a greater percentage of their reduced maximal strength to perform the activities of daily living, and extent and speed of recovery may be very important determinants of whether a necessary activity can be completed successfully, and then repeated. Older women who usually have lower capacities than men must work at a higher percentage of their maximum capacity for a given task, and thus are likely to have a reduced ability to recover and continue with the same or a different activity of daily living.

6.6 Force Control

A generalized slowing of motor control capabilities accompanies aging, despite maintenance of an adequate force, power generating capacity, and endurance; this can significantly affect an individual's success in performing many of the activities of daily living. Impaired motor control can affect the arm and hand muscles, thereby limiting important functions or activities that require appropriate control and accuracy of hand force. Likewise, a reduction of motor control in the lower limb muscles can affect balance and gait, predisposing to falls.

Manual dexterity, pinch force, and target tracking tasks are performed less well and the time required to manipulate small objects increases significantly after 70 years of age.[58,89] Excessive hand grip force during fine motor tasks and greater fluctuations of isometric force have been noted in some,[89,147] but not all studies;[51,58] differences in results may be related to the intensity of force developed. Greater fluctuations in displacement during tracking tasks suggest that there is less steady movement in the finger muscles in old than in young adults.[148] Tasks requiring isometric arm muscle contractions showed no age-related differences in steadiness, but old adults were less steady than young adults when making dynamic contractions.[149] Furthermore, elderly subjects had a reduced ability to change smoothly from continuous concentric to eccentric contractions in the ankle muscles.[150] Thus, age-related changes in the neural strategies associated with force control do seem the same for all muscles and all tasks.

It has been suggested that reduced ability to maintain a constant submaximal force is due, at least partially, to the larger forces exerted by a relatively greater number of low threshold (type I) motor units in aged than in young subjects.[46] This may reflect age-related motor unit remodeling (see previous discussion). The discharge rates of motor units are generally less in aged compared with young adults.[8,51,52] A mean decrease in firing rates might suggest an increased reliance on recruitment to grade force, which could impair force control. In the few studies that have examined motor unit recruitment strategies when hand muscles perform various tasks, older adults have shown either no change[46] or a slight reduction[51] in recruitment thresholds, compared with young adults. Small age-related differences in derecruitment strategies of motor units have also been reported,[58,151] but further studies are required to characterize and understand the relationships between motor unit recruitment and derecruitment strategies and force control. It seems that the decline in force steadiness accompanying aging is not related to differences in coactivation of agonist–antagonist muscles,[152] or to increased motor unit synchronization,[153] but to a greater variability in motor unit discharge rate in old adults,[51,148] at least during low-force contractions Whatever the mechanisms, slowness of movement, reductions in motor skill, impaired coordination, and poor balance, combined with strength loss, cause difficulties for aged humans during everyday activities. It also seems that peripheral vestibular input decreases with advancing age, exacerbating problems of balance.[154]

Injury from falls is one serious consequence of these impairments,[155-157] the risk of which is frequently compounded by the administration of psychotropic drugs.[158] Impaired balance and gait are the two most significant risk factors for limited mobility and falls in the elderly.[159] Few studies have addressed the issue of gender and force control; however, epidemiologic studies suggest that old women are more prone to falls than are old men.[158,160] Laboratory studies indicate that women have longer response times when negotiating sudden turns and stops,[161] and when attempting to recover from a forward fall.[162] These differences may reflect the greater prevalence of physical disability in women, but factors complicating epidemiological studies need to be identified and explored before forming solid conclusions relative to gender. It is clear that increased physical activity and exercise programs can greatly improve mobility and reduce the incidence of falls.[163-165]

6.7 Benefits of Strength Training

Recent reviews have thoroughly summarized the literature supporting the benefits of strength or resistance exercise training for humans as old as 100 years of age.[159,166-170] The main purpose of this section is to evaluate the effects of resistance exercise with regard to gender, mobility, and ability to undertake the activities of daily living. Despite variations in task and measurement techniques, many studies have demonstrated in several muscle groups that, in relative terms, aged humans respond to strength training as well as or better than young people, showing large and functionally important gains in isometric and dynamic strength, power, and force control.[7,89,171,172] Not all of the improvements can be explained by changes in muscle size, especially in the early weeks (<10) of training.[173] Alterations related to specific tension (force), inherent contractile quality, neural modulation, and changes in connective tissue contribute to strength improvements; the absolute or relative impact of these factors has been studied recently.[172,174-177] It has been suggested that aged subjects rely more on neural changes to improve strength than do young subjects, and large changes in neural factors may be observed,[89] although the mechanisms remain to be elucidated.[53] After 10 to 12 weeks of training, the improvements in strength (>100%) and power (>20%) can be remarkable, even in the very old.[178,179]

Because more women live longer but seem to have reduced functional abilities compared with men, there is great interest in determining the effects of strength training on older females and the impact of strength gains on daily function. A recent study reported that after 9 weeks of dynamic resistance exercise training,[177] women aged 65 to 75 years showed similar strength gains to men of the same age. Men and women also showed equal improvements in specific force (muscle quality), but after 31 weeks of detraining, only the women had lost these gains. These results suggest that neural influences or factors other than those related to muscle mass are enhanced by strength training, and that, despite a return to baseline muscle volumes after detraining, old men maintain their strength gains. It remains unclear why this is not the case in women. In a long-term strength training program, men and women aged 60 to 80 years continued to increase their strength throughout a 2-year period; muscles also continued to hypertrophy, but gains in voluntary strength were greater,[171] suggesting that factors other than muscle mass contributed to gains in strength. There were no gender differences for most measures, although there was a trend for greater improvements in the men than the women by the end of the 2-year period. However, when very old men and women (85 to 97 years) were strength trained for 12 weeks, improvements in strength matched increases in muscle CSA.[180] Using twitch interpolation, no improvements in central activation were found, indicating that the strength improvements were due to muscle mass increases. Further studies designed to identify possible neural and other influences are required to elucidate the mechanisms underlying changes in specific force observed in some strength training studies, and whether males respond differently from females.

Men and women aged 65 to 75 years were compared with young adults during 9 weeks of high intensity training studies. The old women proved more susceptible to muscle damage than young women, but old and young men were equally susceptible to exercise-induced damage.[181,182] Reasons for gender difference are unclear. Muscle damage is often related to eccentric contractions, although aged subjects may be less susceptible than previously thought to damage following eccentric contractions.[82,176,183] At higher work loads eccentric strength training can be performed with relatively less cardiovascular and neural stress than concentric contractions; therefore eccentric exercise has been suggested as a very good mode of training for elderly subjects.[91] In a recent study women in their early 70s trained for 7 days, using eccentric loads 50% higher than those used in the standard exercise group.[176] The extra eccentric load doubled strength gains, with lower levels of stress. However, in an animal model, aged muscle showed less adaptive response to eccentric training than muscle in young adults.[184] The utility of eccentric training in aged subjects and whether the different responses observed in animal models are functionally relevant to human exercise training needs to be examined.

Satellite cell populations are not reduced in the elderly relative to young adults, suggesting that recovery from any muscle damage is not impaired with age.[182] Furthermore, biochemical and histochemical markers of muscle fiber growth in response to resistance training do not seem to be affected significantly by increased age,[173,185] although it is unclear whether aged females have less adaptive capacity than males.[186,187] Muscle from older humans has an altered gene expression that may impair the response to resistance training compared with the young.[188] Thus, although current understanding suggests that the muscle tissue of aged men and women has as equal a capacity to respond to resistance training as that of young adults, results from very old rat muscle imply that the myogenic response to resistance exercise is attenuated.[189,190] Further studies are needed to understand these gender and species differences.

It remains unclear whether the training-induced gains in muscle function enhance mobility, activities of daily living, and independence. Some studies report improvements in balance control and gait speed, with a reduced risk of falls, but others suggest that strength exercise must be combined with exercises specific to the task in order to show any improvement.[159,165,191,192] Training for power may enhance overall functional capacity more than training for strength per se,[123] and strength training does not improve flexibility.[168] In women aged 60 to 77 years, improvements in functional abilities were found after 12 weeks of strength training.[193] By contrast, older women (76 to 93 years of age) who were living independently showed substantial improvements in strength and power, but only limited improvements in performance of functional tasks.[179] In a study of dependent men and women in their 80s, functional performance indicators were improved with exercise training, but the improvements did not correlate with strength.[194]

In the frail elderly, strength training has the greatest impact on the most debilitated subjects.[166] One study reported that strength training was the only form of exercise tolerated by debilitated subjects, as few of the participants could perform endurance exercise.[195] Although further studies are required to understand the benefits of resistance exercise training in relation to physical status, age, task, and gender, this mode of training may be preferable to endurance-type exercise because of its many possible benefits to various body systems, and because the ability to endure a physical activity may be limited in old age.

6.8 Conclusions

The loss of strength in old age is substantial and an important determinant of deteriorations in mobility, independence, and quality of life for elderly people. Many studies have described the loss of strength with age (sarcopenia), correlated strength with functional movement and tasks of daily living, and sought to understand the mechanisms associated with strength loss. Although these mechanisms remain to be elucidated, it is clear from the many studies undertaken since 1995 that age-related changes in strength are not the same for all muscle groups, and the degree of strength loss varies during different tasks. Potential training benefits of the apparent relative preservation of eccentric strength need to be explored and understood. The measurement of power may be the most relevant variable to describe muscle function and this measure, in conjunction with an assessment of fatigability, needs to be incorporated into comparative and intervention studies. Gender is being recognized as an important factor in neuromuscular function; studies of sarcopenia should include gender as an independent variable. Thus, one aim of studies in this field is to gain a better understanding of the mechanisms associated with both age-related deteriorations and training-related improvements in strength, as well as the reasons underlying gender differences in these responses. Such research may help to develop the most appropriate exercise and rehabilitation programs to enhance the functional capacity of elderly men and women. Perhaps a greater challenge is to disseminate this information and encourage participation in resistance exercise training before individuals reach old age.[196,197]

Acknowledgments

Supported in part by the Natural Sciences and Engineering Research Council of Canada (NSERC). The authors would like to thank Jennifer M. Jakobi, Ph.D., for expert technical assistance during the preparation of this chapter.

References

1. Lindle, R.S., Metter, E.J., Lynch, N.A., et al., Age and gender comparisons of muscle strength in 654 women and men aged 20–93 years, *J. Appl. Physiol.*, 83, 1581–1587, 1997.
2. Kallman, D.A., Plato, C.C., and Tobin, J.D., The role of muscle loss in the age-related decline of grip strength: cross-sectional and longitudinal perspectives, *J. Gerontol.*, 45, M82–M888, 1990.
3. Amara, C.E., Rice, C.L., Koval, J.J., et al., Factors influencing the decline in strength in older adults aged 55–86 years, (unpublished observations).
4. Malbut-Shennan, K. and Young, A., The physiology of physical performance and training in old age, *Coron. Artery Disease*, 10, 37–42, 1999.
5. Evans, W.J., What is sarcopenia? *J. Gerontol. Biol. Sci.*, 50, 5–8, 1995.
6. Lexell, J., Human aging, muscle mass, and fiber type composition, *J. Gerontol. Biol. Sci.*, 50, 11–16, 1995.
7. Porter, M.M., Vandervoort, A.A., and Lexell, J., Aging of human muscle: structure, function and adaptability, *Scand. J. Med. Sci. Sports*, 129–142, 1995.
8. Roos, M.R., Rice, C.L., and Vandervoort, A.A., Age-related changes in motor unit function, *Muscle Nerve*, 20, 679–690, 1997.
9. Andersen, J.L., Terzis, G., and Kryger, A., Increase in the degree of coexpression of myosin heavy chain isoforms in skeletal muscle fibers of the very old, *Muscle Nerve*, 22, 449–454, 1999.
10. Flanigan, K.M., Lauria, G., Griffin, J.W., et al., Age-related biology and diseases of muscle and nerve, *Neurol. Clin.*, 16, 659–669, 1998.
11. Larsson, L., Li, X.P., and Degens, H., Age-related changes in contractile properties and expression of myosin isoforms in single skeletal muscle cells, *Muscle Nerve*, Suppl. 5, S74–S78, 1997.

12. Pierno, S., Deluca, A., Camerino, C., et al., Chronic administration of taurine to aged rats improves the electrical and contractile properties of skeletal muscle fibers, *J. Pharm. Exp. Ther.*, 286, 1183–1190, 1998.
13. Proctor, D.N., Balagopal, P., and Nair, K.S., Age-related sarcopenia in humans is associated with reduced synthetic rates of specific muscle proteins, *J. Nutr.*, 128, S351–S355, 1998.
14. Renganathan, M., Messi, M.L., and Delbono, O., Dihydropyridine receptor–ryanodine receptor uncoupling in aged skeletal muscle, *J. Membr. Biol.*,157, 247–253, 1997.
15. Thompson, L.V. and Brown, M., Age-related changes in contractile properties of single skeletal fibers from the soleus muscle, *J. Appl. Physiol.*, 86, 881–886, 1999.
16. Larsson, L. and Ramamurthy, B., Aging-related changes in skeletal muscle — mechanisms and interventions, *Drugs Aging*, 17, 303–316, 2000.
17. Guillet, C., Auguste, P., Mayo, W., et al., Ciliary neurotrophic factor is a regulator of muscular strength in aging, *J. Neurosci.*, 19, 1257–1262, 1999.
18. Kullberg, S., Ramirezleon, V., Johnson, H., et al., Decreased axosomatic input to motoneurons and astrogliosis in the spinal cord of aged rats, *J. Gerontol. Biol. Sci.*, 53, B369–B379, 1998.
19. Rossini, P.M., Desiato, M.T., and Caramia, M.D., Age-related changes of motor evoked potentials in healthy human: noninvasive evaluation of central and peripheral motor tracts excitability and conductivity, *Brain Res.*, 593, 14–19, 1992.
20. Engelhardt, J.K., Morales, F.R., Yamuy, J., et al., Cable properties of spinal cord motoneurons in adult and aged cats, *J. Neurophysiol.*, 61, 194–200, 1989.
21. Doherty, T.J., Vandervoort, A.A., and Brown, W.F., Effects of aging on the motor unit: a brief review, *Can. J. Appl. Physiol.*, 18, 331–358, 1993.
22. Smith, D.O. and Rosenheimer, J.L., Factors governing speed of action potential conduction and neuromuscular transmission in aged rats., *Exp. Neurol.*, 83, 358–66, 1984.
23. Roos, M.R., Rice, C.L., Connelly, D.M., et al., Quadriceps muscle strength, contractile properties, and motor unit firing rates in young and old men, *Muscle Nerve*, 22, 1094–1103, 1999.
24. Connelly, D.M., Rice, C.L., Roos, M.R., et al., Motor unit firing rates and contractile properties in tibialis anterior of young and old men, *J. Appl. Physiol.*, 87, 843–852, 1999.
25. De Serres, S.J. and Enoka, R.M., Older adults can maximally activate the biceps brachii muscle by voluntary command, *J. Appl. Physiol.*, 84, 284–291, 1998.
26. Kent-Braun, J.A. and Ng, A.V., Specific strength and voluntary muscle activation in young and elderly women and men, *J. Appl. Physiol.*, 87, 22–29, 1999.
27. Vandervoort, A.A. and McComas, A.J., Contractile changes in opposing muscles of the human ankle joint, *J. Appl. Physiol.*, 61, 361–367, 1986.
28. Dowling, J., Konert, E., Ljucovic, P., et al., Are humans able to voluntarily elicit maximum muscle force? *Neurosci. Lett.*, 179, 25–28, 1994.
29. Strojnik, V., Muscle activation level during maximal voluntary effort, *Eur. J. Appl. Physiol. Occup. Physiol.*, 72, 144–149, 1995.
30. Herbert, R.D. and Gandevia, S.C., Twitch interpolation in human muscles: mechanisms and implications for measurement of voluntary activation, *J. Neurophysiol.*, 82, 2271–2283, 1999.

31. Adams, G.R., Duvoisin, M.R., and Dudley, G.A., Magnetic resonance imaging and electromyography as indexes of muscle function, *J. Appl. Physiol.*, 73, 1578–1583, 1992.
32. Yue, G., Alexander, A.L., Laidlaw, D.H., et al., Sensitivity of muscle proton spin-spin relaxation time as an index of muscle activation, *J. Appl. Physiol.*, 77, 84–92, 1994.
33. Yue, G.H., Ranganathan, V.K., Siemionow, V., et al., Older adults exhibit a reduced ability to fully activate their biceps brachii muscle, *J. Gerontol. Med. Sci.*, 54A, M249–M253, 1999.
34. James, C., Sacco, P., and Jones, D., Loss of power during fatigue of human leg muscles, *J. Physiol.*, 484, 237–246, 1995.
35. Newham, D.J., McCarthy, T., and Turner, J., Voluntary activation of human quadriceps during and after isokinetic exercise, *J. Appl. Physiol.*, 71, 2122–2126, 1991.
36. White, M.J. and Harridge, S.D.R., At high angular velocities voluntary activation limits maximal isokinetic torque generation in elderly and young human triceps surae, *J. Physiol.*, 429, 53P, 1990.
37. Brooks, S.V. and Faulkner, J.A., Skeletal muscle weakness in old age: underlying mechanisms, *Med. Sci. Sports. Exerc.*, 26, 432–439, 1994.
38. Doherty, T.J., Vandervoort, A.A., Taylor, A.W., et al., Effects of motor unit losses on strength in older men and women, *J. Appl. Physiol.*, 74, 868–874, 1993.
39. Galea, V., Changes in motor unit estimates with aging, *J. Clin. Neurophysiol.*, 13, 253–260, 1996.
40. Tomlinson, B.E. and Irving, D., The numbers of limb motor neurons in the human lumbosacral cord throughout life, *J. Neurol. Sci.*, 34, 213–219, 1977.
41. Campbell, M.J., McComas, A.J., and Petito, F., Physiological changes in aging muscles, *J. Neurol. Neurosurg. Psych.*, 36, 174–182, 1973.
42. Carmeli, E. and Reznick, A.Z., The physiology and biochemistry of skeletal muscle atrophy as a function of age, *Proc. Soc. Exp. Biol. Med.*, 206, 103–113, 1994.
43. Ramirez, V. and Ulfhake, B., Anatomy of dendrites in motoneurons supplying the intrinsic muscles of the foot sole in the aged cat: evidence for dendritic growth and neo-synaptogenesis, *J. Compar. Neurol.*, 316, 1–16, 1992.
44. Kadhiresan, V.A., Hassett, C.A., and Faulkner, J.A., Properties of single motor units in medial gastrocnemius muscles of adult and old rats, *J. Physiol.*, 493, 543–552, 1996.
45. Jakobi, J. M., Connelly, D. M., Roos, M. R., et al., Age-related changes of neuromuscular properties in three human limb muscles, in *ALCOA Proceedings: Older Adults and Active Living*, Taylor, A. W., Ecclestone, N. A., Jones G. R., and Paterson, D. H., Eds., Canadian Centre for Activity and Aging, London, Ontario, 1999, 111–121.
46. Galganski, M.E., Fuglevand, A.J., and Enoka, R.M., Reduced control of motor output in a human hand and muscle of elderly subjects during submaximal contractions, *J. Neurophysiol.*, 69, 2108–2115, 1993.
47. Kanda, K. and Hashizume, K., Changes in properties of the medial gastrocnemius motor units in aging rats, *J. Neurophysiol.*, 61, 737, 1989.
48. Brown, M.C., Holland, R.L., and Hopkins, W.G., Motor nerve sprouting, *Ann. Rev. Neurosci.*, 4, 17–42, 1981.
49. Larsson, L. and Ansved, T., Effects of aging on the motor unit, *Prog. Neurobiol.*, 45, 397–458, 1995.

50. Thompson, L.V., Effects of age and training on skeletal muscle physiology and performance, *Phys. Ther.*, 74, 71–81, 1994.
51. Erim, Z., Beg, M.F., Burke, D.T., et al., Effects of aging on motor-unit control properties, *J. Neurophysiol.*, 82, 2081–2091, 1999.
52. Enoka, R.M. and Fuglevand, A.J., Motor unit physiology: some unresolved issues, *Muscle Nerve*, 24, 4–17, 2001.
53. Rice, C.L., Muscle function at the motor unit level: consequences of aging, *Top. Geriatr. Rehabil.*, 15, 70–82, 2000.
54. Luschei, E.S., Ramig, L.O., Baker, K.L., et al., Discharge characteristics of laryngeal single motor units during phonation in young and older adults and in persons with Parkinson's disease, *J. Neurophysiol.*, 81, 2131–2139, 1999.
55. Kernell, D., Bakels, R., and Copray, J.C.V.M., Discharge properties of motoneurones: how are they matched to the properties and use of their muscle units? *J. Physiol.*, 93, 87–96, 1999.
56. Doherty, T.J., Komori, T., Stashuk, D.W., et al., Physiological properties of single thenar motor units in the F-response of younger and older adults, *Muscle Nerve*, 17, 860–872, 1994.
57. Kamen, G., Sison, S.V., Du, C.C.D., et al., Motor unit discharge behavior in older adults during maximal-effort contractions, *J. Appl. Physiol.*, 79, 1908–1913, 1995.
58. Patten, C. and Kamen, G., Adaptations in motor unit discharge activity with force control training in young and older human adults, *Eur. J. Appl. Physiol. Occup. Physiol.*, 83, 128–143, 2000.
59. Kamen, G., Knight, C.A., Laroche, D.P., et al., Resistance training increases vastus lateralis motor unit firing rates in young and old adults, *Med. Sci. Sports Exer.*, 30, S337, 1998.
60. Freund, H.J., Wita, C.W., and Sprung, C., Discharge properties in functional differentiation of single motor units in man, in *Neurophysiology Studied in Man*, Somjen, G.G., Ed., Amsterdam, NL, North Holland, 1972, 305–313.
61. Nelson, R.M., Soderberg, G.L., and Urbscheit, N.L., Comparison of skeletal muscle motor unit discharge characteristics in young and aged humans, *Arch. Gerontol. Geriatr.*, 2, 255–264, 1983.
62. Soderberg, G.L., Minor, S.C., and Nelson, R.M., A comparison of motor unit behaviour in young and aged subjects, *Age Ageing*, 20, 8–15, 1991.
63. Nelson, R.M., Soderberg, G.L., and Urbscheit, N.L., Alteration of motor-unit discharge characteristics in aged humans, *Phys. Ther.*, 64, 29–34, 1984.
64. Duchateau, J. and Hainaut, K., Effects of immobilization on contractile properties, recruitment and firing rates of human motor units. *J. Physiol.*, 422, 55–65, 1990.
65. Semmler, J.G. and Nordstrom, M.A., Motor unit discharge and force tremor in skill- and strength-trained individuals, *Exp. Brain Res.*, 119, 27–38, 1998.
66. Leong, B., Kamen, G., Patten, C., et al., Maximal motor unit discharge rates in the quadriceps muscles of older weight lifters, *Med. Sci. Sports Exerc.*, 31, 1638–1644, 1999.
67. Rich, C. and Cafarelli, E., Submaximal motor unit firing rates after 8 wk of isometric resistance training, *Med. Sci. Sports Exerc.*, 32, 190–196, 2000.
68. Van Cutsem, M., Duchateau, J., and Hainaut, K., Changes in single motor unit behaviour contribute to the increase in contraction speed after dynamic training in humans, *J. Physiol.*, 513, 295–305, 1998.

69. Stanley, S.N. and Taylor, N.A.S., Isokinematic muscle mechanics in 4 groups of women of increasing age, *Eur. J. Appl. Physiol. Occup. Physiol.*, 66, 178–184, 1993.
70. Doherty, T.J. and Brown, W.F., Age-related changes in the twitch contractile properties of human thenar motor units, *J. Appl. Physiol.*, 82, 93–101, 1997.
71. Davies, C.T.M. and White, M.J., Contractile properties of elderly human triceps surae, *Gerontology*, 29, 19–25, 1983.
72. Narici, M.V., Bordini, M., and Cerretelli, P., Effect of aging on human adductor pollicis muscle function, *J. Appl. Physiol.*, 71, 1277–1281, 1991.
73. Polkey, M.I., Harris, M.L., Hughes, P.D., et al., The contractile properties of the elderly human diaphragm, *Am. J. Resp. Crit. Care Med.*, 155, 1560–1564, 1997.
74. Rice, C.L., Cunningham, D.A., Taylor, A.W., et al., Comparison of the histochemical and contractile properties of human triceps surae, *Eur. J. Appl. Physiol.*, 58, 165–170, 1988.
75. Hicks, A.L., Cupido, C.M., Martin, J., et al., Twitch potentiation during fatigue exercise in the elderly: the effects of training, *Eur. J. Appl. Physiol. Occup. Physiol.*, 63, 278–281, 1991.
76. Frontera, W.R., Hughes, V.A., Fielding, R.A., et al., Aging of skeletal muscle: a 12-yr longitudinal study, *J. Appl. Physiol.*, 88, 1321–1326, 2000.
77. Hakkinen, K., Kallinen, M., Linnamo, V., et al., Neuromuscular adaptations during bilateral vs. unilateral strength training in middle-aged and elderly men and women, *Acta Physiol. Scand.*, 158, 77–88, 1996.
78. Jubrias, S.A., Odderson, I.R., Esselman, P.C., et al., Decline in isokinetic force with age — muscle cross-sectional area and specific force, *Pflügers Arch. — Eur. J. Physiol.*, 434, 246–253, 1997.
79. Klitgaard, H., Mantoni, M., Schiaffino, S., et al., Function, morphology and protein expression of aging skeletal muscle: a cross-sectional study of elderly men with different training backgrounds, *Acta Physiol. Scand.*, 140, 41–54, 1990.
80. Phillips, S.K., Woledge, R.C., Bruce, S.A., et al., Study of force and cross-sectional area of adductor pollicis muscle in female hip fracture patients, *J. Am. Geriatr. Soc*, 46, 999–1002, 1998.
81. Phillips, S.K., Bruce, S.A., Newton, D., et al., The weakness of old age is not due to failure of muscle activation, *J. Gerontol. Med. Sci.*, 47, M45–49, 1992.
82. Brooks, S.V. and Faulkner, J.A., Isometric, shortening, and lengthening contractions of muscle fiber segments from adult and old mice, *Am. J. Physiol*, 267, C507–C513, 1994.
83. Gonzalez, E., Messi, M.L., and Delbono, O., The specific force of single intact extensor digitorum longus and soleus mouse muscle fibers declines with aging, *J. Mem. Biol.*, 178, 175–183, 2000.
84. Balagopal, P., Rooyackers, O.E., Adey, D.B., et al., Effects of aging on *in vivo* synthesis of skeletal muscle myosin heavy-chain and sarcoplasmic protein in humans, *Am. J. Physiol. Endocrinol. Metab.*, 36, E790–E800, 1997.
85. Ansved, T. and Edstrom, L., Effects of age on fibre structure, ultrastructure and expression of desmin and spectrin in fast- and slow-twitch rat muscles, *J. Anat.*, 174:61–79, 1991.
86. Delbono, O., Orouke, K.S. and Ettinger, W.H., Excitation calcium release uncoupling in aged single human skeletal muscle fibers, *J. Mem. Biol.*, 148, 211–222, 1995.
87. Lynch, N.A., Metter, E.J., Lindle, R.S., et al., Muscle quality. I. Age-associated differences between arm and leg muscle groups, *J. Appl. Physiol.*, 86, 188–194, 1999.

88. Aoyagi, Y. and Shephard, R.J., Aging and muscle function, *Sports Med.*, 14, 376–396, 1992.
89. Grabiner, M.D.and Enoka, R.M., Changes in movement capabilities with aging, *Exerc. Sport Sci. Rev.*, 23, 65–104, 1995.
90. Rogers, M.A. and Evans, W.J., Changes in skeletal muscle with aging: effects of exercise training, *Exerc. Sport Sci. Rev.*, 21, 65–102, 1993.
91. Vandervoort, A.A. and Symons, J.J., Functional and metabolic consequences of sarcopenia, *Can. J. Appl. Physiol.*, 26, 90–101, 2001.
92. Bemben, M.G., Massey, B.H., Bemben, D.A., et al., Isometric muscle force production as a function of age in healthy 20- to 74-yr-old men, *Med. Sci. Sports Exerc.*, 23, 1302–1310, 1991.
93. Suominen, H., Muscle collagen, aging and exercise, in *Proc. 4th Intl. Congr. Healthy Aging, Activity Sports*, Health Promotion Publication, Heidelberg, Germany, 1996, 91–97.
94. Amara, C.E., Koval, J.J., Johnson, P.J., et al., Modelling the influence of fat-free mass and physical activity on the decline in maximal oxygen uptake with age in older humans, *Exp. Physiol.*, 85, 877–886, 2000.
95. Dutta, C., Commentary on "Effects of strength training and detraining on muscle quality: age and gender comparisons," *J. Gerontol. Biol. Sci.*, 55, B158–B159, 2000.
96. Kent-Braun, J.A., Ng, A.V., and Young, K., Skeletal muscle contractile and noncontractile components in young and older women and men, *J. Appl. Physiol.*, 88, 662–668, 2000.
97. Kent-Braun, J.A. and Ng, A.V., Skeletal muscle oxidative capacity in young and older women and men, *J. Appl. Physiol.*, 89, 1072–1078, 2000.
98. Harris, T., Muscle mass and strength — relation to function in population studies, *J. Nutr.*, 127, S1004–S1006, 1997.
99. Janssen, I., Heymsfield, S.B., Wang, Z.M., et al., Skeletal muscle mass and distribution in 468 men and women aged 18–88 years, *J. Appl. Physiol.*, 89, 81–88, 2000.
100. Baumgartner, R.N., Waters, D.L., Gallagher, D., et al., Predictors of skeletal muscle mass in elderly men and women, *Mech. Ageing Dev.*, 107, 123–136, 1999.
101. Hakkinen, K. and Pakarinen, A., Muscle strength and serum testosterone, cortisol and SHBG concentrations in middle-aged and elderly men and women, *Acta Physiol. Scand.*, 148, 199–207, 1993.
102. Metter, E.J., Conwit, R., Tobin, J., et al., Age-associated loss of power and strength in the upper extremities in women and men, *J. Gerontol. Biol. Sci.*, 52, B267–B276, 1997.
103. Phillips, S.K., Rook, K.M., Siddle, N.C., et al., Muscle weakness in women occurs at an earlier age than in men, but strength is preserved by hormone replacement therapy, *Clin. Sci.*, 84, 95–98, 1993.
104. Rice, C.L., Cunningham, D.A., Paterson, D.H., et al., Strength in an elderly population, *Arch. Phys. Med. Rehabil.*, 70, 391–397, 1989.
105. Young, A., Stokes, M. and Crowe, M., Size and strength of the quadriceps muscle of old and young women, *Eur. J. Clin. Invest.*, 14, 282–287, 1984.
106. Young, A., Stokes, M. and Crowe, M., The size and strength of the quadriceps muscles of old and young men, *Clin. Physiol.*, 5,145–154, 1985.
107. Christ, C.B., Boileau, R.A., Slaughter, M.H., et al., Maximal voluntary isometric force production characteristics of six muscle groups in women aged 25 to 74 years, *Am. J. Hum. Biol.*, 4, 537–545, 1992.

108. Hunter, S.K., Thompson, M.W. and Adams, R.D., Relationships among age-associated strength changes and physical activity level, limb dominance, and muscle group in women, *J. Gerontol. Biol. Sci.*, 55, B264–B273, 2000.
109. Murray, M.P., Duthie Jr, E.H., Gambert, S.R., et al., Age-related differences in knee muscle strength in normal women, *J. Gerontol.*, 40, 275–280, 1985.
110. Samson, M.M., Meeuwsen, I.B., Crowe, A., et al., Relationships between physical performance measures, age, height and body weight in healthy adults, *Age Ageing*, 29, 235–242, 2000.
111. Faulkner, J.A. and Brooks, S.V., Muscle fatigue in old animals: unique aspects of fatigue in elderly humans, in *Fatigue: Neurological and Muscular Mechanisms,* Gandevia, S. C., Enoka, R. M., McComas, A. J., et al., Eds., Plenum Press, New York, 384, 1995, 471–479.
112. Bassey, E.J., Measurement of muscle strength and power, *Muscle Nerve*, Suppl. 5, S44–S46, 1997.
113. Martin, J.C., Farrar, R.P., Wagner, B.M., et al., Maximal power across the life span, *J. Gerontol. Biol. Sci.*, 55, M311–M316, 2000.
114. Metter, E.J., Lynch, N., Conwit, R., et al., Muscle quality and age: cross-sectional and longitudinal comparisons, *J. Gerontol. Biol. Sci.*, 54, B207–B218, 1999.
115. Marsh, G.D., Paterson, D.H., Govindasamy, D., et al., Anaerobic power of the arms and legs of young and older men, *Exp. Physiol.*, 84, 589–597, 1999.
116. Izquierdo, M., Ibanez, J., Gorostiaga, E., et al., Maximal strength and power characteristics in isometric and dynamic actions of the upper and lower extremities in middle-aged and older men, *Acta Physiol. Scand.*, 167, 57–68, 1999.
117. Conley, K.E., Jubrias, S.A., and Esselman, P.C., Oxidative capacity and aging in human muscle, *J. Physiol.*, 526, 203–210, 2000.
118. Brown, M., Fisher, J.S., and Salsich, G., Stiffness and muscle function with age and reduced muscle use, *J. Orthop. Res*, 17, 409–414, 1999.
119. Evans, W.J., Exercise strategies should be designed to increase muscle power, *J. Gerontol. Biol. Sci.*, 55, M309–M310, 2000.
120. Bassey, E.J., Fiatarone, M.A., O'Neill, E.F., et al., Leg extensor power and functional performance in very old men and women, *Clin. Sci.*, 82, 321–327, 1992.
121. Kostka, T., Arsac, L.M., Patricot, M.C., et al., Leg extensor power and dehydroepiandrosterone sulfate, insulin-like growth factor-i and testosterone in healthy active elderly people, *Eur. J. Appl. Physiol.*, 82, 83–90, 2000.
122. Guralnik, J.M., Simonsick, E.M., Ferrucci, L., et al., A short physical performance battery assessing lower extremity function: association with self-reported disability and prediction of mortality and nursing home admission, *J. Gerontol.*, 49, M85–M94, 1994.
123. Foldvari, M., Clark, M., Laviolette, L.C., et al., Association of muscle power with functional status in community-dwelling elderly women, *J. Gerontol. Med. Sci.*, 55, M192–M199, 2000.
124. Andersen-Ranberg, K., Christensen, K., Jeune, B., et al., Declining physical abilities with age: a cross-sectional study of older twins and centenarians in Denmark, *Age Ageing*, 28, 373–377, 1999.
125. Bigland-Ritchie, B., Rice, C. L., Garland, S. J., et al., Task-dependent factors in fatigue of human voluntary contractions, in *Fatigue: Neurological and Muscular Mechanisms*, Gandevia, S. C., Enoka, R. M., McComas, A. J., et al., Eds., Plenum Press, New York, 1995, 361–380.
126. Bemben, M.G., Age-related alterations in muscular endurance, *Sports Med.*, 25, 259–269, 1998.

127. Enoka, R.M. and Stuart, D.G., Neurobiology of muscle fatigue, *J. Appl. Physiol.*, 72, 1631–1648, 1992.
128. Makrides, L., Heigenhauser, G.J.F., McCartney, N., et al., Maximal short term exercise capacity in healthy subjects aged 15–70 years, *Clin. Sci.*, 69, 197–205, 1985.
129. Overend, T.J., Cunningham, D.A., Paterson, D.H., et al., Physiological responses of young and elderly men to prolonged exercise at critical power, *Eur. J. Appl. Physiol.*, 64, 187–193, 1992.
130. Bemben, M.G., Massey, B.H., Bemben, D.A., et al., Isometric intermittent endurance of four muscle groups in men aged 20–74 years, *Med. Sci. Sports Exerc.*, 28, 145–154, 1996.
131. Hicks, A.L., Cupido, C.M., Martin, J., et al., Muscle excitation in elderly adults: effects of training, *Muscle Nerve*, 15, 87–93, 1992.
132. Laforest, S., St-Pierre, D.M., Cyr, J., et al., Effects of age and regular exercise on muscle strength and endurance, *Eur. J. Appl. Physiol.*, 60, 104–111, 1990.
133. Anianson, A., Grimby, G., Hedberg, M., et al., Muscle function in old age, *J. Rehab. Med.*, Suppl. 6, 43–49, 1978.
134. Ditor, D.S. and Hicks, A.L., The effect of age and gender on the relative fatigability of the human adductor pollicis muscle, *Can. J. Physiol. Pharm.*, 78, 781–790, 2000.
135. Hara, Y., Akaboshi, K., Masakado, Y., et al., Physiologic decrease of single thenar motor units in the f-response in stroke patients, *Arch. Phys. Med. Rehab.*, 81, 418–423, 2000.
136. Bilodeau, M., Erb, M.D., Nichols, J.M., et al., Fatigue of elbow flexor muscles in younger and older adults, *Muscle Nerve*, 24, 98–106, 2001.
137. Petrofsky, J.S. and Lind, A.R., Aging, isometric strength and endurance, and cardiovascular responses to static effort, *J. Appl. Physiol.*, 38, 91–95, 1975.
138. Smolander, J., Aminoff, T., Korhonen, I., et al., Heart rate and blood pressure responses to isometric exercise in young and older men, *Eur. J. Appl. Physiol. Occup. Physiol.*, 77, 439–444, 1998.
139. Larsson, L. and Karlsson, J., Isometric and dynamic endurance as a function of age and skeletal muscle characteristics, *Acta Physiol. Scand.*, 104, 129–136, 1978.
140. Allman, B.L. and Rice, C.L., Incomplete recovery of voluntary isometric force after fatigue is not affected by old age, *Muscle Nerve*, in press, 2001.
141. Pagala, M.K., Ravindran, K., Namba, T., et al., Skeletal muscle fatigue and physical endurance of young and old mice, *Muscle Nerve*, 21, 1729–1739, 1998.
142. Hill, F., Stewart, A.W. and Verrier, C.S., An aging-associated decline in force production after repetitive contractions by rat skinned skeletal muscle fibres, *Tiss. Cell*, 29, 585–588, 1997.
143. Kovalenko, S.A., Kopsidas, G., Kelso, J.M., et al., Deltoid human muscle mtDNA is extensively rearranged in old age subjects, *Biochem. Biophys. Res. Commun.*, 232, 147–152, 1997.
144. Hicks, A.L. and McCartney, N., Gender differences in isometric contractile properties and fatigability in elderly human muscle, *Can. J. Appl. Physiol.*, 21, 441–454, 1996.
145. Tiidus, P.M., Bestic, N.M. and Tupling, R., Estrogen and gender do not affect fatigue resistance of extensor digitorum longus muscle in rats, *Physiol. Res.*, 48, 209–213, 1999.

146. Li, Z., Krause, D.N., Doolen, S., et al., Ovariectomy eliminates sex differences in rat tail artery response to adrenergic nerve stimulation, *Am. J. Physiol.*, 272, H1819–H1825
147. Kinoshita, H. and Francis, P.R., A comparison of prehension force control in young and elderly individuals, *Eur. J. Appl. Physiol. Occup. Physiol.*, 74, 450–460, 1996.
148. Laidlaw, D.H., Bilodeau, M. and Enoka, R.M., Steadiness is reduced and motor unit discharge is more variable in old adults, *Muscle Nerve*, 23, 600–612, 2000.
149. Graves, A.E., Kornatz, K.W. and Enoka, R.M., Older adults use a unique strategy to lift inertial loads with the elbow flexor muscles, *J. Neurophysiol.*, 83, 2030–2039, 2000.
150. Connelly, D.M. and Vandervoort, A.A., Effects of isokinetic strength training on concentric and eccentric torque development in the ankle dorsiflexors of older adults, *J. Gerontol. Biol. Sci.*, 55, B465–B472, 2000.
151. Kamen, G. and De Luca, C.J., Unusual motor unit firing behavior in older adults, *Brain Res.*, 482, 136–140, 1989.
152. Burnett, R.A., Laidlaw, D.H. and Enoka, R.M., Coactivation of the antagonist muscle does not covary with steadiness in old adults, *J. Appl. Physiol.*, 89, 61–71, 2000.
153. Semmler, J.G., Steege, J.W., Kornatz, K.W., et al., Motor-unit synchronization is not responsible for larger motor-unit forces in old adults, *J. Neurophysiol.*, 84, 358–366, 2000.
154. Strupp, M., Arbusow, V., Pereira, C.B., et al., Subjective straight-ahead during neck muscle vibration: effects of aging, *Neuroreport*, 10, 3191–3194, 1999.
155. Nardone, A., Siliotto, R., Grasso, M., et al., Influence of aging on leg muscle reflex responses to stance perturbation, *Arch. Phys. Med. Rehab.*, 76, 158–165, 1995.
156. Smith, B.N., Segal, R.L. and Wolf, S.L., Long latency ankle responses to dynamic perturbation in older fallers and nonfallers, *J. Am. Geriatr. Soc.*, 44, 1447–1454, 1996.
157. Thelen, D.G., Muriuki, M., James, J., et al., Muscle activities used by young and old adults when stepping to regain balance during a forward fall, *J. Electromyo. Kin.*, 10, 93–101, 2000.
158. Kannus, P., Parkkari, J., Koskinen, S., et al., Fall-induced injuries and deaths among older adults, *JAMA*, 281, 1895–1899, 1999.
159. Daley, M.J. and Spinks, W.L., Exercise, mobility and aging, *Sports Med.*, 29, 1–12, 2000.
160. Lipsitz, L.A., Jonsson, P.V., Kelley, M.M., et al., Causes and correlates of recurrent falls in ambulatory frail elderly, *J. Gerontol.*, 46, M114–M122, 1991.
161. Cao, C., Schultz, A.B., Ashton-Miller, J.A., et al., Sudden turns and stops while walking — kinematic sources of age and gender differences, *Gait Posture*, 7, 45–52, 1998.
162. Wojcik, L.A., Thelen, D.G., Schultz, A.B., et al., Age and gender differences in single-step recovery from a forward fall, *J. Gerontol. Med. Sci.*, 54, M44–M50, 1999.
163. Butler, R.N., Davis, R., Lewis, C.B., et al., Physical fitness — benefits of exercise for the older patient — part 2 of a round table discussion, *Geriatrics*, 53, 46, 1998.
164. Kasprisin, J.E. and Grabiner, M.D., Joint angle-dependence of elbow flexor activation levels during isometric and isokinetic maximum voluntary contractions, *Clin. Biomech.*, 15, 743–749, 2000.

165. Wolfson, L., Whipple, R., Derby, C., et al., Balance and strength training in older adults — intervention gains and Tai Chi maintenance, *J. Am. Geriatr. Soc.*, 44, 498–506, 1996.
166. Connelly, D.M., Resisted exercise training of institutionalized older adults for improved strength and functional mobility: a review, *Top. Geriatr. Rehab.*, 15, 6–28, 2000.
167. Hurley, B.F. and Hagberg, J.M., Optimizing health in older persons: aerobic or strength training? *Exerc. Sport Sci. Rev.*, 26, 61–89, 1998.
168. Hurley, B.F. and Roth, S.M., Strength training in the elderly — effects on risk factors for age-related diseases, *Sports Med.*, 30, 249–268, 2000.
169. Tseng, B.S., Marsh, D.R., Hamilton, M.T., et al., Strength and aerobic training attenuate muscle wasting and improve resistance to the development of disability with aging, *J. Gerontol. Biol. Sci.*, 50, 113–119, 1995.
170. Mazzeo, R.S., Cavanagh, P., Evans, W.J., et al. Exercise and physical activity for older adults, *Med. Sci. Sports Exerc.*, 30, 992–1008, 1998.
171. McCartney, N., Hicks, A.L., Martin, J., et al., A longitudinal trial of weight training in the elderly — continued improvements in year 2, *J. Gerontol. Biol. Sci.*, 51, B425–B433, 1996.
172. Tracy, B.L., Ivey, F.M., Hurlbut, D., et al., Muscle quality. II. Effects of strength training in 65- to 75-yr-old men and women, *J. Appl. Physiol.*, 86, 195–201, 1999.
173. Porter, M.M., The effects of strength training on sarcopenia, *Can. J. Appl. Physiol.*, 26, 123–141, 2001.
174. Enoka, R.M., Neural strategies in the control of muscle force, *Muscle Nerve Suppl.*, 5, S66–S69, 1997.
175. Hakkinen, K., Alen, M., Kallinen, M., et al., Neuromuscular adaptation during prolonged strength training, detraining and re-strength training in middle-aged and elderly people, *Eur. J. Appl. Physiol. Occup. Physiol.*, 83, 51–62, 2000.
176. Hortobagyi, T. and DeVita, P., Favorable neuromuscular and cardiovascular responses to 7 days of exercise with an eccentric overload in elderly women, *J. Gerontol. Biol. Sci.*, 55, B401–B410, 2000.
177. Ivey, F.M., Tracy, B.L., Lemmer, J.T., et al., Effects of strength training and detraining on muscle quality: age and gender comparisons, *J. Gerontol. Biol. Sci.*, 55, B152–B157, 2000.
178. Fiatarone, M.A., Marks, E.C., Ryan, N.D., et al., High-intensity strength training in nonagenarians. Effects on skeletal muscle, *JAMA*, 263, 3029–3034, 1990.
179. Skelton, D.A., Young, A., Greig, C.A., et al., Effects of resistance training on strength power and selected functional abilities of women aged 75 and older, *J. Am. Ger. Soc.*, 43, 1081–1087, 1995.
180. Harridge, S.D.R., Kryger, A. and Stensgaard, A., Knee extensor strength, activation, and size in very elderly people following strength training, *Muscle Nerve*, 22, 831–839, 1999.
181. Roth, S.M., Martel, G.F., Ivey, F.M., et al., Ultrastructural muscle damage in young vs. older men after high-volume, heavy-resistance strength training, *J. Appl. Physiol.*, 86, 1833–1840, 1999.
182. Roth, S.M., Martel, G.F., Ivey, F.M., et al., High-volume, heavy-resistance strength training and muscle damage in young and older women, *J. Appl. Physiol.*, 88, 1112–1118, 2000.
183. Money, J., Dudek, R., Fraser, D., et al., Absence of damage in aged human skeletal muscle after acute training with an eccentric overload, *Med. Sci. Sports Exerc.*, 30, S335, 1998.

184. McBride, T., Increased depolarization, prolonged recovery and reduced adaptation of the resting membrane potential in aged rat skeletal muscles following eccentric contractions, *Mech. Ageing Dev.*, 115, 127–138, 2000.
185. Trappe, S., Williamson, D., Godard, M., et al., Effect of resistance training on single muscle fiber contractile function in older men, *J. Appl. Physiol.*, 89, 143–152, 2000.
186. Yarasheski, K.E., Pak-Loduca, J., Hasten, D.L., et al., Resistance exercise training increases mixed muscle protein synthesis rate in frail women and men ≧76 years old, *Am. J. Physiol. Endocrinol. Met.*, 40, E118–E125, 1999.
187. Ivey, F.M., Roth, S.M., Ferrell, R.E., et al., Effects of age, gender, and myostatin genotype on the hypertrophic response to heavy resistance strength training, *J. Gerontol. Med. Sci.*, 55, M641–M648, 2000.
188. Jozsi, A.C., Dupont-Versteegden, E.E., Taylor-Jones, J.M., et al., Aged human muscle demonstrates an altered gene expression profile consistent with an impaired response to exercise, *Mech. Ageing Dev.*, 120, 45–56, 2000.
189. Blough, E.R. and Linderman, J.K., Lack of skeletal muscle hypertrophy in very aged male Fischer 344× brown Norway rats, *J. Appl. Physiol.*, 88, 1265–1270, 2000.
190. Tamaki, T., Uchiyama, S., Uchiyama, Y., et al., Limited myogenic response to a single bout of weight-lifting exercise in old rats, *Am. J. Physiol.*, 278, C1143–C1152, 2000.
191. Taaffe, D.R. and Marcus, R., Musculoskeletal health and the older adult, *J. Rehab. Res. Dev.*, 37, 245–254, 2000.
192. Salem, G.J., Wang, M.Y., Young, J.T., et al., Knee strength and lower- and higher-intensity functional performance in older adults, *Med. Sci. Sports Exerc.*, 32, 1679–1684, 2000.
193. Hunter, G.R., Treuth, M.S., Weinsier, R.L., et al., The effects of strength conditioning on older women's ability to perform daily tasks, *J. Am. Geriatr. Soc.*, 43, 756–760, 1995.
194. Carmeli, E., Reznick, A.Z., Coleman, R., et al., Muscle strength and mass of lower extremities in relation to functional abilities in elderly adults, *Gerontology*, 46, 249–257, 2000.
195. Meuleman, J.R., Brechue, W.F., Kubilis, P.S., et al., Exercise training in the debilitated aged: strength and functional outcomes, *Arch. Phys. Med. Rehab.*, 81, 312–318, 2000.
196. Brown, M., Strength training and aging, *Top. Geriatr. Rehab.*, 15, 1–5, 2000.
197. Roubenoff, R., Sarcopenia and its implications for the elderly, *Eur. J. Clin. Nutr.*, 54,S40–S47, 2000.
198. Hortobagyi, T., Zheng, D., Weidner, M., et al., The influence of aging on muscle strength and muscle fiber characteristics with special reference to eccentric strength, *J. Gerontol. Biol. Sci.*, 50, B399–B406, 1995.
199. Poulin, M.J., Vandervoort, A.A., Paterson, D.H., et al., Eccentric and concentric torques of knee and elbow extension in young and older men, *Can. J. Sport Sci.*, 17, 3–7, 1992.
200. Vandervoort, A.A., Kramer, J.F., and Wharran, E.R., Eccentric knee strength of elderly females, *J. Gerontol. Biol. Sci.*, 45, B125–B128, 1990.
201. Cunningham, D.A., Morrison, D., Rice, C.L., et al., Aging and isokinetic plantar flexion, *Eur. J. Appl. Physiol.*, 56, 24–29, 1987.

202. Klein, C., Cunningham, D.A., Paterson, D.H., et al., Fatigue and recovery of contractile properties in young and elderly men, *Eur. J. Appl. Physiol.*, 57, 684–690, 1988.
203. Porter, M.M., Vandervoort, A.A. and Kramer, J.F., Eccentric peak torque of the plantar and dorsiflexors is maintained in older women, *J. Gerontol. Biol. Sci.*, 52, B125–B131, 1997.
204. Klein, C.S., Rice, C.L. and Marsh, G.D., Normalized force, activation, and coactivation in the arm muscles of young and old men, *J. Appl. Physiol.*, in press.

7

Aging and Sarcopenia: Influences of Gender and Physical Activity

Mark A. Tarnopolsky and Gianni Parise

CONTENTS

0-8493-1027-X/02/$0.00+$1.50

7.1 Introduction

The process of aging is inevitable in all living organisms. The fundamental mechanisms behind aging are multifactorial, involving genetic background as well as environmental modulation (see also Chapter 3). Arguments for the dominant genetic component of aging come from studies of a rare genetic condition (progeria, Hutchinson–Guilford syndrome) where rapid aging leads to premature death from conditions usually associated with advanced aging, such as atherosclerosis.[1] The recent discovery of the *Indy* gene has demonstrated a near doubling of the life span in *Drosophila* who harbor mutations in one of the gene copies.[2] Mutations in the insulin signaling pathways of worms (*Caenorhabditis Elegans*) are also associated with a prolonged life span.[3] In addition, females of many species have longer life span and a lower mortality rate than males.[4] Together, these data could suggest that aging is genetically determined and that humans have little control over the process. At the opposite end of the spectrum are studies showing that dietary restriction[5,6] and exercise[6-10] can enhance longevity significantly, thus providing evidence that genetic background can be modified. Although gender is genetically determined, the administration of sex hormones may influence age-related declines in secretion of these hormones.

In a given individual, aging reflects a complex interrelationship between genes and environment, and one factor may be more or less dominant. A number of structural and ultimately functional outcomes of the aging process may be amenable to exogenous influences. For example, a 70-year-old will never hold the world record for the 100-m sprint (an inevitable consequence of aging); nevertheless, a 70-year-old person who has cross-country skied for 40 years is likely to be in much better physical shape than a 35-year-old overweight smoker who has performed no physical activity since adolescence. Although regular physical activity can attenuate the loss of function with aging, there remains an overall age-related decline in functional capacity, even in well-trained athletes.[11] Overall, there is a reduction in total muscle and bone mass from age 30 to senescence (see Chapters 6 and 9). This may involve genetic factors, together with the cumulative influences of oxidative stress, physical activity, nutritional status, and exposure to environmental stressors. This chapter focuses upon possible factors underlying loss of muscle and bone mass (sarcopenia) that occurs with aging and an evaluation of exercise as a countermeasure to this process. The roles of gender and the sex hormones as modulators of sarcopenia are also examined.

An understanding of the mechanisms behind sarcopenia and the development of appropriate countermeasures are important, since significant public health issues surround this phenomenon.[12] From an epidemiological perspective, the prevalence of sarcopenia ranges from 6 to 24%, (depending on definition of the condition).[13,14] Prevalence increases with age, to as much as 50% in persons over the age of 80.[14] As the population ages, it is thus important to consider economic, gender, and race factors influencing the development of preventive strategies.

7.2 Muscle Structural and Functional Decline

7.2.1 Myofibrillar Changes with Age

The etiology of sarcopenia is poorly understood. A pronounced change in body composition occurs with age, so that a loss in lean mass is "replaced" by an increased proportion of connective tissue and fat.[15] This change may account for some of the decreases in muscle strength and function. However, since the myofibril is the contractile apparatus for muscle, much of the age-related loss in muscle strength, mass, and function probably should be attributed to alterations of myofibrillar protein with age.

The most consistently reported age-related change in muscle morphology is a decrease in type II fiber cross-section.[16-23] Some researchers have also suggested that the relative proportion of type II muscle fibers decreases with age[21,24] while the proportion of type I fibers increases.[25,26] In support of the hypothesis that fiber-type transitions occur with age, single fiber analysis reveals that older adults have a higher proportion of fibers showing a coexistence of myosin heavy chain type I and IIA, and type IIA and IIB, as compared to young adults.[25] The age-related shift in fiber type affects whole muscle performance; the increased proportion of type I fibers augments resistance to fatigue, but the reduced proportion of type II fibers reduces peak torque.[27]

Along with the shift in myosin heavy chain muscle isoforms toward slower fibers, there is a deterioration in the quality of individual muscle fibers, defined as the force developed per unit of muscle mass (specific tension), independent of fiber-type.[28] The maximal force developed by single type I and type IIA fibers is greater in young than in old men, even after correcting for cross-sectional area. Type IIA fibers are stronger than type I fibers in both young and old men, but the strength of type IIA fibers does not differ from that of type I fibers in older women.[28] The discrepancy between men and women suggests that age-related sarcopenia may be regulated by different factors in the two sexes. An action of estrogen remains an intriguing potential mechanism underlying the observed gender differences in muscle function, as discussed in greater detail later in this chapter. Taken together, these observations suggest a general trend toward an age-related decrease in muscle strength, through decreases in the proportion and size of type II fiber, and an increase in the proportion of type I fibers. More importantly, these observations suggest that, in the elderly, transitions occur between type I and type II fibers, and that contractile proteins may become less efficient with age. Furthermore, age-related changes in the myofibril appear to be regulated by different factors in men and women. More research is needed to decipher these potential gender differences.

7.2.2 Functional Decline with Age

One of the most common consequences of sarcopenia is a decrease in physical function. Falls are a primary cause of injury, morbidity, and mortality in the elderly, commonly related to a weakening of the ankle, knee, and hip muscles.[29] Typically, there is a profound reduction in maximum voluntary torque in both upper and lower body muscles. For example, the maximum voluntary isometric torque produced by knee extensors and elbow flexors was 35% lower in older (69-year-old) vs. younger (28-year-old) men.[30] Muscle power, the ability to produce force rapidly, also decreases with age, to an even greater extent than peak torque, with resulting impairments in physical function.[31] This change may be explained by a combination of losses in muscle mass and alterations in muscle morphology — predominantly a decrease in the proportion and cross-sectional area of type II muscle fibers.

Some recent work using dynamic contractions has demonstrated a linear age-related decrease in arm and leg muscle quality of similar magnitude in men and women.[32] Others, however, have reported no age-related differences in the isometric strength of the knee extensors and ankle dorsiflexors if peak muscle force was expressed as a function of cross-sectional area.[33,34] In support of the latter observations are data showing that age-related decreases in strength can be almost fully explained by muscle atrophy.[35] A 12-year longitudinal study of men from age 65 to 77 demonstrated a 20 to 30% decrease in the strength of knee and elbow extensors and flexors at both slow and fast angular velocities of contraction. Computerized tomography revealed decreases in the cross-sectional area of all thigh muscles combined (–14.7%), of the quadriceps femoris muscle (–16.1%), and of the flexor muscles (–14.9%), corresponding to a 1.4% decrease in muscle cross-sectional area per year.[35] Together, these observations suggest that the loss of muscle cross-sectional area with age accounts for as much as 90% of the observed loss of strength in men. Discrepant observations with respect to changes in muscle quality during aging can be attributed to several factors. First and foremost are the methods used to estimate muscle mass. For example, when muscle mass was estimated using creatinine excretion, no decline in muscle quality was observed, but when cross-sectional area was determined in the same subjects, a linear decline in muscle quality was calculated.[36] A second consideration is the gross structure of the muscle tested. For example, if a pennate muscle is assessed, the determination of cross-sectional area underestimates the force-generating capacity of the muscle. Finally, the measure of strength used may provide differing results, as seen when using dynamic vs. isometric measures of strength.[32,34,36] All of these factors aside, however, single fiber analysis suggests that the contractile proteins may become less effective with age, resulting in a loss of functional capacity.[28]

Despite discrepancies in the literature, the loss of function appears related to a decrease in peak torque, reflecting both losses in muscle mass and decreases in muscle quality. The mechanisms underlying these structural and functional changes are complex and incompletely understood; they form the focus of the following section.

7.3 Cellular Aspects of Aging

The fundamental mechanisms behind sarcopenia and aging are complex, multifactorial, and inseparable. Senescence can be observed at the cellular level or at the level of the whole organism. Ultimately, sarcopenia needs to be understood at the organism and functional level, but to do this one must understand underlying cellular mechanisms. A classic example of senescence comes from the observation, made many decades ago, that cultured primary cell lines undergo a finite number of replications (between 30 and 50), termed the Hayflick phenomenon.[37,38] A reduction in the number of cell cycles to death has been observed in fibroblast cultures obtained from elderly vs. young patients; this seems to be related to mitochondrial alterations and is correlated with telomere shortening.[39-41] Normal cell development and growth involves a form of cell death termed apoptosis (or preprogrammed cell death); the inhibition of preprogrammed cell death can lead to neoplasia. It may be that senescence and death have evolved as prices to be paid to allow a complex cellular organizational structure.

7.3.1 Oxidative Stress and Mitochondrial Changes

A number of cellular theories of aging involve the production of free radicals or reactive oxygen species. Free radicals are short-lived and highly reactive compounds that have an unpaired electron. Their accumulation results in damage to lipids, protein and DNA, and modifications of structure, with an ultimate deterioration in function. The concentration of free radicals in a given tissue is a function of the rate of free radical generation and the activity of antioxidant enzymes that protect the tissue by converting reactive oxygen species to less reactive compounds. Examples of reactive oxygen species include peroxynitrite, superoxide, the hydroxyl radical, and hydrogen peroxide. Specific enzymes which remove free radicals include copper/zinc superoxide dismutase(Cu/ZnSOD; cytosolic SOD-1), intramitochondrial manganese superoxide dismutase (MnSOD; mitochondrial SOD-2), mitochondrial and cytosolic glutathione peroxidase, and catalase. Reactive oxygen species can be generated in the cell from xanthine oxidase, complex I, and complex III of the electron transport chain and from ferrous iron via the Fenton reaction.[42] Potential consequences of reactive oxygen species-induced damage include disturbances in fundamental processes such as the fidelity of DNA replication (8-OH-2-deoxy-guanosine), altered secondary and tertiary protein structure (protein carbonyls), and alterations in membrane integrity and permeability (lipid hydroperoxides). If aging reflects a lifetime accumulation of free radicals, then supplementation with antioxidants or an overexpression/up-regulation of antioxidant enzymes would be expected to enhance longevity.

The observation that rodents live longer on an energy restricted diet has attracted much interest.[5,6] The hypothesis developed from this observation was that, as basal metabolic rate was reduced, the flux through the free radical producing complexes I and III of the electron transport chain was reduced. More recently, a group of researchers studying *Drosophila* found that some of the insects were living a great deal longer than others. A search in these animals revealed a gene termed *Indy* ("**I**'m **n**ot **d**ead **y**et"),[2] which encoded a protein homologous with a dicarboxylate transporter. *Drosophila* harboring a mutation in this gene in one of their alleles had twice the average life span of the species. The cellular consequences of the *Indy* gene mutations were suggested to represent a form of cellular starvation. Nevertheless, the biological viability of these animals, in terms of movement, reproduction, egg production, etc. was similar to the wild type of *Drosophila*.[2]

Although in theory energy restriction and *Indy* protein mutations both lead to a decreased flux through complexes I and III of the electron transport chain (thus reducing reactive oxygen species generation), this has not yet been proven conclusively; indeed, experiments manipulating antioxidant enzymes in animal systems have yielded conflicting results. Studies in mice found that longevity was enhanced only if a cocktail of antioxidants was given early in development.[43] The overexpression of Cu/Zn superoxide dismutase (an antioxidant) is responsible for a familial form of amyotrophic lateral sclerosis,[44] a mutation that results in increased production of the hydroxyl radical.[45] In *Drosophila*, the overexpression of Cu/Zn superoxide dismutase increased life span only if there was also an overexpression of catalase (to remove the excess hydroxyl radical).[46] On the other hand, superoxide dismutase-2 (Mn-superoxide dismutase) knockout mice show a severe phenotype, with death at approximately 1 week of age.[47] Clearly, the balance between pro- and antioxidant pathways must be well regulated. A major alteration in either arm of this balance can lead to significant cellular dysfunction and ultimately to cell death. Some studies suggest that the pro-oxidant effects of aging are predominant;[48] however, antioxidant enzyme concentrations also decrease with aging.[48-50] Future studies need to measure the effects of aging and physical activity on the concentration and activity of antioxidant enzymes in humans.

One of the major targets of free radical attack is the DNA found in the mitochondrial matrix, which represents approximately 1% of total DNA. Mitochondrial DNA is a 16.5-kD structure with a paucity of introns (intragenic regions of DNA not expressed ultimately in a mature RNA molecule). The small number of introns and the primitive nature of DNA repair mechanisms provide an ideal target for free radical attack.[51] Oxidative damage and resultant DNA mutations occur at a much higher frequency in mitochondrial DNA than in nuclear DNA.[52-54] Mitochondrial DNA deletions are found more frequently in tissues from the elderly than in those from young individuals.[55,56] The "common deletion" is a 5-kD segment of DNA between the ATPase-8 and ND-5 subunits. In parallel with an age-related increase in the number of deletions, there is an increase in the number of cells (COX-negative fibers) that stain negatively for cytochrome oxidase. Cytochrome oxidase-negative skeletal muscle fibers show a clonal expansion of mitochondrial DNA deletions and an increase in oxidative stress markers.[57] The progressive accumulation of mitochondrial point mutations and DNA rearrangements (deletions/duplications) may serve as a positive feedback cycle, altering mitochondrial complexes I and III, which are the main intracellular sites of reactive oxygen species generation.[57] The mitochondria play an important role in the activation of apoptosis through the release of cytochrome-c; this substance interacts with Apaf-1 and caspase-9 to form the apoptosome, which activates downstream effector caspases (cysteine endopeptidases) such as caspase-3. Part of this activation process involves an opening of the mitochondrial permeability transition by free radicals (predominantly peroxynitrate).[58] Apoptosis plays a role not only in the death of neurons[59] and immune cells,[60] but also in muscle atrophy.[61] Aging is associated with increased apoptosis in some cell types,[59] but there have been no studies to determine whether aging is associated with an increase in skeletal muscle apoptosis and thus sarcopenia.

Endurance exercise increases the flux of oxygen through the mitochondria, causing an increase in free radical production. In resistance exercise there is also a period of ischemia–reperfusion known to induce free radical generation.[62,63] In humans, both acute endurance exercise and acute resistance exercise result in the production of free radicals (as measured by protein carbonyls, malondialdehyde, and lipid hydroperoxides).[64,65] Given the cotemporal and possibly mechanistic relationship between reactive oxygen species and aging, it would at first appear that vigorous physical activity should accelerate aging and decrease life span. The high energy intake of athletes, as well as the increased basal metabolic rate, would also seem unfavorable, given animal data showing that energy restriction and a reduction in basal metabolic rate correlate with a prolonged life span. However, animal studies have also found that physical activity is associated with an increase in longevity.[6,7] Interestingly, exercise and dietary energy restriction are not additive in their ability to extend longevity.[6] Humans who participate in vigorous physical activities have an enhanced life span.[9,10] The explanation seems to be that the organism strives for homeostasis, and increased production of free radicals leads to a compensatory upregulation of antioxidant enzyme protein expression. Several studies have shown that the activity of enzymes such as superoxide dismutase-1 is increased in skeletal muscle following long-term exercise training.[66,67] In contrast, other investigators have found that only superoxide dismutase-2 activity was increased in the soleus muscle after training — a far smaller change than the increase in marker enzymes of the citric acid cycle.[68] A fruitful future area of investigation will be to tease out the temporal patterning in which enzymes are affected by different types of exercise and to relate this to the pro- and antioxidant capacity of aging skeletal muscle.

7.3.2 Telomeres

Another critical target for reactive oxygen species is the telomere. Telomeres consist of stretches of TTAGG motif repeats at the ends of each chromosome. The telomeres are required for chromosomal replication and are removed sequentially by an enzyme-mediated process catalyzed by the enzyme telomerase. After several rounds of telomere shortening, no further chromosomal replication is possible, and growth is arrested.[39] Telomere length is reduced as age advances.[69,70] The telomeres are particularly sensitive to reactive oxygen species, and they can be damaged by both hydrogen peroxide and hydroxyl radical. Telomeres are drastically shorter in progeria, a condition where premature aging and death occur.[69,70] To date, no studies have examined whether physical activity has any acute or chronic effect on telomeres or telomerase, particularly in satellite cells.

7.3.3 Protein Turnover — Links to Oxidative Stress?

Although there are some suggestive cotemporal relationships, no direct relationship has been established between reactive oxygen species and sarcopenia. In general, aged animals show a decrease in the expression of skeletal muscle mRNA encoding for proteins involved in protein turnover and energy metabolism.[71] There is an increase in reactive oxygen species as demonstrated by protein carbonyl accumulation with immobilization; this is attenuated by growth hormone administration.[72] Denervation increases apoptosis in skeletal muscle,[61] but whether apoptosis occurs in response to the more modest age-related loss of motor units remains unclear.[73] For the elderly person with a condition such as osteoarthritis, immobility and aging may combine to promote sarcopenia.

At the physiological level, reactive oxygen species would have either to increase protein degradation or to decrease protein synthesis in order to affect muscle mass per se. Conceivably, reactive oxygen species could affect DNA (8-OH-2-deoxy-guanosine), reducing mRNA transcription. However, mitochondrial DNA mRNA transcripts are maintained in elderly compared to young rats, in spite of a reduction in mitochondrial DNA copy number with aging (perhaps reflecting an enhanced mRNA transcript stability).[74] In humans, there is a reduction in high abundance mRNAs encoding for subunits of the electron transport chain; there are also fewer fast myosin isoforms in the elderly compared to the young,[75] suggesting that translational factors could play a role in sarcopenia. Oxidized proteins could also undergo structural or catalytic alterations, leading to a decrease in the translational efficiency of proteins, an alteration in post-translational modifications, or proteolysis.

Several studies have shown a lower fractional synthetic rate of mixed muscle protein in the elderly as compared to young men and women.[76-79] More specifically, the rates of both myofibrillar (actin/myosin) and mitochondrial protein synthesis were reduced in elderly individuals.[78,80] There does not appear to be a reduction in the rate of synthesis of sarcoplasmic proteins with aging.[78] From a functional standpoint, reductions in the myofibrillar fractional synthetic rate have been correlated with the functional measure of knee strength.[78] The age-related reduction in the basal muscle fractional synthetic rate is associated with a lesser abundance of the mRNA species involved in electron transport chain and myofibrillar gene expression.[75]

An acute bout of resistance exercise stimulates both mixed muscle[76,79,81,82] and myosin-specific[82] fractional synthetic rate. Young and elderly subjects show a similar increase in mixed and protein-specific fractional synthetic rate,[82-84] although absolute levels are still marginally lower in the elderly.[83] The mechanism behind the acute, exercise-mediated increase in muscle fractional synthetic rate is thought to involve translational or post-translational mechanisms.[85]

Studies comparing protein breakdown in response to resistance exercise in young and elderly subjects[76,83] have found no between-group differences in whole body proteolysis or 3-methylhistidine excretion (the latter an indirect measure of myofibrillar proteolysis). Future studies should compare the acute and chronic adaptive protein breakdown responses to resistance exercise, using newer methods to determine the fractional breakdown rate of mixed muscle protein.[81] Given that oxidative stress is increased in the skeletal muscle of the elderly, it could be hypothesized that an increase in oxidatively modified proteins would increase the flux though the ubiquitin–proteosome pathway, thus increasing proteolysis.[86] This may be overly simplistic, since senescent fibroblast cell lines have attenuated proteolysis that can lead to the accumulation of defective oxidatively modified proteins.[37,87]

From the standpoint of aerobic exercise, a link between reactive oxygen species and a decrease in aerobic power and aerobic enzyme activity is more straightforward than the potential links between oxidative stress and sarcopenia. The aforementioned increase in mitochondrial deletions and point mutations could lead to defects in the mitochondrial encoded protein subunits that make up the electron transport chain, ultimately affecting electron flux and subsequent oxygen consumption. This hypothesis is not inconceivable, given that the mitochondrion is the main site of free radical generation.[42] The maximal activity of mitochondrial enzymes in skeletal muscle is lower in elderly than in young individuals.[88] Some have argued that this difference is related to physical inactivity and is not an effect of aging per se, based upon the finding of similar electron transport chain enzyme activities in Masters athletes as compared to young sedentary individuals.[89] Others have found a decline in maximal oxygen intake in elderly male athletes despite their training; however, the decline was less rapid than that observed in sedentary subjects.[11,90] Antioxidant enzyme activity also increases in response to endurance exercise in rats.[91-93] There is need for a comprehensive study comparing the adaptability of electron transport chain enzymes, aerobic power, activity of antioxidant enzymes, and free radical production in young and elderly individuals in order to determine whether the adaptability of these systems is altered with aging in humans.

7.4 Exercise as a Countermeasure for Sarcopenia

7.4.1 Cross-Sectional Studies of Athletes and Nonathletes

Evidence is accumulating that progressive resistance exercise is an efficacious, nonpharmacological treatment for age-related losses in muscle mass, quality, and function. The benefits of regular physical activity throughout the life span have been a major focus of exercise physiologists for many decades. Difficulty in understanding the benefits of exercise during aging lies with the research models that have been used. Many investigations have examined the effects of relatively short (8 to 12 weeks) bouts of exercise training; the obvious limitation of this type of model is the short time period for observations. Furthermore, some irreversible age-related changes may already have occurred when a study is initiated, and thus the potential attenuation of the aging process may not be apparent with such a research design. There are also major difficulties associated with conducting a sustained longitudinal study; hence, despite limitations of a cross-sectional design, comparisons of sedentary individuals and Masters athletes may provide the most helpful data on the long-term effects of physical activity upon the aging process.

One cross-sectional study reported that sedentary older adults (69 years old) demonstrated lower maximal isometric torque of the knee extensors (–44%) and elbow flexors (–32%), slower speed of movement of knee extensors and elbow flexors (–25%), smaller cross-sectional area of the quadriceps and biceps (–24%), and lower specific tensions in the quadriceps (–27%) and elbow flexor muscles (–14%). Furthermore, a higher proportion of myosin heavy chain type I (27%) and type IIA (39%) was found in the *vastus lateralis* of older sedentary men as compared to young sedentary men.[30] Habitually trained older men demonstrated similar results to sedentary young men with respect to dynamic strength, maximum voluntary isometric strength, muscle cross-sectional area, specific tension, power, and proportion of myosin heavy chain isoforms. These results suggest that an active lifestyle during aging is able to preserve a muscle function similar to that of sedentary young adults. Similar results have been reported with respect to aerobic exercise and aging. Mitochondrial function has been reported to decline in the elderly, but this may be secondary to disease or muscle disuse.[89] Brierley et al.[89] demonstrated that oxidative metabolism was poorly correlated with chronological age, but strongly correlated with markers of physical activity. In other words, a physically active older adult displays healthy mitochondrial function, whereas a sedentary older adult of the same age displays reduced mitochondrial function. In order to allow for this confounding factor and present a true picture of aging with respect to mitochondrial function, Brierley et al.[94] examined young and elderly athletes, finding that mitochondrial respiratory chain function did not differ significantly between the two groups. Although aerobic power has many determinants, even physically active older males show a decline over an 8-year follow-up.[11] Nevertheless, the decline was about twice as great for a sedentary cohort followed over the same time period.[11] Taken together, these results suggest that, if sustained over a lifetime, regular physical activity has a significant protective effect on muscle strength, function, and oxidative capacity. Benefits appear to relate not only to function, but also to longevity.[9,10]

7.4.2 Prospective Studies of Resistance Exercise Training

The ability to increase the rate of muscle protein synthesis following an exercise session is thought to be a major determinant of exercised-induced hypertrophy and strength. Muscle protein synthesis rate is stimulated in the postexercise period, and may remain elevated for up to 48 h in young men.[81,95] Acute resistance exercise induces a similar stimulation of mixed and myosin heavy chain protein synthesis in 23- to 32-year-old, 63- to 66-year-old, and 78- to 83-year-old men and women.[76,79,82] Thus, adults retain the ability to stimulate the processes responsible for protein synthesis until very old age. This finding justifies the use of resistance exercise, not only as a preventive measure, but also as a potential therapy to restore muscle mass, strength, and function during old age.

An increasing pool of literature suggests that resistance exercise training can induce muscle hypertrophy and increase muscle protein synthesis, strength, mass, and quality, thus improving physical function in older adults. Two weeks of whole-body resistance training were sufficient to increase mixed (182%) and myosin heavy chain (105%) protein synthesis in men and women aged 78 to 83 years old to the levels found in young men and women, with no apparent gender difference in this response.[76,82] The stimulation of muscle protein synthesis in the elderly appears to be mediated by post-transcriptional events.[85] In 62- to 75-year-old men and women, the myofibrillar protein synthesis rate (isolated from the mixed muscle fraction using centrifugation) was increased 30% following three bouts of resistance exercise, with no compensatory increase in total RNA, actin, or myosin heavy chain mRNA.[85] Taken together, these results suggest that older adults preserve the ability to increase muscle protein synthesis following resistance exercise training. Increases in the rate of protein synthesis are mediated by improved translational efficiency of mRNAs, and it appears that men and women can stimulate protein synthesis in a similar fashion.

Based on these results, it stands to reason that regular resistance exercise training is a viable treatment for age-related sarcopenia in men and women. Whole-body resistance exercise training has resulted in a significant increase in muscle strength, mass, and protein synthesis rates in older men and women.[84] Elderly subjects (76 to 92 years old) participated in whole-body resistance exercise training 3 days per week for 3 months, at 65 to 100% of 1-repetition maximal force. At the end of training, the mixed muscle protein synthesis rate had increased significantly in both men and women. The isokinetic strength (at an angular velocity of 60°/s) increased by 10% in women and 23% in men, with parallel gains in muscle mass of 1.0 and 2.2 kg, respectively. Based on the increases in muscle mass (1 to 2 kg), it must be assumed that increases in muscle protein synthesis were counterbalanced by similar increases in muscle protein breakdown; otherwise the increases in muscle mass would have been much greater.[84] The accumulation of lean mass apparently differed between men and women; the mechanism underlying this phenomenon remains unclear, although evidence is mounting that estrogen may be a key hormone for maintaining muscle strength in women.[96]

It was originally thought that older adults lost the capacity for exercise-induced hypertrophy. Moritani and De Vries[97] reported that 8 weeks of progressive resistance exercise training increased muscle strength similarly in young and elderly men; nevertheless, muscle hypertrophy did not occur in the elderly men. They concluded that, in the elderly, exercise-induced gains in muscle strength were mediated through improvements in motor unit recruitment and activation. In partial support of this view, Fiatarone et al.[98-100] reported that resistance exercise training increased maximum voluntary thigh muscle strength in physically frail elderly men and women, but the increase in thigh muscle cross-sectional area was much smaller than the increase in strength. This suggests that the large training-induced increase in muscle strength was due primarily to neural adaptation, with insignificant contributions from an increase in muscle mass. However, as discussed earlier, muscle protein synthesis is stimulated in elderly men and women in response to an acute exercise bout.[76,79,84] The relative lack of hypertrophy in these studies may simply reflect an augmented muscle protein breakdown in the elderly following an exercise session. The difficulty in attaining an accurate kinetic measure of muscle protein breakdown has impeded progress in understanding this phenomenon. Another potential explanation for increases in strength with a relative lack of hypertrophy in older adults following exercise training may be that the elderly have a larger capacity for neural adaptation during resistance training. The neuromuscular junction undergoes degeneration with muscle disuse and aging; coupled with the fact that neural adaptation may precede muscle hypertrophy in response to a training stimulus,[101] this may indicate that elderly men and women undergo a longer period of neural adaptation than do young men and women in the early stages of a resistance exercise program. The elderly thus may not show significant muscle hypertrophy over relatively short periods of training. However, if the muscle protein synthesis rate remains elevated in elderly men and women during a resistance exercise program, then it stands to reason that prolonged involvement in the program will increase muscle mass and induce hypertrophy. A 2-year longitudinal trial of resistance exercise training (2 times/wk for 2 years at 80% of the 1-repetition maximal force) increased leg press (32%) and military press (90%) 1-repetition maximum in 60- to 80-year-old men and women. The knee extensor muscle cross-sectional area increased by 8.7% in the trained subjects, whereas no change was observed in nonexercising control subjects.[102]

Along with improvements in absolute strength and muscle mass, resistance training may increase muscle quality. Tracy and colleagues[103] reported that 9 weeks of unilateral leg training increased the maximal voluntary muscle force of knee extensors by 28% and leg muscle mass by 12% in twenty-three 65- to 75-year-old men and women. Knee extensor muscle quality increased by 14% after training, suggesting that resistance training, perhaps through an increased stimulation of muscle protein turnover, had improved the quality of contractile proteins. Furthermore, the muscle power of the elderly, here defined as the ability to contract at high velocity, improved following resistance training.[104]

Given the growing proportion of elderly men and women in society, it is important that functional ability be improved by interventions designed to attenuate sarcopenia. Functional benefits of resistance exercise training were evaluated in a large-scale trial of 72- to 98-year-old physically frail nursing home residents (37 men, 63 women).[100] Lower body resistance exercise training increased muscle strength (113%) and gait velocity (12%), whereas these same variables remained unchanged in a nonexercising control group. The resistance exercise program increased stair climbing power (28%), the level of spontaneous physical activity, and thigh muscle cross-sectional area (2.7%).

The mechanisms responsible for improvements in strength and function are less well understood. Muscle plasticity, including increases in protein synthesis,[76,79,82,84] and changes in fiber type,[30,105] is a strong candidate for explanations of the increases in strength and function that follow resistance training. Histochemical techniques show significant alterations in muscle morphology in the elderly subsequent to resistance training. Predominant changes are an increase in type II fibers and an increase of muscle fiber area. Twelve weeks of whole-body resistance exercise were sufficient to increase type II muscle fiber area in the vastus lateralis of 64- to 86-year-old men[106] and 60- to 72-year-old men.[107] Similarly, 12 weeks of unilateral resistance exercise training of the elbow flexors increased type II muscle fiber area (by 30%) in 60- to 70-year-old men, and increased 1-repetition maximal force (by 48%) in their elbow flexors.[108] Recent studies have also shown that 12 weeks of progressive resistance exercise training may reduce myosin heavy chain coexpression in single muscle fibers, with a predominant increase in myosin heavy chain type I expression,[105] and increased muscle cell size, strength, contractile velocity, and power in both slow- and fast-twitch single fibers.[109]

Clearly, long-term training studies in both men and women are needed, which look at protein structure and composition, together with other molecular, histologic, physiologic, and functional outcomes in young and elderly persons participating in both resistance and endurance exercise.

7.5 Sex Hormone and Gender Influences on the Adaptability of Skeletal Muscle to Resistance Training

7.5.1 Effect of Sex Hormones on Protein Turnover

A number of hormones can influence muscle protein synthesis and/or degradation, thus affecting net protein accretion. Included in this list are cortisol, insulin-like growth factor-1, insulin, growth hormone, and dihydroepiandrostenedione.[110-112] The focus of this chapter, however, is on an evaluation of the predominant male and female sex steroids, testosterone and 17β-estradiol, respectively.

17β-estradiol is a steroid hormone produced by the ovaries and the adrenal cortex. Typical concentrations are <180 pmol/L in males, and 70 to 2900 pmol/L in menstruating females (values depending on the menstrual cycle phase). 17β-estradiol has an effect on the development of secondary sex characteristics, bone formation, and, particularly in females, muscle mass. At the cellular level, 17β-estradiol induces the transcription of a number of proteins mediating the aforementioned functions, and has secondary effects as an antioxidant.[113,114] No gender differences are apparent in mixed muscle fractional synthesis rate[81] or whole body protein synthesis;[115,116] however, it has been found that leucine oxidation is lower in females compared to males.[115,116] It remains unclear whether this difference is due to estradiol per se, but it suggests that an increase in proteolysis or amino acid oxidation may accompany estradiol withdrawal at menopause. The effect of 17β-estradiol on osteoblast function has been well described, and there is a clear relationship between the decrease in estrogen at menopause and the rapid phase of bone mineral content loss which occurs at that time.[96] Estrogen replacement therapy provides an effective treatment for osteoporosis and the maintenance of bone mineral content.[117-119] The effects of 17β-estradiol on the maintenance of muscle mass are less well described;[120] however, the decrease in fat-free mass that occurs at menopause is cotemporal with the decrease in estradiol.[96,121,122] The striking reduction in muscle strength occurring over the perimenopausal period can be prevented by estrogen replacement therapy.[96] Some evidence exists that the effect of estradiol on muscle mass is regulated indirectly via factors such as insulin-like growth factor-1, leptin, and growth hormone.[123]

The anabolic effects of testosterone have been characterized more extensively. Testosterone is a steroid-based hormone produced from the Leydig cells of the testes and the adrenal cortex. Circulating concentrations of testosterone in males are approximately tenfold greater than in females. Males show a less dramatic and later-onset decrease in testosterone concentration analogous to the female menopause — sometimes termed the "andropause."[110] Given the cotemporal association between age-related loss of skeletal muscle mass and decline in testosterone, a causal link was suspected and supplementation trials were proposed.

Anecdotally, testosterone has been used for decades to augment muscle mass, as evidenced by anabolic steroid abuse in the sporting arena. Scientific investigations have more recently demonstrated that testosterone treatment increases protein synthesis and thus augments fat-free mass. Griggs and colleagues demonstrated that testosterone administration over a 3-month period significantly increased lean body mass and muscle protein synthesis in healthy sedentary males[124] Another study demonstrated that 10 weeks of testosterone administration increased strength and muscle size relative to men receiving placebo treatment.[125] At the protein turnover level, Ferrando and colleagues demonstrated that 5 days of testosterone heptanoate administration yielded a twofold increase in fractional synthesis rate, with no change in fractional breakdown rate.[126] Arterio-venous balance studies demonstrated that testosterone did not increase amino acid transport, and it was hypothesized that the increase in net protein synthesis was due to a reutilization of intracellular amino acids.[126] Increases in muscle strength and mass have been demonstrated following testosterone replacement in hypogonadal males.[127,128] Whether routine testosterone replacement should be used to prevent sarcopenia in elderly men requires further investigation, particularly in view of the theoretical risk of prostate hypertrophy and cancer.[129]

7.5.2 Resistance Exercise ± Hormone Replacement Therapy in the Elderly

Resistance training increases muscle mass and strength, improves function, and increases bone mass in both males and females (see earlier discussion). The question of a possible interactive effect between hormone replacement therapy and resistance exercise is not well characterized in the elderly. Acute resistance exercise results in an increase in free testosterone, growth hormone, and insulin-like growth factor in men.[130-132] The increase in free testosterone after acute exercise is greater in younger vs. older males.[131,132] A 10-week resistance training program increased free testosterone levels in both young and elderly males, yet basal and exercise-stimulated levels were higher in the young men.[132] Thus, it appears that acute and chronic resistance exercise provides stimuli that increase testosterone concentrations and contribute to the beneficial effects of this type of exercise on strength and muscle mass in the elderly.

To date, the authors are not aware of any prospective studies examining whether combinations of hormone replacement therapy and resistance exercise are beneficial in enhancing gains of muscle mass and strength in the elderly. In young men, there were interactive effects of testosterone and exercise; gains of fat-free mass, muscle size, and strength were greater in a testosterone plus resistance exercise group than in a nonexercising group that received testosterone treatment.[125] A recent study in hypogonadal men with HIV wasting found that resistance exercise, testosterone administration, and a combination of both treatments yielded similar increases in muscle strength and mass.[133] It is possible that, if an elderly male were hypogonadal, testosterone replacement would enhance muscle strength and mass gains during a resistance exercise program;[127,128] however, the safety, efficacy, and cost of such a strategy remain to be determined. In theory, 17β-estradiol hormone replacement therapy for postmenopausal females may also have a synergistic effect in combination with resistance training, but this remains to be fully characterized.[122]

7.6 Conclusions

Aging is a complex and inevitable process, genetically determined and environmentally modified. The mechanisms underlying aging are complex and not fully elucidated. The effects of aging and potential countermeasures must be evaluated with these fundamental characteristics in mind. The fundamental biological processes involved in aging include oxidative stress, preprogrammed cell death, and telomere shortening. Environmental influences can accelerate or retard the aging process to some degree, but some decline in function appears inevitable. One consequence of aging is the process of sarcopenia, which involves a loss of bone and muscle mass. As a result of this loss, there is a decrease in functional capacity that ultimately leads to dependency and heavy costs for personal care.

Regular physical activity is an important countermeasure that can attenuate and reverse sarcopenia. Resistance exercise is the most effective direct countermeasure, but even walking is beneficial. Secretion of the sex hormones declines with advancing age and there is a cotemporal increase in the prevalence of sarcopenia. The benefits of hormone replacement therapy in countering bone loss are well established in females, but whether such treatment should be recommended to counter sarcopenia in either men or women remains unclear.

Future studies should examine the protective and rehabilitative potential of both hormone replacement therapy and exercise in the age-related sarcopenia. Such studies must examine basic molecular, physiological, and functional outcomes in order to understand underlying mechanisms and to develop novel intervention strategies.

References

1. Abdenur, J.E., Brown, W.T., Friedman, S., et al., Response to nutritional and growth hormone treatment in progeria, *Metabolism*, 46, 851–856, 1997.
2. Rogina, B., Reenan, R.A., Nilsen, S.P. et al., Extended life-span conferred by cotransporter gene mutations in *Drosophila, Science*, 290, 2137–2140, 2000.
3. Morris, J.Z., Tissenbaum, H.A., and Ruvkun, G., A phosphatidylinositol-3-OH kinase family member regulating longevity and diapause in *Caenorhabditis elegans, Nature*, 382, 536–539, 1996.
4. Janghorbani, M., Hedley, A.J., Jones, R.B., et al., Gender differential in all-cause and cardiovascular disease mortality, *Int. J. Epidemiol.*, 22, 1056–1063, 1993.
5. Weindruch, R., Walford, R.L., Fligiel, S., et al., The retardation of aging in mice by dietary restriction: longevity, cancer, immunity and lifetime energy intake, *J. Nutr.*, 116, 641–654, 1986.
6. Holloszy, J.O. and Schechtman, K.B., Interaction between exercise and food restriction: effects on longevity of male rats, *J. Appl. Physiol.* 70, 1529–1535, 1991.
7. Holloszy, J.O., Exercise increases average longevity of female rats despite increased food intake and no growth retardation, *J. Gerontol.*, 48, B97–B100, 1993.
8. Fortes, C., Forastiere, F., Farchi, S., et al., Diet and overall survival in a cohort of very elderly people, *Epidemiology*, 211, 440–445, 2000.
9. Lee, I.M., Hsieh, C.C., and Paffenbarger, R.S., Exercise intensity and longevity in men. The Harvard alumni health study, *JAMA*, 273, 1179–1184, 1995.
10. van Saase, J.L., Noteboom, W.M., and Vandenbroucke, J.P., Longevity of men capable of prolonged vigorous physical exercise: a 32-year follow up of 2259 participants in the Dutch eleven cities ice skating tour, *Br. Med. J.*, 301, 1409–1411, 1990.
11. Rogers, M.A., Hagberg, J.M., Martin, W.H., et al., Decline in $\dot{V}O_{2max}$ with aging in master athletes and sedentary men, *J. Appl. Physiol.*, 68, 2195–2199, 1990.
12. Dutta, C., Significance of sarcopenia in the elderly, *J. Nutr.*, 127, 992S-993S, 1997.
13. Melton, L.J., Khosla, S., Crowson, C.S., et al., Epidemiology of sarcopenia, *J. Am. Geriatr. Soc.*, 48, 625–630, 2000.
14. Baumgartner, R.N., Koehler, K.M., Gallagher, D., et al., Epidemiology of sarcopenia among the elderly in New Mexico, *Am. J. Epidemiol.*, 147, 755–763, 1998.
15. Forsberg, A.M., Nilsson, E., Werneman, J., et al., Muscle composition in relation to age and sex, *Clin. Sci. (Colch.)*, 81, 249–256, 1991.
16. Aniansson, A., Hedberg, M., Henning, G.B., et al., Muscle morphology, enzymatic activity, and muscle strength in elderly men: a follow-up study, *Muscle Nerve*, 9, 585–591, 1986.
17. Coggan, A.R., Spina, R.J., King, D.S., et al., Histochemical and enzymatic comparison of the gastrocnemius muscle of young and elderly men and women, *J. Gerontol.*, 47, B71–B76, 1992.
18. Grimby, G. and Saltin, B., The aging muscle, *Clin. Physiol.*, 3, 209–218, 1983.
19. Grimby, G., Danneskiold-Samsoe, B., Hvid, K., et al., Morphology and enzymatic capacity in arm and leg muscles in 78–81 year old men and women, *Acta Physiol. Scand.*, 115, 125–134, 1982.
20. Klitgaard, H., Mantoni, M., Schiaffino, S., et al., Function, morphology and protein expression of aging skeletal muscle: a cross-sectional study of elderly men with different training backgrounds, *Acta Physiol. Scand.*, 140, 41–54, 1990.

21. Larsson, L., Sjodin, B., and Karlsson, J., Histochemical and biochemical changes in human skeletal muscle with age in sedentary males, age 22–65 years, *Acta Physiol. Scand.*, 103, 31–39, 1978.
22. Lexell, J., Henriksson-Larsen, K., Winblad, B., et al., Distribution of different fiber types in human skeletal muscles: effects of aging studied in whole muscle cross sections, *Muscle Nerve*, 6, 588–595, 1983.
23. Tomonaga, M., Histochemical and ultrastructural changes in senile human skeletal muscle, *J. Am. Geriatr. Soc.*, 25, 125–131, 1977.
24. Jakobsson, F., Borg, K., and Edstrom, L., Fibre-type composition, structure and cytoskeletal protein location of fibres in anterior tibial muscle. Comparison between young adults and physically active aged humans, *Acta Neuropathol. (Berl.)*, 80, 459–468, 1990 (Abstract).
25. Larsson, L., Histochemical characteristics of human skeletal muscle during aging, *Acta Physiol. Scand.*, 117, 469–471, 1983.
26. Larsson, L., Grimby, G., and Karlsson, J., Muscle strength and speed of movement in relation to age and muscle morphology, *J. Appl. Physiol.*, 46, 451–456, 1979.
27. Cupido, C.M., Hicks, A.L., and Martin, J., Neuromuscular fatigue during repetitive stimulation in elderly and young adults, *Eur. J. Appl. Physiol.* 65, 567–572, 1992.
28. Frontera, W.R., Suh, D., Krivickas, L.S., et al., Skeletal muscle fiber quality in older men and women, *Am. J. Physiol.*, 279, C611–C618, 2000.
29. Province, M.A., Hadley, E.C., Hornbrook, M.C., et al., The effects of exercise on falls in elderly patients. A preplanned meta- analysis of the FICSIT trials. Frailty and Injuries: cooperative studies of intervention techniques, *JAMA*, 273, 1341–1347, 1995.
30. Klitgaard, H., Mantoni, M., Schiaffino, S., et al., Function, morphology and protein expression of aging skeletal muscle: a cross-sectional study of elderly men with different training backgrounds, *Acta Physiol. Scand.*, 140, 41–54, 1990.
31. Martin, J.C., Farrar, R.P., Wagner, B.M., et al., Maximal power across the life span, *J. Gerontol.*, 55, M311–M316, 2000.
32. Lynch, N.A., Metter, E.J., Lindle, R.S., et al., Muscle quality. I. Age-associated differences between arm and leg muscle groups, *J. Appl. Physiol.*, 86, 188–194, 1999.
33. Hakkinen, K., Kraemer, W.J., Kallinen, M., et al., Bilateral and unilateral neuromuscular function and muscle cross-sectional area in middle-aged and elderly men and women, *J. Gerontol.*, 51, B21–B29, 1996.
34. Kent-Braun, J.A. and Ng, A.V., Specific strength and voluntary muscle activation in young and elderly women and men, *J. Appl. Physiol.*, 87, 22–29, 1999.
35. Frontera, W.R., Hughes, V.A., Fielding, R.A., et al., Aging of skeletal muscle: a 12-yr longitudinal study, *J. Appl. Physiol.*, 88, 1321–1326, 2000.
36. Metter, E.J., Lynch, N., Conwit, R., et al., Muscle quality and age: cross-sectional and longitudinal comparisons, *J. Gerontol.*, 54, B207–B218, 1999.
37. Bradley, M.O., Hayflick, L., and Schimke, R.T., Protein degradation in human fibroblasts (WI-38). Effects of aging, viral transformation, and amino acid analogs, *J. Biol. Chem.*, 251, 3521–3529, 1976.
38. Houck, J.C., Sharma, V.K., and Hayflick, L., Functional failures of cultured human diploid fibroblasts after continued population doublings, *Proc. Soc. Exp. Biol. Med.*, 137, 331–333, 1971.

39. Harley, C.B., Human aging and telomeres, *Ciba Found. Symp.*, 211, 129–139; discussion 139–144, 1997.
40. Martens, U.M., Chavez, E.A., Poon, S.S., et al., Accumulation of short telomeres in human fibroblasts prior to replicative senescence, *Exp. Cell Res.*, 256, 291–299, 2000.
41. Tresini, M., Pignolo, R.J., Allen, R.G., et al., Effects of donor age on the expression of a marker of replicative senescence (EPC-1) in human dermal fibroblasts, *J. Cell. Physiol.*, 179, 11–17, 1999.
42. Raha, S. and Robinson, B.H., Mitochondria, oxygen free radicals, disease and aging, *Trends Biochem. Sci.*, 25, 502–508, 2000.
43. Bezlepkin, V.G., Sirota, N.P., and Gaziev, A.I., The prolongation of survival in mice by dietary antioxidants depends on their age by the start of feeding this diet, *Mech. Ageing Dev.*, 92, 227–234, 1996.
44. Siddique, T., Nijhawan, D., and Hentati, A., Molecular genetic basis of familial ALS, *Neurology*, 47, S27–S34; discussion S34–S35, 1996.
45. Liu, R., Narla, R.K., Kurinov, I., et al., Increased hydroxyl radical production and apoptosis in PC12 neuron cells expressing the gain-of-function mutant G93A SOD1 gene, *Radiat. Res.*, 151, 133–141, 1999.
46. Orr, W.C. and Sohal, R.S., Extension of life-span by overexpression of superoxide dismutase and catalase in *Drosophila melanogaster, Science*, 263, 1128–1130, 1994.
47. Melov, S., Coskun, P., Patel, M., et al., Mitochondrial disease in superoxide dismutase 2 mutant mice, *Proc. Natl. Acad. Sci. USA*, 96, 846–851, 1999.
48. Sohal, R.S. and Orr, W.C., Relationship between antioxidants, prooxidants, and the aging process. *Ann. N.Y. Acad. Sci.*, 663, 74–84, 1992.
49. Semsei, I., Rao, G., and Richardson, A., Expression of superoxide dismutase and catalase in rat brain as a function of age, *Mech. Ageing Dev.*, 58, 13–19, 1991.
50. Sohal, R.S., Arnold, L., and Orr, W.C., Effect of age on superoxide dismutase, catalase, glutathione reductase, inorganic peroxides, TBA-reactive material, GSH/GSSG, NADPH/NADP+ and NADH/NAD+ in *Drosophila melanogaster, Mech. Ageing Dev.*, 56, 223–235, 1990.
51. Simon, D.K. and Johns, D.R., Mitochondrial disorders: clinical and genetic features, *Ann. Rev. Med.*, 50, 111–127, 1999.
52. Barja, G. and Herrero, A., Oxidative damage to mitochondrial DNA is inversely related to maximum life span in the heart and brain of mammals, *FASEB J.*, 14, 312–318, 2000.
53. Wei, Y.H., Lu, C.Y., Lee, H.C., et al., Oxidative damage and mutation to mitochondrial DNA and age-dependent decline of mitochondrial respiratory function, *Ann. N.Y. Acad. Sci.* 854, 155–170, 1998.
54. Yakes, F.M. and Van Houten, B., Mitochondrial DNA damage is more extensive and persists longer than nuclear DNA damage in human cells following oxidative stress, *Proc. Natl. Acad. Sci. USA*, 94, 514–519, 1997.
55. Lezza, A.M., Boffoli, D., Scacco, S., et al., Correlation between mitochondrial DNA 4977-bp deletion and respiratory chain enzyme activities in aging human skeletal muscles, *Biochem. Biophys. Res. Commun.*, 205, 772–779, 1994.
56. Lezza, A.M., Mecocci, P., Cormio, A., et al., Mitochondrial DNA 4977 bp deletion and OH8dG levels correlate in the brain of aged subjects but not Alzheimer's disease patients, *FASEB J.*, 13, 1083–1088, 1999.
57. Brierley, E.J., Johnson, M.A., Lightowlers, R.N., et al., Role of mitochondrial DNA mutations in human aging: implications for the central nervous system and muscle, *Ann. Neurol.*, 43, 217–223, 1998.

58. Stachowiak, O., Dolder, M., Wallimann, T., et al., Mitochondrial creatine kinase is a prime target of peroxynitrite- induced modification and inactivation, *J. Biol. Chem.*, 273, 16694–16699, 1998.
59. Adams, J.D., Mukherjee, S.K., Klaidman, L.K., et al., Apoptosis and oxidative stress in the aging brain, *Ann. N.Y. Acad. Sci.*, 786, 135–151, 1996.
60. Haslett, C., Lee, A., Savill, J.S., et al., Apoptosis (programmed cell death) and functional changes in aging neutrophils. Modulation by inflammatory mediators, *Chest*, 99, 6S, 1991.
61. Tews, D.S. and Goebel, H.H., Apoptosis-related proteins in skeletal muscle fibers of spinal muscular atrophy, *J. Neuropathol. Exp. Neurol.*, 56, 150–156, 1997.
62. Grisotto, P.C., dos Santos, A.C., Coutinho-Netto, J., et al., Indicators of oxidative injury and alterations of the cell membrane in the skeletal muscle of rats submitted to ischemia and reperfusion, *J. Surg. Res.*, 92, 1–6, 2000.
63. Gute, D.C., Ishida, T., Yarimizu, K., et al., Inflammatory responses to ischemia and reperfusion in skeletal muscle, *Mol. Cell. Biochem.*, 179, 169–187, 1998.
64. Ji, L.L., Leeuwenburgh, C., Leichtweis, S., et al., Oxidative stress and aging. Role of exercise and its influences on antioxidant systems, *Ann. N.Y. Acad. Sci.*, 854, 102–117, 1998.
65. Sen, C.K., Atalay, M., Agren, J., et al., Fish oil and vitamin E supplementation in oxidative stress at rest and after physical exercise, *J. Appl. Physiol.*, 83, 189–195, 1997.
66. Navarro-Arevalo, A. and Sanchez-del-Pino, M.J., Age and exercise-related changes in lipid peroxidation and superoxide dismutase activity in liver and soleus muscle tissues of rats, *Mech. Ageing Dev.*, 104, 91–102, 1998.
67. Pereira, B., Costa Rosa, L.F., Safi, D.A., et al., Superoxide dismutase, catalase, and glutathione peroxidase activities in muscle and lymphoid organs of sedentary and exercise-trained rats, *Physiol. Behav.*, 56, 1095–1099, 1994.
68. Higuchi, M., Cartier, L.J., Chen, M., et al., Superoxide dismutase and catalase in skeletal muscle: adaptive response to exercise, *J. Gerontol.*, 40, 281–286, 1985.
69. Harley, C.B. and Villeponteau, B., Telomeres and telomerase in aging and cancer, *Curr. Opin. Genet. Dev.* 5, 249–255, 1995.
70. Harley, C.B., Futcher, A.B., and Greider, C.W., Telomeres shorten during aging of human fibroblasts, *Nature*, 345, 458–460, 1990.
71. Lee, C.K., Klopp, R.G., Weindruch, R., et al., Gene expression profile of aging and its retardation by caloric restriction, *Science*, 285, 1390–1393, 1999.
72. Carmeli, E., Hochberg, Z., Livne, E., et al., Effect of growth hormone on gastrocnemius muscle of aged rats after immobilization: biochemistry and morphology, *J. Appl. Physiol.*, 75, 1529–1535, 1993.
73. Doherty, T.J. and Brown, W.F., The estimated numbers and relative sizes of thenar motor units as selected by multiple point stimulation in young and older adults, *Muscle Nerve*, 16, 355–366, 1993.
74. Barazzoni, R., Short, K.R., and Nair, K.S., Effects of aging on mitochondrial DNA copy number and cytochrome c oxidase gene expression in rat skeletal muscle, liver, and heart, *J. Biol. Chem.* 275, 3343–3347, 2000.
75. Welle, S., Bhatt, K., and Thornton, C.A., High-abundance mRNAs in human muscle: comparison between young and old, *J. Appl. Physiol.*, 89, 297–304, 2000.
76. Yarasheski, K.E., Zachwieja, J.J., and Bier, D.M., Acute effects of resistance exercise on muscle protein synthesis rate in young and elderly men and women, *Am. J. Physiol.*, 265, E210–E214, 1993.

77. Welle, S., Bhatt, K., and Thornton, C., Polyadenylated RNA, actin mRNA, and myosin heavy chain mRNA in young and old human skeletal muscle, *Am. J. Physiol.*, 270, E224–E229, 1996.
78. Balagopal, P., Rooyackers, O.E., Adey, D.B., et al., Effects of aging on *in vivo* synthesis of skeletal muscle myosin heavy-chain and sarcoplasmic protein in humans, *Am. J. Physiol.*, 273, E790–E800, 1997.
79. Welle, S., Thornton, C., Jozefowicz, R., et al., Myofibrillar protein synthesis in young and old men, *Am. J. Physiol.*, 264, E693–E698, 1993.
80. Rooyackers, O.E., Adey, D.B., Ades, P.A., et al., Effect of age on *in vivo* rates of mitochondrial protein synthesis in human skeletal muscle, *Proc. Natl. Acad. Sci. USA*, 93, 15364–15369, 1996.
81. Phillips, S.M., Tipton, K.D., Aarsland, A., et al., Mixed muscle protein synthesis and breakdown after resistance exercise in humans, *Am. J. Physiol.*, 273, E99–E107, 1997.
82. Hasten, D.L., Pak-Loduca, J., Obert, K.A., et al., Resistance exercise acutely increases MHC and mixed muscle protein synthesis rates in 78–84 and 23–32 years olds, *Am. J. Physiol.*, 278, E620–E626, 2000.
83. Welle, S., Thornton, C., and Statt, M., Myofibrillar protein synthesis in young and old human subjects after three months of resistance training, *Am. J. Physiol.*, 268, E422–E427, 1995.
84. Yarasheski, K.E., Pak-Loduca, J., Hasten, D.L., et al., Resistance exercise training increases mixed muscle protein synthesis rate in frail women and men ≧76 years old, *Am. J. Physiol.*, 277, E118–E125, 1999.
85. Welle, S., Bhatt, K., and Thornton, C.A., Stimulation of myofibrillar synthesis by exercise is mediated by more efficient translation of mRNA, *J. Appl. Physiol.*, 86, 1220–1225, 1999.
86. Mitch, W.E. and Goldberg, A.L., Mechanisms of muscle wasting. The role of the ubiquitin-proteasome pathway, *N. Engl. J. Med.*, 335, 1897–1905, 1996.
87. Sitte, N., Merker, K., Von Zglinicki, T., et al., Protein oxidation and degradation during cellular senescence of human BJ fibroblasts: part I — effects of proliferative senescence, *FASEB J.*, 14, 2495–2502, 2000.
88. Pastoris, O., Boschi, F., Verri, M., et al., The effects of aging on enzyme activities and metabolite concentrations in skeletal muscle from sedentary male and female subjects, *Exp. Gerontol.*, 35, 95–104, 2000.
89. Brierley, E.J., Johnson, M.A., James, O.F., et al., Effects of physical activity and age on mitochondrial function, *Q. J. Med.*, 89, 251–258, 1996.
90. Shephard, R.J., Kavanagh, T., Mertens, D.J., et al., Personal health benefits of Masters athletics competition, *Br. J. Sports Med.*, 29, 35–40, 1995.
91. Powers, S.K., Criswell, D., Lawler, J., et al., Influence of exercise and fiber type on antioxidant enzyme activity in rat skeletal muscle, *Am. J. Physiol.*, 266, R375–R380, 1994.
92. Hammeren, J., Powers, S., Lawler, J., et al., Exercise training-induced alterations in skeletal muscle oxidative and antioxidant enzyme activity in senescent rats, *Int. J. Sports Med.*, 13, 412–416, 1992.
93. Kanaley, J.A. and Ji, L.L,. Antioxidant enzyme activity during prolonged exercise in amenorrheic and eumenorrheic athletes, *Metabolism*, 40, 88–92, 1991.
94. Brierley, E.J., Johnson, M.A., Bowman, A., et al., Mitochondrial function in muscle from elderly athletes, *Ann. Neurol.*, 41, 114–116, 1997.

95. Chesley, A., MacDougall, J.D., Tarnopolsky, M.A., et al., Changes in human muscle protein synthesis after resistance exercise, *J. Appl. Physiol.*, 73, 1383–1388, 1992.
96. Phillips, S.K., Rook, K.M., Siddle, N.C., et al., Muscle weakness in women occurs at an earlier age than in men, but strength is preserved by hormone replacement therapy, *Clin. Sci. (Colch.)*, 84, 95–98, 1993.
97. Moritani, T. and deVries, H.A., Potential for gross muscle hypertrophy in older men, *J. Gerontol.*, 35, 672–682, 1980.
98. Fiatarone, M.A., Marks, E.C., Ryan, N.D., et al., High-intensity strength training in nonagenarians. Effects on skeletal muscle, *JAMA*, 263, 3029–3034, 1990.
99. Fiatarone, M.A. and Evans, W.J., The etiology and reversibility of muscle dysfunction in the aged, *J. Gerontol.*, 48, Spec No: 77–83, 1993.
100. Fiatarone, M.A., O'Neill, E.F., Ryan, N.D., et al., Exercise training and nutritional supplementation for physical frailty in very elderly people, *N. Engl. J. Med.*, 330, 1769–1775, 1994.
101. Sale, D.G., Neural adaptation to resistance training, *Med. Sci. Sports Exerc.*, 20, S135–S145, 1988.
102. McCartney, N., Hicks, A.L., Martin, J., et al., A longitudinal trial of weight training in the elderly: continued improvements in year 2, *J. Gerontol.*, 51, B425–B433, 1996.
103. Tracy, B.L., Ivey, F.M., Hurlburt, D, et al., Muscle quality. II. Effects of strength training in 65- to 75-yr-old men and women, *J. Appl. Physiol.*, 86, 195–201, 1999.
104. Jozsi, A.C., Campbell, W.W., Joseph, L., et al., Changes in power with resistance training in older and younger men and women, *J. Gerontol.*, 54, M591–M596, 1999.
105. Williamson, D.L., Godard, M.P., Porter, D.A., et al., Progressive resistance training reduces myosin heavy chain coexpression in single muscle fibers from older men, *J. Appl. Physiol.*, 88, 627–633, 2000.
106. Charette, S.L., McEvoy, L., Pyka, G., et al., Muscle hypertrophy response to resistance training in older women, *J. Appl. Physiol.*, 70, 1912–1916, 1991.
107. Frontera, W.R., Meredith, C.N., O'Reilly, K.P., et al., Strength conditioning in older men: skeletal muscle hypertrophy and improved function, *J. Appl. Physiol.*, 64, 1038–1044, 1988.
108. Brown, A.B., McCartney, N., and Sale, D.G., Positive adaptations to weightlifting training in the elderly, *J. Appl. Physiol.*, 69, 1725–1733, 1990.
109. Trappe, S., Williamson, D., Godard, M., et al., Effect of resistance training on single muscle fiber contractile function in older men, *J. Appl. Physiol.*, 89, 143–152, 2000.
110. Lamberts, S.W., van den Beld, A.W., and van der Lely, A.J., The endocrinology of aging, *Science*, 278, 419–424, 1997.
111. Harman, S.M. and Tsitouras, P.D., Reproductive hormones in aging men. I. Measurement of sex steroids, basal luteinizing hormone, and Leydig cell response to human chorionic gonadotropin, *J. Clin. Endocrinol. Metab.*, 51, 35–40, 1980.
112. Berr, C., Lafont, S., Debuire, B., et al., Relationships of dehydroepiandrosterone sulfate in the elderly with functional, psychological, and mental status, and short-term mortality: a French community-based study, *Proc. Natl. Acad. Sci. USA*, 93, 13410–13415, 1996.
113. Hernandez, I., Delgado, J.L., Diaz, J., et al., 17beta-estradiol prevents oxidative stress and decreases blood pressure in ovariectomized rats, *Am. J. Physiol.*, 279, R1599–R1605, 2000.

114. Behl, C., Widmann, M., Trapp, T., et al., 17-beta estradiol protects neurons from oxidative stress-induced cell death *in vitro*, *Biochem. Biophys. Res. Commun.*, 216, 473–482, 1995.
115. McKenzie, S., Phillips, S.M., Carter, S.L., et al., Endurance exercise training attenuates leucine oxidation and BCOAD activation during exercise in humans, *Am. J. Physiol.*, 278, E580–E587, 2000.
116. Volpi, E., Lucidi, P., Bolli, G.B., et al., Gender differences in basal protein kinetics in young adults, *J. Clin. Endocrinol. Metab.*, 83, 4363–4367, 1998.
117. McKeever, C., McIlwain, H., Greenwald, M., et al., An estradiol matrix transdermal system for the prevention of postmenopausal bone loss, *Clin. Therap.*, 22, 845–857, 2000.
118. Cooper, C., Stakkestad, J.A., Radowicki, S., et al., Matrix delivery transdermal 17beta-estradiol for the prevention of bone loss in postmenopausal women. The international study group, *Osteoporos. Internat.*, 9, 358–366, 1999.
119. Weiss, S.R., Ellman, H., and Dolker, M., A randomized controlled trial of four doses of transdermal estradiol for preventing postmenopausal bone loss. Transdermal estradiol investigator group, *Obstetr. Gynecol.*, 94, 330–336, 1999.
120. van den Beld, A.W., de Jong, F.H., Grobbee, D.E., et al., Measures of bioavailable serum testosterone and estradiol and their relationships with muscle strength, bone density, and body composition in elderly men, *J. Clin. Endocrinol. Metab.*, 85, 3276–3282, 2000.
121. Dionne, I.J., Kinaman, K.A., and Poehlman, E.T., Sarcopenia and muscle function during menopause and hormone-replacement therapy, *J. Nutr. Health Aging*, 4, 156–161, 2000.
122. Poehlman, E.T., Toth, M.J., Fishman, P.S., et al., Sarcopenia in aging humans: the impact of menopause and disease, *J. Gerontol.*, 50, Spec. No.: 73–77, 1995.
123. Roubenoff, R., Rall, L.C., Veldhuis, J.D., et al., The relationship between growth hormone kinetics and sarcopenia in postmenopausal women: the role of fat mass and leptin, *J. Clin. Endocrinol. Metab.*, 83, 1502–1506, 1998.
124. Griggs, R.C., Kingston, W., Jozefowicz, R.F., et al., Effect of testosterone on muscle mass and muscle protein synthesis, *J. Appl. Physiol.*, 66, 498–503, 1989.
125. Bhasin, S., Storer, T.W., Berman, N., et al., The effects of supraphysiologic doses of testosterone on muscle size and strength in normal men, *N. Engl. J. Med.*, 335, 1–7, 1996.
126. Ferrando, A.A., Tipton, K.D., Doyle, D., et al., Testosterone injection stimulates net protein synthesis but not tissue amino acid transport, *Am. J. Physiol.*, 275, E864–E871, 1998.
127. Bhasin, S., Storer, T.W., Berman, N., et al., Testosterone replacement increases fat-free mass and muscle size in hypogonadal men, *J. Clin. Endocrinol. Metab.*, 82, 407–413, 1997.
128. Brodsky, I.G., Balagopal, P., and Nair, K.S., Effects of testosterone replacement on muscle mass and muscle protein synthesis in hypogonadal men — a clinical research center study, *J. Clin. Endocrinol. Metab.*, 81, 3469–3475, 1996.
129. Bhasin, S. and Tenover, J.S., Age-associated sarcopenia — issues in the use of testosterone as an anabolic agent in older men, *J. Clin. Endocrinol. Metab.*, 82, 1659–1660, 1997.
130. Kraemer, R.R., Kilgore, J.L., Kraemer, G.R., et al., Growth hormone, IGF-I, and testosterone responses to resistive exercise, *Med. Sci. Sports Exerc.*, 24, 1346–1352, 1992.

131. Kraemer, W.J., Hakkinen, K., Newton, R.U., et al., Acute hormonal responses to heavy resistance exercise in younger and older men, *Eur. J. Appl. Physiol.*, 77, 206–211, 1998.
132. Kraemer, W.J., Hakkinen, K., Newton, R.U., et al., Effects of heavy-resistance training on hormonal response patterns in younger vs. older men, *J. Appl. Physiol.*, 87, 982–992, 1999.
133. Bhasin, S., Storer, T.W., Javanbakht, M., et al., Testosterone replacement and resistance exercise in HIV-infected men with weight loss and low testosterone levels, *JAMA*, 283, 763–770, 2000.

8

Aging, Gender, and Susceptibility to Muscle Damage and Overtraining

Peter M. Tiidus

CONTENTS

0-8493-1027-X/02/$0.00+$1.50

8.1 Introduction

Physiological reactions to, and mechanisms associated with exercise-induced muscle damage and subsequent repair processes have been well characterized in young adults. This chapter examines evidence from human- as well as animal-based studies linking aging with an increased susceptibility to exercise-induced muscle damage and an impairment of muscle repair and adaptation processes. Further, the possible physiological mechanisms associated with such age-related changes are discussed.

Gender differences in susceptibility to muscle damage and postexercise inflammation have also been reported recently. This chapter further examines the evidence for and potential mechanisms behind such differences. It concludes with a look at the potential interaction of age and gender in susceptibility to exercise-induced muscle damage and the potential for physical training to modify these responses.

8.2 Exercise-Induced Muscle Damage and Repair Processes

8.2.1 Mechanisms of Exercise-Induced Muscle Damage

Exercise-induced muscle damage is a common consequence of unaccustomed physical activity, overtraining, or eccentrically biased muscle contractions. Muscle damage may be caused by excessive tension on muscle fibers, myofibrils, and sarcomeres, which can result in sarcomere and Z-line disruption, as well as damage to connective tissues and structural proteins such as desmin.[1,2] Eccentric muscle actions are particularly damaging, since a smaller cross section of the muscle is activated to provide the same tension as that induced by a concentric contraction.[3] Relative changes in muscle length during contraction also contribute to muscle damage, the injury associated with eccentric contractions being greater at longer rather than shorter muscle lengths.[4] It is hypothesized that, during muscle contractions causing excessive strain, the "weaker" or more damage-susceptible sarcomeres become overstretched and damaged.[4] This type of damage should not result in any specific focal location for muscle damage, since damage-susceptible muscle fibers could theoretically occur throughout a muscle. Consistent with this hypothesis, histochemically determined ultrastructural evidence indicates that damaged sarcomeres are indeed randomly scattered throughout an exercise-damaged muscle rather than concentrated in any particular location.[5,6]

In addition to mechanically induced muscle damage, exercise may result in oxygen radical or other chemically induced muscle structural and membrane disruption.[7,8] During prolonged exercise, oxygen radicals are inadvertently generated from mitochondrial electron transport "leakage" or from xanthine dehydrogenase-induced generation of oxygen radicals.[7] These oxygen radicals may be responsible for exercise-induced peroxidation of membrane lipids, macromolecules, and other peroxidation-related muscle structural damage.[7,8] Postexercise muscle inflammation is also characterized by oxygen radical generation from invading neutrophils and macrophages and by hypochlorous acid generated by neutrophil myeloperoxidase activity.[9] These processes, although necessary to help degrade and remove damaged muscle tissue and macromolecules, may also contribute to damage and disruption of muscle cells associated with the inflammatory response in the days following exercise.[10]

8.2.2 Reactions to Muscle Damage: Inflammation and Repair

Physical activity resulting in damage to skeletal muscle is followed by well-described physiological reactions collectively known as the "acute phase response."[1] As described earlier, engagement in unaccustomed physical exercise or overtraining can result in damage to muscle ultrastructure, contractile elements, and sarcolemma. In rapid response to muscle damage, several whole-body and muscle-specific reactions take place. Evans and Cannon have noted an exercise-induced systemic activation of the inflammation-mediating complement system analogous to that seen with foreign infection.[1] Of specific importance to muscle damage is the activation of membrane-attack complexes and anaphylatoxins (i.e., C3a, C4a, and C5a) that activate mast cells, neutrophils, and monocytes. In addition, circulating levels of neutrophils, macrophages, and inflammation-mediating cytokines all increase within hours following an acute exercise bout.[11,12] All of these systemic changes ultimately influence muscular inflammatory and repair responses to exercise-induced damage.

In the muscle itself, exercise-induced mechanical or chemical disruption of the muscle sarcolemma or sarcoplasmic reticulum can result in a loss of muscle calcium homeostasis and an increase in cellular calcium levels.[4,13] Increases in circulating creatine kinase (CK) activity due to increased macromolecule leakage across disrupted muscle membranes is seen as an indicator of exercise-induced muscle membrane damage.[1,4] This membrane-damage-induced increase in intracellular calcium will lead to the production of inflammatory mediators such as those resulting from initiation of the arachadonic acid cascade.[1,14] In addition, increased calcium levels will activate lysosomal and nonlysosomal proteases such as calpain, which will in turn initiate degeneration of specific Z-line and structural and functional muscle proteins.[14,15] Some byproducts of muscle protein degeneration may serve as chemoattractants to initiate immediate postexercise neutrophil adhesion to and infiltration into skeletal muscle.[1,15] Neutrophils have been directly and indirectly observed in human and animal skeletal muscle within

1 hour postexercise and have continued to be observed in muscle up to 5 days postexercise.[15,17]

Within 24 hours of exercise-induced damage, further muscle infiltration by macrophages takes place.[18] Macrophages are the primary leukocytes associated with post-24-hour muscle damage and repair processes. St. Pierre and Tidball noted in animal models that different macrophage subpopulations were associated with different stages of muscle recovery following damage.[19] In addition to their role in helping remove damaged tissue via phagocytosis, macrophages help to initiate a number of steps in the muscle repair process. These include stabilization of the extracellular connective tissue matrix, and secretion of inflammation-mediating cytokines such as interleukin-1 (IL-1) and tumor necrosis factor-alpha (TNF-α).[1]

A further critical step in the muscle repair process, also initiated directly by macrophages, is the activation of muscle satellite cells. Satellite cells function as stem cells and provide myoblasts for muscle regeneration.[20] Macrophages secrete basic fibroblast growth factor (bFGF), which acts as one of several stimulants for the proliferation and differentiation of satellite cells.[21] The infiltration of muscle by macrophages following damage, and their influence in the activation and proliferation of satellite cells followed by their incorporation into damaged muscle, is critical to the muscle repair and regeneration process. Without macrophage infiltration, muscle repair does not proceed.[22]

Muscle damage also leads to the synthesis of specific heat shock proteins (HSPs).[4] Heat shock proteins such as HSP72 act as chaperones, assisting in the proper folding and incorporation of newly synthesized proteins into appropriate myofibrillar structures during the repair process.[23] Thus the upregulation of their synthesis is critical to the appropriate repair of muscle damage.

A primary overt manifestation of exercise-induced muscle damage is a prolonged loss of muscle strength. Loss of the ability to generate muscle force is thought to be related directly to damage-induced disruption of muscle ultrastructure, contractile elements, and membrane function and it is a sensitive indicator of overall muscle damage and recovery.[24,25] In humans, muscle force declines by up to 40% immediately following damaging exercise and, depending on the degree of damage, it may take upwards of 4 to 14 days to recover fully.[26] The sensation of delayed-onset muscle soreness (DOMS) is often present following muscle damage. The soreness sensation is usually not felt until 12 to 24 hours following muscle damage; it peaks around 24 to 48 hours postdamage and usually resolves within 4 to 5 days.[1,26] It is likely that inflammation- and edema- related events associated with muscle damage and repair contribute to the degree of soreness.[14]

Muscle appears to adapt following a single exposure to damaging exercise, such that a second exposure within several weeks will result in significant attenuation of DOMS sensation, strength loss, and indicators of membrane damage.[27]

8.3 Modification of Muscle Damage and Repair Mechanisms with Aging

8.3.1 Age-Related Differences in Postexercise Muscle Damage and Recovery

Evidence from both animal and human models suggests that there are age-related differences in the susceptibility of skeletal muscle to exercise-induced damage and ability for post-damage repair. One such difference is in the amount of work required to induce muscle damage. Studies from Faulkner's laboratory have demonstrated that when young (2 to 3 months), adult (11 to 12 months) and old (26 to 27 months) mice were administered the same 5-minute protocol of eccentric muscle contractions, muscles from the old mice exhibited a greater degree of injury (as determined by loss of isometric force) than muscles from young or adult mice.[28] However, administration of the eccentric protocol for 15 minutes resulted in further damage to the young and adult mice so their degree of isometric strength loss was now at the level seen in aged animals.[24] It is likely that a population of injury-susceptible muscles or sarcomeres exists[13] and in older animals these fibers are more prone to injury early in eccentric contractions.[24] Longer application of eccentric contractions results in the eventual injury of an equivalent number of muscle fibers in younger animals, without further increasing the degree of injury in the old animals. Others have not always demonstrated an age-related difference in the degree of postexercise muscle damage between old and young rats, but these discrepancies may in part be explained by the number of contractions performed.

Human studies have also tended to demonstrate a greater degree of exercise-induced muscle damage in elderly than in younger adults. Manfredi et al.[29] reported that following eccentric exercise, older (59 to 63 years) untrained males exhibited significantly greater muscle damage than younger (20 to 30 years) males. From electron and light microscopic examination of muscle biopsies, they determined that the older males exhibited extensive focal damage and edema in over 90% of muscle fibers immediately postexercise, compared with damage to 5 to 50% damaged fibers in younger males.[29] Although not comparing results directly to younger adults, others have also reported significant myofibrillar and Z-line damage in muscles from older adults following acute exercise.[30] As well, Fielding et al. noted higher rates of protein breakdown in muscles from older compared to younger men following eccentric exercise.[31] Postexercise serum creatine kinase (CK) activities are either similar between younger and older males[29] or lower in older males.[17] Fielding et al.[17] have suggested that lower values in older adults may reflect a reduced ability to translocate muscle CK into the plasma following muscle damage, rather than a lesser degree of muscle membrane damage.

Confounding reports of age-related differences in muscle damage, a recent study by Roth et al.[32] found no difference in electron microscope-quantified muscle damage between older (65 to 75 years) and younger (20 to 30 years) males following 9 weeks of strength training. One interpretation of these findings may be that, although an acute bout of eccentric exercise induces significantly more damage to untrained muscle in older males, this difference is eliminated with regular training. More studies are needed to confirm this possibility, but these observations suggest that training may be important in reducing the degree of exercise-induced damage in elderly muscle. A further study by the same group saw significantly higher levels of muscle damage in older compared to younger females who had performed the same strength training program.[33] This controversial finding will be discussed in more detail in Section 8.5.

Most animal and human studies agree that recovery from acute exercise-induced muscle damage is impaired in older subjects. Brooks and Faulkner reported that, when muscles from old (26 to 27 months) and younger (2 to 3 months) mice were injured to the same degree by eccentric contractions, the recovery was significantly delayed in older animals.[24] Specifically, in the younger mice, isometric muscle force had recovered fully 28 days postexercise, whereas older mice had achieved only an 84% recovery at this stage. Even following 60 days of recovery, muscles from older mice had not completely regained their pre-injury isometric force production.[24] They concluded that "although the overall pattern of injury and regeneration appeared to be similar for young and old mice, in old mice the timing of these processes was delayed...."[24] Similarly, McBride et al.[34] reported a delayed recovery of twitch and tetanic force in tibialis anterior muscles from aged compared to adult rats following damage caused by eccentric contractions. Older humans have also been reported to exhibit a delayed recovery in muscle force following acute eccentric exercise when compared to younger subjects.[35] To date, no studies have reported histological data quantifying different rates of muscle repair in older vs. younger subjects.

In addition to slower recovery rates in aged muscle, McBride et al.[34] reported a lack of protective adaptation in muscles injured by eccentric contraction. Young adult rats (6 months) were subjected to a second bout of eccentric muscle contractions after 2 weeks of recovery from an initial bout of eccentric muscle contractions. As is commonly seen in young humans,[1] the muscles from the young animals manifested adaptations to the initial muscle injury, so the second bout of eccentric contractions induced little further damage (as evidenced by maintenance of pre-exercise muscle force generation).[34] In contrast, muscles from older animals were less successful in inducing protective adaptations, so a second bout of eccentric contractions still induced a significant loss of contractile force.[34] This suggests that, in addition to slower muscle repair, the quality of muscle repair may be compromised in older animals.

8.3.2 Physiological Mechanisms Accounting for Age-Related Differences in Postexercise Muscle Damage and Recovery

Numerous factors may account for the impaired ability of aged muscle to withstand potentially damaging exercise and to recover optimally from damage. As discussed in Chapter 4, muscle sarcopenia is apparently an inevitable part of aging. The age-related death of motor nerves and the subsequent loss of muscle fibers, particularly fast type II fibers, can account for much of the loss of strength reported with aging.[36-38] Age-related loss of muscle fibers is accompanied by a decrease in randomness of fiber type distribution within muscles and increased fiber type grouping, particularly as some denervated type II muscle fibers may be reinnervated by type I motor nerves.[37-39] This would account for some of the loss of muscle force and power with aging. Since smaller, weaker, and functionally compromised muscles may be more susceptible to exercise-related damage than larger and stronger muscles, the decrease in overall muscle strength associated with aging may be an important factor in causing the susceptibility of older muscle to exercise-induced injury. Since strength training significantly augments muscle mass and strength even in the elderly,[40] regular training could be an important prophylactic against exercise-induced muscle damage in older adults. In support of this suggestion, Brooks et al.[41] reported that muscles from old rats that had been exposed to a 6-week stretch-conditioning program were more resistant to damage induced by stretch than muscles from unconditioned animals. Thus, despite some initial impairment of muscle repair and adaptation processes, muscle in elderly animals still seems robust enough eventually to adapt to and develop protection from resistance exercise training. McBride et al.[34] attributed the relative lack of adaptation to eccentric exercise-induced muscle damage in older animals to a lack of muscular activity (their animals were confined to cages). Since physical activity induces muscle adaptations which minimize exercise-induced muscle damage in humans,[1,4] it is possible that an age-related reduction in habitual physical activity may play a role in making older muscle more susceptible to exercise-induced damage, in addition to any intrinsic, age-related changes in muscle quality.

In addition to mechanical factors, chemical events, particularly those related to oxygen radical-induced peroxidation may play a role in exercise-induced muscle damage.[7,21] Although research data are very limited, there is some evidence that exercise-induced oxidative damage is greater in older animals and humans than in the young.[42] Zerba et al.[28] treated old and young mice with the antioxidant free radical scavenger polyethylene glycol superoxide dismutase (PEG-SOD) 24 hours prior to and 24 and 48 hours after lengthening-induced muscle injury. Three days postinjury, maximum tetanic muscle force was significantly more attenuated in older than younger mice. Treatment with PEG-SOD reduced the amount of muscle damage (as indicated by loss of muscle force) in both young and older animals. Some researchers have interpreted these data as evidence that older animals are more susceptible to peroxidative postexercise muscle damage, but more research is needed to confirm this conclusion.[42] In most tissues, aging appears to result in diminished antioxidant enzyme activities.[7] However, muscle from old animals tends to have levels as high as or higher than the levels of antioxidant enzymes and other intracellular antioxidants such as glutathione and vitamin E in younger animals.[7,43] Despite possibly having higher levels of antioxidant enzymes, muscles from older rats do not appear any better protected from exercise-induced lipid peroxidation than muscles from younger animals.[44] The antioxidant enzymes animals may be less effective in preventing *in vivo* peroxidation than in younger animals, due to unexplained conditions.[44] Training studies with older animals have not produced any clear evidence of positive muscle antioxidant adaptations as a result of exercise training.[7] Thus, possible differences in protection against exercise-induced oxidative damage or ability for antioxidant adaptation to training in older vs. younger muscle remains controversial.

In addition to the quality of aged muscle, another potential factor in the ability to resist exercise-induced damage and to optimize repair is the quality of muscle repair-related factors external to the muscle. Carlson and Faulkner[45] cross transplanted extensor digitorum longus (EDL) muscles within and between young and old rats. Muscles from old and young rats demonstrated an equal ability to repair themselves when transplanted into young animals. However, muscles from young and old rats showed significant impairments in the repair process when transplanted into older animals. This model demonstrated that the age of the host had a more important influence on muscle repair than the age of the muscle per se.[45] In support of this suggestion, a recent study reported no influence of age on the ability of muscle satellite cells to activate and proliferate in response to resistance training in rats,[46] implying that age does not diminish the intrinsic ability of muscle satellite cells to respond to muscle damage. Thus the intrinsic ability of older muscle to repair muscle damage or to induce a satellite cell-mediated muscle hypertrophy in response to resistance training may not be impaired in older individuals. Indeed, as discussed in Chapter 6, the ability of skeletal muscle to respond to strength training does not seem to be greatly impaired by age. Hence, age-related systemic factors may be more important than the age of the muscle itself in attenuating postdamage muscle recovery.

Carlson and Faulkner[45] suggested that, in their muscle transplantation model, age-related deficiencies in reinnervation and revascularization of transplanted muscle may have been important to deficiencies in regenerative ability seen in older animals. However, as previously discussed, there is evidence for impaired recovery of muscle in older animals following exercise-induced injury in circumstances where reinnervation and revascularization are not factors in muscle recovery. Other systemic factors, possibly related to control of systemic inflammatory reactions or levels of circulating hormones (such as testosterone or cortisol) may be important influences in muscle repair in older animals.[24] However, little experimental data have been gathered on these possibilities as yet.

Aging is associated with increased levels of circulating inflammatory markers such as tumor necrosis factor alpha (TNF-α), interleukin-6 (IL-6) and C-reactive protein.[47] Abnormally high levels of inflammation are often seen as factors in suboptimal responses to disease or infection in aged subjects.[47] Hence, a supranormal systemic inflammatory stimulus may be a factor delaying postexercise muscle repair in older individuals. Despite this possibility, older humans (61 to 72 years) demonstrate a significantly lower increase in circulating neutrophil levels than younger (20 to 32 years) adults following eccentric exercise;[48] the reasons for this diminished neutrophilia remain unknown. Cannon et al.[48,49] have suggested that the phenomenon may be related to a diminished antioxidant capacity in older individuals, since vitamin E supplements increased postexercise neutrophilia in older but not younger males. Melatonin is an important circulating antioxidant which is significantly lower in older compared to younger adults, and it may account for some of the diminished antioxidant capacity in the blood of older adults.[50] Cannon et al.[48] have not seen age-related differences in systemic complement system response (as determined by plasma des-Arg-C3a levels) following eccentric exercise, hence excluding this as a factor in explaining age-diminished postexercise neutrophilia. Since neutrophil activation and infiltration into damaged skeletal muscle are important in ultimate muscle repair, a diminished circulating neutrophilia could have important consequences for postdamage muscle recovery. However, more research is required before such cause and effect relationships are firmly established.

Impaired muscle protein synthesis rates have also been reported in older animals.[37] As previously discussed, this does not appear greatly to impair positive muscle adaptations to resistance training in older adults. A recent study reported that muscle from very old (36 months) male hybrid rats was unable to hypertrophy in response to synergist ablation.[51] Although this is an unphysiological model, it suggests that some aspect of muscle hypertrophy-related adaptation is impaired in extreme old age. Muscle hypertrophy and muscle repair processes are both mediated by satellite cell proliferation.[37] Hence, these findings could extend to the repair process as well. Again, more research is needed before any such conclusions can be reached.

8.4 Modification of Muscle Damage and Repair Mechanisms by Gender

8.4.1 Gender-Related Differences in Postexercise Muscle Damage and Recovery

A growing body of evidence has pointed to gender-related differences in exercise-induced muscle damage and inflammation-related responses. The earliest and best documented differences in muscle damage-related indices between genders are in the magnitude of postexercise creatine kinase (CK) leakage from muscle. The level of circulating CK activity has often been used as an indirect marker of muscle damage.[4] Circulating CK activity is a relatively poor quantifier of structural muscle damage, but it can be a sensitive marker of muscle sarcolemmal membrane disruption.[4,21] As early as 1979, Shumate et al.[52] showed that 24 hours postexercise, adult males had approximately sixfold higher elevations in serum CK activity than females. Clarkson and Sayers[4] reviewed several human studies which reported these types of postexercise gender differences in serum CK activities. Bär and colleagues performed several rat studies which found similar gender-based differences in postexercise serum CK activities.[21] Collectively, these studies suggest that females are less prone to exercise-induced muscle sarcolemmal membrane disruption — a gender difference in postexercise membrane stability with possible implications for responses to muscle damage. As discussed in Section 8.1, membrane disruption influences numerous muscle degenerative and inflammatory processes following exercise-induced damage. Postexercise gender differences in these responses may relate in part to the gender difference in postexercise muscle sarcolemmal stability. This possibility is discussed further in the next section.

A small but growing number of studies have examined potential gender-based differences in morphological indices of postexercise muscle damage. Using a downhill running rodent model, Komulainen et al.[53] reported gender differences in damage to specific muscle structural proteins (desmin, actin, dystrophin, etc.) as well as differences in the degree and onset of muscle fiber swelling and necrosis at various times up to 96 hours postexercise. Following exercise, histopathological changes associated with loss of sub-membrane dystrophin and desmin and disorganization of actin and fiber swelling occurred earlier and, to a greater extent, in male than in female rats.[53,54] This study also found beta-glucoronidase (a lysosomal enzyme indicative of exercise-induced muscle damage)[55] activities twice as high in male animals as in females at 48 hours postexercise.[53] An earlier study also reported significantly more disruption of muscle banding patterns 48 hours postexercise in male than in female rats.[56]

As previously noted, the production of heat shock proteins (HSPs) is a characteristic and important response to exercise-induced muscle damage and repair.[4] Paroo et al.[57] have found significantly higher muscle levels of HSP72 24 hours postexercise in male than in female rats, and estrogen administration diminishes the postexercise HSP72 response of male animals to levels seen in females. Reports on both humans and animals have noted that females conserve protein better than males during and following exercise.[58] However, it is unknown whether lesser protein catabolism relates to a reduction in exercise-induced muscle damage, in addition to the better understood ability of females to conserve carbohydrates during exercise.

Not all studies have found gender differences in exercise-induced muscle structural damage. Van der Meulen et al.[59] reported no gender differences in morphological indices of muscle damage in rats 72 hours postexercise. St.

Pierre-Schnieder et al.[60] saw a similar number of necrotic and damaged muscle fibers in female and male mice 24 hours following eccentric contraction-induced injury. The only study to report the effects of eccentric exercise on histological indices of muscle damage in humans found little difference between genders 48 hours postexercise.[61] The reasons for these differing results are not known, but may relate to the type of exercise performed or to how long after initiation of exercise the muscle was examined.

Muscle leukocyte invasion shows more consistent gender differences in response to muscle-damaging exercise. Determination of tissue myeloperoxidase (MPO) activity provides an accurate indication of muscle neutrophil infiltration.[62] Using this index, Tiidus and Bombardier[63] inferred significantly greater muscle neutrophil infiltration 24 hours following uphill running exercise in male compared to female rats. Others also have reported that histological evidence of muscle macrophage infiltration up to 7 days following eccentric exercise is delayed and attenuated in female compared to male mice.[60] Muscle leukocyte infiltration 48 hours following eccentrically induced muscle damage is also less in female than in male human subjects.[62]

8.4.2 Physiological Mechanisms Underlying Gender-Related Differences in Postexercise Muscle Damage and Recovery

Much of the evidence explaining gender differences in postexercise muscle damage and inflammation points to the involvement of the female hormone estrogen.[54,56,64] A series of studies by Amelink, Bär and colleagues have demonstrated that estrogen can influence muscle sarcolemmal membrane stability significantly, as evidenced by *in vivo* and *in vitro* CK leakage in rats.[65-69] For example, the *in vitro* rate of CK loss from contraction-damaged, isolated soleus muscles was twice as great in ovariectomized female rats as in ovariectomized females pretreated with estrogen.[65] In addition, serum CK activities following treadmill running were significantly lower in male rats treated with daily estrogen injections when compared to untreated male controls.[67]

The ability of estrogen to protect muscle sarcolemmal membrane from exercise-induced disruption is thought to be related to its antioxidant and membrane stabilizing properties.[21,54,64] Sugioka et al.[70] found that unlike other natural steroids (i.e., testosterone), estrogens have significant antioxidant properties, due to the presence of a hydroxyl group on their "A" ring. *In vitro* physiological concentrations of estrogen can inhibit superoxide production directly, acting as a peroxidative chain and breaking antioxidant for both lipids and DNA.[71] Estrogen may also interact directly with muscle membranes, increasing their stability in ways similar to the actions of cholesterol or vitamin E.[64,68] Relatively few studies have examined the potential influence of estrogen or gender on oxygen radical-induced peroxidation during actual whole-body exercise. Dernback et al.[72] reported lower circulating levels of lipid peroxidation byproducts in female compared to male elite rowers during a 30-day heavy training cycle. However, Tiidus et al.[73] found little difference in immediate postexercise muscle indices of oxidative stress in male rats with or without estrogen supplementation. Estrogen and other gender-related factors may also contribute to gender differences in tissue levels of the antioxidant vitamins C and E and the antioxidant peptide glutathione.[73,74] Hence, although gender differences in tissue antioxidant potential, partially due to estrogen, may exist, their importance in influencing exercise-induced peroxidative muscle damage is still undefined.

Despite this uncertainty, a role for estrogen in influencing postexercise muscle leukocyte infiltration and inflammation is beginning to emerge. To determine the influence of estrogen on gender differences in postexercise muscle neutrophil infiltration, Tiidus and Bombardier[63] injected male rats with estrogen daily for 14 days. The estrogen injected males had attenuated 24-hr postexercise muscle neutrophil levels, similar to those seen in females and significantly lower than those seen in muscles from normal males.[63] In a follow-up study, ovariectomized female rats were implanted with either a placebo or an estrogen replacement pellet for 14 days prior to running exercise.[75] One hour postexercise, muscle neutrophil infiltration (as determined by MPO activities and histochemical staining) was again attenuated in estrogen-implanted females compared to the ovariectomized females.[75] As previously noted, others have also recently reported lower posteccentric exercise muscle leukocyte levels in female mice and humans compared to males.[60,61]

It has been recently suggested that this estrogen-mediated, gender-based difference in postexercise muscle neutrophil infiltration may be due to the potential membrane stabilizing and/or antioxidant properties of estrogen.[54] Belcastro et al.[16] have argued, based on experimental data[74] that exercise-induced muscle sarcolemmal damage will disrupt intramuscular calcium homeostasis and thereby activate calpain, a nonlysosomal protease. Calpain will catalyze specific protein degradation, resulting in production of specific peptide fragments that can act rapidly as chemoattractants for neutrophil adhesion and infiltration into muscle. This would explain the previously reported immediate postexercise increases in muscle neutrophil infiltration.[74] If, as previously discussed, estrogen can influence muscle membrane stability, this could conceivably diminish exercise-induced disruption of muscle calcium homeostasis and thus attenuate exercise-induced calpain activation. Less activation of calpain would, in turn, reduce the synthesis of neutrophil chemoattractants and ultimately attenuate postexercise neutrophil infiltration.[54] In support of this suggestion, estrogen administration to ovariectomized female rats has recently been found to result in diminished 1-hour postexercise muscle calpain activation,[75] with reduced muscle neutrophil infiltration when compared to that seen in ovariectomized rats with no estrogen supplementation.[75]

Although this suggestion may explain diminished neutrophil infiltration immediately postexercise, it is unlikely to account fully for attenuated muscle leukocyte levels reported 2 to 7 days postexercise.[60,61] St. Pierre-Schneider et al.[60] have suggested that the attenuation of muscle leukocyte (primarily macrophage) infiltration up to 7 days following eccentric exercise may reflect the ability of estrogen to limit the availability of other endothelial adhesion molecules such as its inhibition of the IL-1-induced expression of endothelial cell adhesion factor. Further research is necessary to elucidate potential estrogen-related mechanisms.

The ultimate consequences of altered postexercise muscle leukocyte infiltration for muscle damage and repair are as yet unknown. In addition to helping remove damaged tissues, neutrophil infiltration and activation can induce further damage to healthy tissue as an unavoidable consequence of their oxygen radical and hypochlorous acid production.[9,77] On the other hand, inhibition of muscle inflammatory response and macrophage infiltration inhibits muscle repair.[18,22] St. Pierre-Schneider et al.[60] have suggested that the attenuated invasion of macrophages into injured muscles of female mice may result in slower removal of damaged tissue and slower activation of satellite cells and muscle repair processes. On the other hand, Tiidus et al.[75] have noted that, in other tissue damage models, an attenuation of neutrophil invasion has generally reduced collateral damage of healthy tissue with enhancement of ultimate healing. No data are yet available from either humans or animals which follow the time course of exercise- induced muscle damage through to eventual healing in a gender comparative model. Hence, whether females are afforded greater protection from postexercise muscle inflammatory damage and/or are delayed in muscle healing rates as a consequence of their higher estrogen levels is not yet firmly established.

8.5 Interactions of Age and Gender in Exercise-Induced Muscle Damage and Repair

Relatively little is known about the effects of aging on potential gender differences in exercise-induced muscle damage. As previously noted, both elderly males and females have the capacity to respond to resistance exercise by increasing muscle size and strength and aging-related loss of muscle mass accounts for most of the loss of muscle strength in the elderly.[36,38,78] Hence, any age-related loss of muscle protection from or adaptability to exercise-induced damage does not seem large enough to hinder greatly ultimate adaptation to strength training in either gender. However, some studies have suggested that estrogen may influence muscle strength in females and that some of the loss of muscle strength in aging females may be due to postmenopausal reductions in estrogen levels.[79,80] The mechanisms responsible for the potential muscle strength enhancement by estrogen are unknown.

If estrogen does protect skeletal muscle from exercise-induced damage, the reduction in estrogen levels in older postmenopausal females may render their muscles noticeably more susceptible to damage than the muscles of older males.[64] Indirect support for such a proposition may be inferred from the comparatively lower incidence of cardiac disease in premenopausal females compared to matched age males.[81] The cardioprotective effects of estrogen are lost with reductions in circulating estrogen levels in postmenopausal women, as their incidence of heart disease then rises to that of males.[81] At least a part of this cardioprotective effect of estrogen may reflect its ability to protect cardiac muscle from oxidative stress.[71]

Roth et al. [32,33] have found more evidence of ultrastructural damage in skeletal muscles of older (65 to 75 years) women than in younger (20 to 30 years) women following a 9-week resistance training program, whereas no such differences existed following training in males of comparable ages. Following training, the older females displayed significantly more signs of ultrastructural muscle damage than younger females, as well as both younger and older males. Roth et al. interpreted these findings to indicate that, possibly due to a loss of estrogen, older females were relatively more susceptible to resistance training-induced muscle damage than younger females or comparable age males.[33] Even though older males have an equivalent loss of testosterone, this hormone may not be as critical to protecting muscle from exercise-induced damage in males as estrogen is in females. It would be of interest to determine if estrogen replacement therapy can prevent such differences in exercise-induced muscle damage in older females.

Despite their relatively greater degree of susceptibility to muscle damage, older females in these and other studies were still able to adapt positively to the training program.[33,40] Thus, the degree of exercise-induced muscle damage incurred by older females, although possibly greater than that seen in older males, does not seem to impair positive adaptive responses to resistance training. Nevertheless, more research is needed to determine the physiological implications of the potentially greater susceptibility of older females to exercise-induced muscle damage.

8.6 Conclusions

The elderly appear to be more susceptible to exercise-induced muscle damage than younger adults. In addition, following such damage, there seems to be a relative impairment in muscle repair and adaptation in the sedentary elderly. Nevertheless, evidence suggests that the ability of older muscle to adapt to a resistance training program remains robust, and the physiological mechanisms associated with muscle repair and hypertrophy are still able to function even in older adults.

Estrogen may afford younger adult females relatively more protection against exercise-induced and postexercise inflammation-induced muscle damage than males have. However, their muscles may lose this protection and become even more susceptible to exercise-induced damage than males of comparable age, consequent upon reductions in circulating estrogen levels following menopause. Nevertheless, regular physical activity may still ultimately engender positive protective muscle adaptations in the aged of both genders, albeit more slowly than in younger adults. Thus regular resistance exercise may be one of the best intrinsic methods of protecting muscles from exercise-induced muscle damage and helping to normalize the rate and quality of muscle repair processes and adaptation to muscular activity in older individuals.

References

1. Evans, W. and Cannon, J., Metabolic effects of exercise-induced muscle damage, in *Exercise and Sports Sciences Reviews 19*, Holloszy, J.O., Ed., Williams & Wilkins, Baltimore, MD, 1991, 99–125.
2. Friden, J. and Leiber, R.L., Structural and mechanical basis of exercise-induced muscle injury, *Med. Sci. Sports Exerc.*, 24, 521–530, 1992.
3. Enoka, R.M., Eccentric contractions require unique activation strategies by the nervous system, *J. Appl. Physiol.*, 81, 2339–2346, 1996.
4. Clarkson, P.M. and Sayers, S.P., Etiology of exercise-induced muscle damage, *Can. J. Appl. Phyiol.*, 24, 234–348, 1999.
5. Talbot, J.A. and Morgan, D.L., Quantitative analysis of sarcomere nonuniformities in active muscle following stretch, *J. Muscle Res. Cell. Motility*, 17, 261–268, 1996.
6. Fridén, J., Sjörström, M., and Ekblom, B., Myofibrillar damage following intense eccentric exercise in man, *Int. J. Sports Med.*, 4, 170–176, 1983.
7. Ji, L.L., Exercise and oxidative stress: role of the cellular antioxidant systems, in *Exercise and Sports Sciences Reviews* 23, Holloszy J.O. Ed., Williams & Wilkins, Baltimore, MD, 1995, 135–166.
8. Clanton, T.L., Zuo, L., and Klawitter, P., Oxidants and skeletal muscle function: physiological and pathophysiological implications, *P.S.E.B.M.*, 222, 253–262, 1999.
9. Tiidus, P.M., Radical species in inflammation and overtraining, *Can. J. Physiol. Pharmacol.*, 76, 533–538, 1998.
10. Ward, P., Warren, J., and Johnson, K., Oxygen radicals, inflammation, and tissue injury, *Free Rad. Biol. Med.*, 5, 403–408, 1988.
11. Nehlsen-Cannarella, S., Cellular responses to moderate and heavy exercise, *Can. J. Physiol. Pharmacol.*, 76, 485–489, 1998.
12. Pedersen, B.K., Ostrowski, K., Rohde, T., et al., The cytokine response to strenuous exercise, *Can. J. Physiol. Pharmacol.*, 76, 505–511, 1998.
13. Armstrong, R.B., Initial events in exercise-induced muscular injury, *Med. Sci. Sports Exerc.*, 22, 429–435, 1990.
14. MacIntyre, D., Reid, W., and McKenzie, D., Delayed muscle soreness: the inflammatory response to muscle injury and its clinical implications, *Sports Med.*, 20, 24–40, 1995.
15. Belcastro, A.N., Shewchuk, L., and Raj, D.A., Exercise-induced muscle injury: a calpain hypothesis, *Mol. Cell Biochem.*, 179, 135–145, 1998.

16. Belcastro, A.N., Arthur, G.D., Albisser, T.A., et al., Heart, liver and skeletal muscle myeloperoxidase activity during exercise, *J. Appl. Physiol.*, 80, 1331–1335, 1996.
17. Fielding, R., Manfredi, T., Ding, W., et al., Acute phase response to exercise III. Neutrophils and IL-1 accumulation in skeletal muscle, *Am. J. Physiol.*, 265, R166–R172, 1993.
18. Tidball, J.G., Inflammatory cell response to acute muscle injury, *Med. Sci. Sports Exerc.*, 27, 1022–1032, 1995.
19. St. Pierre, B. and Tidball, J.G., Differential response of macrophage subpopulations to soleus muscle reloading after rat hindlimb suspension, *J. Appl. Physiol.*, 77, 290–296, 1994.
20. Schultz, E., Satellite cell behavior during skeletal muscle growth and regeneration, *Med. Sci. Sports Exerc.*, 21, S181–S186, 1989.
21. Bär, P.R., Reijneveld, J., Wokke, J., et al., Muscle damage induced by exercise: nature, prevention and repair, in *Muscle Damage*, Salmons, S., Ed., Oxford University Press, Oxford, 1997, 1–27.
22. Carlson, B.M. and Faulkner, J.A., The regeneration of skeletal muscle fibers following injury: a review, *Med. Sci. Sports Exerc.*, 15, 187–193, 1983.
23. Kilgore, J.L., Musch, T.I., and Ross, C.R., Physical activity, muscle and HSP70 response, *Can. J. Appl. Physiol.*, 23, 245–260, 1998.
24. Brooks, S.V. and Faulkner, J.A., Contraction-induced injury: recovery of skeletal muscles in young and old mice, *Am. J. Physiol.*, 258, C436–C442, 1990.
25. Warren, G.L., Lowe, D., Inman, O., et al., Estradiol effect on anterior crural muscles — tibial bone relationship and susceptibility to injury, *J. Appl. Physiol.*, 80, 1660–1665, 1996.
26. Ebbeling, C. and Clarkson, P.M., Exercise-induced muscle damage and adaptation, *Sports Med.*, 7, 207–234, 1989.
27. Clarkson, P.M., Nosaka, K., and Braun, B., Muscle function after exercise-induced muscle damage and rapid adaptation, *Med. Sci. Sports Exerc.*, 24, 512–520, 1992.
28. Zerba, E., Komorowski, T.E., and Faulkner, J.A., Free radical injury to skeletal muscles of young, adult, and old mice, *Am. J. Physiol.*, 258, C429–C435, 1990.
29. Manfredi, T.G., Fielding, R.A., O'Reilly, K.P. et al., Plasma creatine kinase activity and exercise-induced muscle damage in older men, *Med. Sci. Sports Exerc.*, 23, 1028–1034, 1991.
30. Scelsi, R., Marchetti, C., and Poggi, P., Histochemical and ultrastructural aspects of m. vastus lateralis in sedentary old people (age 65–89), *Acta Neuropathol.*, 51, 99–104, 1980.
31. Fielding, R.A., Meredeth, C., O'Reilly, K. et al., Enhanced protein breakdown after eccentric exercise in young and older men, *J. Appl. Physiol.*, 71, 674–670, 1991.
32. Roth, S., Martel, G., Ivey, F., et al., Ultrastructural muscle damage in young vs. older men after high-volume, heavy-resistance strength training, *J. Appl. Physiol.*, 86, 1833–1840, 1999.
33. Roth, S., Martel, G., Ivey, F., et al., High- volume, heavy-resistance strength training and muscle damage in young and older women, *J. Appl. Physiol.*, 88, 1112–1118, 2000.
34. McBride, T.A., Gorin, F.A., and Carlsen, R.C., Prolonged recovery and reduced adaptation in aged rat muscle following eccentric exercise, *Mech. Ageing Dev.*, 83, 185–200, 1995.

35. Clarkson, P.M. and Dedrick, M.E., Exercise-induced muscle damage, repair and adaptation in old and young subjects, *J. Gerontol.*, 43, M91–M96, 1988.
36. Brooks, S.V. and Faulkner, J.A., Skeletal muscle weakness in old age: underlying mechanisms, *Med. Sci. Sports Exerc.*, 26, 432–439, 1994.
37. Hughes, S.M. and Schiaffino, S., Control of muscle fibre size: a crucial factor in aging, *Acta Physiol. Scand.*, 167, 307–312, 1999.
38. Frontera, W., Hughes, V., Fielding, R., et al., Aging of skeletal muscle: a 12-yr longitudinal study, *J. Appl. Physiol.*, 88, 1321–1326, 2000.
39. Lexell, J. and Downhan, D.Y., The occurrence of fibre-type grouping in healthy human muscle: a quantitative study of cross-sections of whole vastus lateralis from men between 15 and 83 years, *Acta Neuropathol.*, 81, 377–381, 1991.
40. Fiatarone-Singh, M., Ding, W., Manfredi, T. et al., Insulin-like growth factor I in skeletal muscle after weight-lifting exercise in frail elders, *Am. J. Physiol.*, 277, E135–E143, 1999.
41. Brooks, S.V., Koh, T., Rashes, S., et al., Conditioning of skeletal muscles in adult and old animals for protection from contraction-induced injury. *Proc. CSEP Ann. Sci. Conf.*, 2000, 34–35, 2000.
42. Poidori, M., Mecocci, P., Cherubini, A., et al., Physical activity and oxidative stress during aging, *Int. J. Sports Med.*, 21, 154–157, 2000.
43. Leeuwenburgh, C., Fiebig, R., Chandwaney, R., et al., Aging and exercise training in skeletal muscle: response of glutathione and antioxidant enzyme systems, *Am. J. Physiol.*, 267, R439–R445, 1994.
44. Starnes, J., Cantu, G., Farrer, R.P., et al., Skeletal muscle lipid peroxidation in exercise and food restricted rats during aging, *J. Appl. Physiol.*, 67, 69–75, 1989.
45. Carlson, B. and Faulkner, J.A., Muscle transplantation between young and old rats: age of host determines recovery, *Am. J. Physiol.*, 256, C1262–C1266, 1989.
46. Roth, S., Martel, G., Ivey, F., et al., Satellite cell response to nine weeks of strength training in young and older men and women, *Med. Sci. Sports Exerc.*, 32, S294 (1459), 2000.
47. Pedersen, B.K., Bruunsgaard, H., Ostrowski, K., et al., Cytokines in aging and exercise, *Int. J. Sports Med.*, 21, S4–S9, 2000.
48. Cannon, J.G., Fiatarone, M., Fielding, R., et al., Aging and stress-induced changes in complement activation and neutrophil mobilization, *J. Appl. Physiol.*, 76, 2616–2620, 1994.
49. Cannon, J.G., Orencole, S., Fielding, R., et al., Acute phase response to exercise: interaction of age and vitamin E on neutrophils and muscle enzyme release, *Am. J. Physiol.*, 259, R1214–R1219, 1990.
50. Reiter, R.J., Melatonin: lowering the high price of free radicals, *N.I.P.S.*, 15, 246–250, 2000.
51. Blough, E.R. and Linderman, J.K., Lack of skeletal muscle hypertrophy in very aged male Fischer 344 × brown Norway rats, *J. Appl. Physiol.*, 88, 1265–270, 2000.
52. Shumate, J.B., Brooke, M.H., Carroll, J. et al., Increased serum creatine kinase after exercise: a sex linked phenomenon, *Neurology*, 29, 902–904, 1979.
53. Komulainen, J., Koskinen, S., Kalliokoski, R., et al., Gender differences in skeletal muscle fibre damage after eccentrically biased downhill running in rats, *Acta Physiol. Scand.*, 165, 57–63, 1999.
54. Tiidus, P.M., Estrogen and gender effects on muscle damage, inflammation, and oxidative stress, *Can. J. Appl. Physiol.*, 25, 274–287, 2000.
55. Salminen, A. and Kihlström, M., Lysosomal changes in mouse skeletal muscle during repair of exercise injuries, *Muscle Nerve*, 8, 269–279, 1985.

56. Amelink, G.J., Van der Waal, W.A., Wokke, J.H., et al., Exercise induced muscle damage in the rat: the effect of vitamin E deficiency, *Pflügers Arch. — Eur. J. Physiol.*, 419, 304–309, 1991.
57. Paroo, Z., Tiidus, P.M., and Noble, E.G., Estrogen attenuates HSP 72 expression in acutely exercised male rodents, *Eur. J. Appl. Physiol.*, 80, 180–184, 1999.
58. Phillips, S.M., Protein metabolism and exercise: potential sex-based differences, in *Gender Differences in Metabolism; Practical and Nutritional Implications*, Tarnopolsky, M., Ed., CRC Press, Boca Raton FL, 1999, 155–178.
59. Van der Meulen, J.H., Kuipers, H., and Drukker, J., Relationship between exercise-induced muscle damage and enzyme release in rats, *J. Appl. Physiol.*, 71, 999–1104, 1991.
60. St. Pierre-Schneider, B., Correia, L.A., and Cannon, J.G., Sex differences in leukocyte invasion of injured murine skeletal muscle, *Res. Nurs. Health*, 22, 243–251, 1999.
61. Stupka, N., Lowther, S., Chorneyko, K., et al., Gender differences in muscle inflammation following eccentric exercise, *J. Appl. Physiol.*, 89, 2325–2332, 2001.
62. Xiao, F., Eppiheimer, M., Willis, B., et al., Complement-mediated lung injury and neutrophil retention after intestinal ischemia–reperfusion, *J. Appl. Physiol.*, 82, 1459–1465, 1997.
63. Tiidus, P.M. and Bombardier, E., Estrogen attenuates postexercise myeloperoxidase activity in skeletal muscle of male rats, *Acta Physiol. Scand.*, 166, 85–90, 1999.
64. Tiidus, P,M., Can estrogens diminish exercise-induced muscle damage?, *Can. J. Appl. Physiol.*, 20, 26–38, 1995.
65. Amelink, G. J. and Bär, P.R., Exercise induced muscle protein leakage in the rat: effects of hormonal manipulation, *J. Neurol. Sci.*, 76, 61–65, 1986.
66. Amelink, G.J., Kamp, H.H., and Bär, P.R., Creatine kinase isoenzyme profiles after exercise in the rat: sex-linked differences in leakage of CK-MM, *Pflügers Arch. — Eur. J. Physiol.*, 412, 417–421, 1988.
67. Amelink, G.J., Koot, R.W., Erich, W.B., et al., Sex-linked variation in creatine kinase release, and its dependence on estradiol can be demonstrated in an *in vitro* rat skeletal muscle preparation, *Acta Physiol. Scand.*, 138, 115–124, 1990.
68. Koot, R.W., Amelink, G.J., Blankenstein, M.A., et al., Tamoxifen and estrogen both protect the rat muscle against physiological damage, *J. Steroid Biochem. Mol. Biol.*, 40, 689–695, 1991.
69. Bär, P.R., Rodenburg, A.J., Koot, R.W., et al., Exercise-induced muscle damage: recent developments, *Basic Appl. Myo.*, 4, 5–16, 1994.
70. Sugioka, K., Shimosegawa, Y., and Nakano, M., Estrogens as natural antioxidants of membrane phospholipid peroxidation, *FEBS Lett.*, 210, 37–39, 1987.
71. Ayers, S., Abplanalp, W., Lui, J.H., et al., Mechanisms involved in the protective effect of estradiol-17 on lipid peroxidation and DNA damage, *Am. J. Physiol.*, 274, E1002–E1008, 1998.
72. Dernbach, A., Sherman, W., Simonsen, J., et al., No evidence of oxidative stress during high-intensity rowing, *J. Appl. Physiol.*, 74, 2140–2145, 1993.
73. Tiidus, P.M., Bombardier, E., Hidiroglou, N., et al., Estrogen administration, postexercise tissue oxidative stress and vitamin C status in male rats, *Can. J. Physiol. Pharmacol.*, 76, 952–960, 1998.
74. Tiidus, P.M., Bombardier, E., Hidiroglou, N., et al., Gender and exercise influence on tissue antioxidant vitamin status in rats, *J. Nutr. Sci. Vitaminol.*, 45, 701–710, 1999.

75. Tiidus, P.M., Holden, D., Bombardier, E., et al., Estrogen effect on postexercise muscle neutrophil level and calpain activity, *Can. J. Physiol Pharmacol.*, 79, 400–406, 2001.
76. Raj, D., Booker, T., and Belcastro, A.N., Striated muscle calcium-stimulated cysteine protease (calpain-like) activity promotes myeloperoxidase activity with exercise, *Pflügers Arch. — Eur. J. Physiol.*, 435, 804–809, 1998.
77. Walden, D., McCutchan, J., Enquist, E., et al., Neutrophils accumulate and contribute to skeletal muscle dysfunction after ischemia–reperfusion, *Am. J. Physiol.*, 259, H1809–H1812, 1990.
78. Lemmer, J., Hurlbut, D., Martel, G., et al., Age and gender responses to strength training and detraining, *Med. Sci. Sports Exerc.*, 32, 1505–1512, 2000.
79. Sarwar, R., Beltran-Niclos, B., and Rutherford, O.M., Changes in muscle strength, relaxation rate and fatigability during the human menstrual cycle, *J. Physiol.*, 493, 267–272, 1996.
80. Phillips, S.K., Rook, K., Siddle, R. et al., Muscle weakness in women occurs at an earlier age than in men, but strength is preserved by hormone replacement therapy, *Clinical Sci.*, 84, 95–98, 1993.
81. Stampfer, M., Colditz, G., Willett, W., et al., Postmenopausal estrogen therapy and cardiovascular disease, *N. Eng. J. Med.*, 325, 756–762, 1991.

9

Aging of Joints and Skeletal System: Influence of Gender and Physical Activity

Charlotte F. Sanborn and Maureen J. Simmonds

CONTENTS

9.1 Introduction

Osteoarthritis, rheumatoid arthritis, and osteoporosis are some of the most common skeletal disorders in the elderly. Osteoarthritis is primarily a degenerative disease of the joints, rheumatoid arthritis is a systemic autoimmune inflammatory disease of the joints, but osteoporosis is a disease of the bones. These skeletal diseases are major health problems, characterized by significant morbidity, mortality, and economic burden. Over half of the older population is afflicted by arthritis, and approximately one-third of postmenopausal women will experience an osteoporotic fracture in their lifetime.[1] The numbers of those impacted and the associated medical costs

0-8493-1027-X/02/$0.00+$1.50

will only be magnified as the proportion of elderly people grows and the projected rise in life expectancy develops.[1]

It is difficult to distinguish between the normal aging process and pathologies of the joints and skeletal system due to disease or activity and other aspects of lifestyle. Osteoporotic fractures should not be viewed as an inevitable consequence of aging, nor should the gradual deterioration of bone tissue with advancing years be thought of as a disease.[2] Likewise, distinguishing between disease processes and disease consequences of arthritis and normal aging is complex. This chapter examines the underlying physiological, biochemical, and biomechanical mechanisms in the joint and skeletal systems, and how pathology, age, gender, and physical activity influence them.

9.2 Definitions and Prevalence

9.2.1 Rheumatoid/Osteoarthritis

Arthritis is a generic term that includes more than 100 different degenerative and inflammatory conditions of the joints, most of them chronic. Joints generally consist of bone, cartilage, and connective tissue. Hyaline cartilage covers the articulating surface of the bone. This cartilage consists of type II collagen, chondrocytes, and proteoglycans. Proteoglycans are high molecular weight glycoproteins that retain water and provide resiliency of the cartilage. Essentially, the collagen provides tensile strength and the proteoglycans, distensibility. A capsule that is reinforced by ligaments on the outer surface and lined by synovial membrane on its inner surface surrounds the joint. The synovial membrane secretes the synovial fluid that lubricates the joint. Under normal conditions, the joint surfaces are congruent. Joint movements occur with minimal friction and joint loads (compressive and shear) that occur with regular activity pose no problem. Although osteoarthritis and rheumatoid arthritis have vastly different etiologies, both can result in joint destruction, whereby congruence is reduced and friction increased. The joint may become painful, stiff, and less able to withstand normal forces. Both rheumatoid arthritis and osteoarthritis lead to physical dysfunction and may also lead to disability. Chronic conditions, including different forms of arthritis, are highly prevalent in the older population and frequently associated with joint degeneration, pain, stiffness, and loss of mobility. Prevalence estimates of pain from these conditions range from 10 to 71%.[3-6] Disability estimates also vary widely, ranging from 5 to 90%.[7,8]

Osteoarthritis is primarily a degenerative condition, characterized initially by focal and progressive hyaline (articular) cartilage loss. The disease process can ultimately affect the whole joint and its surrounding structures. This most common form of arthritis affects approximately 16 to 23 million Americans older than 60 years of age; it is also one of the more debilitating diseases

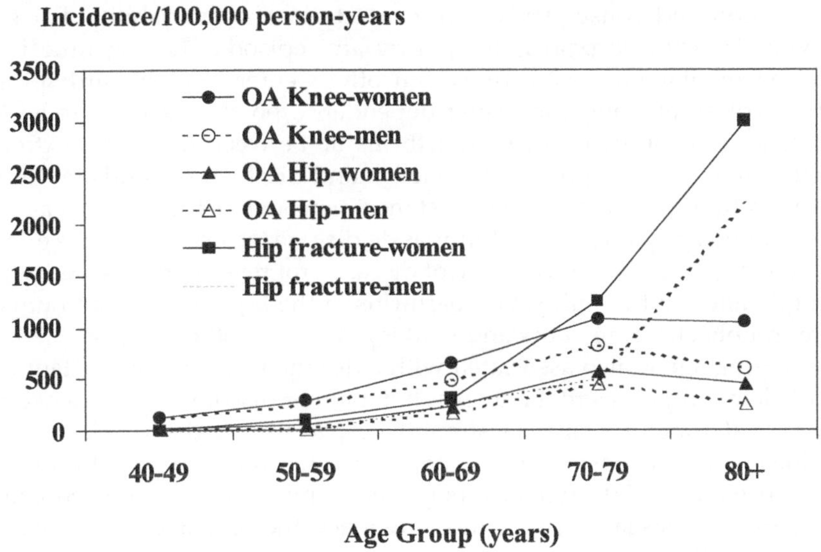

FIGURE 9.1
Incidence rates of knee and hip osteoarthritis (OA) and proximal femur (hip) fractures for men and women. (From References 9 and 17.)

in the U.S. More than 80% of people over the age of 75 years have clinical osteoarthritis and more than 80% of people over the age of 50 have radiologic evidence of the condition. Before the age of 50 years, the prevalence of osteoarthritis in most joints is higher in men than in women. After the age of 50 years, the prevalence of osteoarthritis in women's hands, knees, and feet increases relative to that of men (see Figure 9.1). Osteoarthritis also occurs in younger individuals who have undergone trauma.[9]

Rheumatoid arthritis is the second most common type of arthritis. It is an autoimmune systemic disease destructive to joints, and can be extremely debilitating. Rheumatoid arthritis affects women more frequently than men, regardless of age. The disease generally occurs between the ages of 20 to 50 years. The prevalence rate of rheumatoid arthritis is approximately 1 to 2% of adults. Rheumatoid arthritis affects 2.1 million Americans, approximately 1.5 million women compared to 600,000 men. The prevalence of rheumatoid arthritis increases with age and is found in about 10% of adults older than 65 years of age. A variant of rheumatoid arthritis, elderly onset rheumatoid arthritis has its onset at age 60 years or older and has a more equal gender distribution.[10]

The most common type of pain experienced by the elderly is that associated with degenerative joint conditions. In 1994, the U.S. Centers for Disease Control and Prevention (CDC) reported that, by the year 2000, arthritis would show the largest increase in new patients of any disease in the U.S. Although arthritis is one of the most widely experienced health-related problems, and is incredibly costly in both human and economic terms, its presentation and consequences are characterized by variability. For some individuals, arthritic pain is temporary and episodic, having little if any effect on regular physical activity, but others enter a downward spiral of distress, disability, and increasing dependence on the health care system. The majority of individuals with arthritis lie between these two extremes; whether they become physically inactive and disabled depends on myriad factors in multiple domains. For instance, personal factors such as age and gender influence pain and disability, as do disease factors such as the number and type of joints affected, the rate of disease progression, pain severity, joint strength, and joint mobility. Osteoarthritis of the hip and knee accounts for more trouble climbing stairs and walking than any other disease.[11]

Increasing age is also associated with a decline in several important musculoskeletal properties that may result in pain or discomfort with a decrease in physical function. Muscle strength, especially in the trunk and legs, declines with increasing age especially after the age of 60 years (see Chapters 6 and 7). Lifestyle factors related to physical activity, occupational demands, and social support also influence the extent of disability and resulting quality of life. Arthritis affects individuals during their working life and can thus cause a considerable economic burden in terms of lost work time, early retirement, and disability payments. The associations between arthritis and joint stiffness, muscle weakness, and obesity have been recognized for many years, but only recently has it been recognized that these are often consequences of inactivity secondary to arthritis rather than part of the disease process per se. Moreover, it appears that, in many instances, obesity actually antedates osteoarthritis. The CDC has recently emphasized the importance of treating arthritis early and aggressively and, in the case of rheumatoid arthritis, before cartilage destruction has occurred.[12]

9.2.2 Osteoporosis

The definition of osteoporosis, simply stated, is a skeletal disorder where one is predisposed to an increased risk of fracture because of compromised bone strength.[2] Osteoporosis is generally categorized as primary or secondary, based on the absence or presence of clinical disorders. Primary osteoporosis, also referred to as involutional osteoporosis, has been separated further into two entities: postmenopausal osteoporosis (type I) and senile or age-related osteoporosis (type II).[13,14] The low bone mass (osteopenia) associated with exercise-related amenorrhea (athletic amenorrhea) has been described as a variant of primary osteoporosis because it presents underlying hormone deficiencies similar to those seen in postmenopausal osteoporosis.[13]

Secondary osteoporotic bone loss is the result of a specific, defined clinical disorder. It falls into several categories: genetic disorders, hypogonadal states, endocrine disorders, gastrointestinal diseases, hematologic disorders, connective tissue disease, nutritional deficiencies, side effects of drugs (for example, glucocorticoid-induced osteoporosis), hypogonadism, and celiac disease.[2] The focus of this chapter is on primary or involutional osteoporosis.

Since bone mineral density (BMD) has a direct and strong relationship to fracture incidence, the World Health Organization (WHO) has devised the following operational definitions:

- Osteopenia (low bone mass): BMD between 1 and 2.5 standard deviations (SD) below the young normal mean
- Osteoporosis: BMD more than 2.5 standard deviations below the mean for young white adults
- Established osteoporosis: history of one or more fragility fractures[15]

The WHO diagnostic criteria for osteoporosis are based exclusively on bone mass and have several limitations. Bone mineral density can be used to assess an individual's prospective, long-term risk of fracture; however, bone mineral density does not predict the presence or absence of an osteoporotic fracture accurately.[13] The applicability of this approach to men and nonwhite women also remains unknown. Finally, a finding of current low bone density does not provide any information regarding the amount of peak bone mass attained, the subsequent degree of bone loss, or the quality of bone that remains.[13]

Although the WHO operational definition of osteoporosis has its limitations, it has fostered better estimates of prevalence, including figures for men and nonwhite women.[1] Some comparisons have failed to control adequately for habitual physical activity, diet, and social class; nevertheless, the prevalence of osteoporosis and the incidence of established osteoporosis (fractures) seem to vary by sex, race, and ethnicity. Much of the difference in fracture rates appears to be explained by differences in bone mineral density (reflecting both peak bone mass acquisition and rate of bone loss), bone geometry, and other factors such as risk of falls.[2,16]

Of all the fracture sites, hip fractures have by far the most profound impact from both the individual and the public health perspective. The incidence of proximal femoral fractures rises exponentially with age in most populations. After menopause, the incidence in women is approximately twice that in men[17] (see Figure 9.1). A far greater proportion of women who sustain a hip fracture become functionally dependent in daily living activities (10%) in comparison to those with vertebral fractures (4%) and distal forearm fractures (1%).[1] Furthermore, hip fractures are the predominant cause of deaths from osteoporotic fractures, accounting for a major share of the medical cost. The estimated lifetime risks of a hip fracture for white women and men in the U.S. are 13 to 18% and 6%, respectively.[1,18] High lifetime hip fracture rates (approximately 14% and 5%, respectively) have also been reported in Swedish women and men; these rates could easily double if life expectancy increases as projected.[1] Although the WHO definition of osteoporosis was established for white women, because of insufficient data for other population groups, bone loss from the proximal femur is similar for women of all races. The prevalence of hip fractures appears to be lower in Hispanic women (12%), black women (8%), and Asian women compared to white women.[1,18] The observed differences were originally attributed to the high BMD in black women. However, when bone density is adjusted for bone size, race-specific differences in bone density are reduced or eliminated.[1] Also, Asian women have a lower BMD than white women, so a higher hip fracture incidence would have been expected in Asians. These findings suggest that low BMD is not the only possible explanation and perhaps biomechanical differences or reduced risk of falling may be involved.[16] The prevalence of vertebral fractures appears to be comparable among women of different races.[1]

9.3 Etiology and Risk Factors

9.3.1 Rheumatoid/Osteoarthritis

Osteoarthritis is a complex disease that can be defined either by symptoms or by pathology.[9] The disease process affects the whole joint and its surrounding structures and is characterized initially by focal and progressive loss of hyaline cartilage. As the cartilage becomes damaged, there is not only progressive thinning of the tissue but also a decrease in proteoglycan synthesis and a destructive cascade of action by metalloproteinases and lysosomal proteases. The joint synovium becomes moderately inflamed, and there are concomitant changes in subchondral bone that include increased thickening (sclerosis) and osteophyte formation. Osteoarthritis is generally characterized by an asymmetrical involvement of large weight bearing joints. Lax ligaments, weakened muscles, and pain with joint use complete the main features of this disease.

Discussion at a recent National Institutes of Health (NIH) conference considered the question whether osteoarthritis was a single disease or comprised many distinct disorders with a final common pathway.[9] The consensus statement provided evidence that osteoarthritis comprises several distinct entities, including the fact that osteoarthritis in the knee and hip appears to be associated with different risk factors than osteoarthritis of the spine. Genetic and/or systemic factors appear to be more important in "generalized osteoarthritis." One classification system divides individuals with osteoarthritis according to whether the cause is known (secondary) or unknown (primary). Another classification system specific to the hip divides individuals according to whether the disease leads to bone hypertrophy and osteophyte formation or to atrophy.[9] Although osteoarthritis is generally considered a degenerative rather than an inflammatory disease, there is clearly an inflammatory component with systemic effects.[19]

Systemic risk factors for osteoarthritis appear to include ethnicity, hormonal status, bone density, nutritional status, genetics, and certain biochemical markers. The literature is contradictory regarding the influence of ethnicity. When comparing osteoarthritis of the hip and knee between African American males and females and white males and females, the NHANES I survey reported a higher prevalence of knee osteoarthritis in African American women (but not in men), but no ethnic differences in the prevalence of osteoarthritis of the hip.[20,21] In contrast, the Johnston County Osteoarthritis Project, a survey from the rural south of the U.S., found no difference in the prevalence of knee osteoarthritis between African American and white individuals but a higher prevalence of hip osteoarthritis in African American males compared to whites.[9,22] The contradictory findings suggest that factors other than ethnicity play a role; these probably include lifestyle and socioeconomic factors.

Genetic factors have been examined in twin studies, and appear to account for 50% of osteoarthritis in the hands and hips.[23] It seems likely that genetic factors affect disease occurrence in many joints, although it is also possible that there are specific genes for specific sites.[9] Elucidation of the genes responsible for osteoarthritis at specific sites may clarify the existence of distinct osteoarthritis disease entities. Hormones, especially an estrogen deficiency, have been implicated in osteoarthritis; however, studies examining the potential role of estrogen in prevention or progression of osteoarthritis are contradictory. Again, this suggests that other factors such as a healthy lifestyle are involved in disease prevention.[9] There appears to be an inverse relationship between the incidence of osteoarthritis and osteoporosis. Women with knee and hip osteoarthritis and osteophyte formation have greater bone density and lose bone more slowly around menopause than do their nonosteoarthritic peers.[24,25] The association between obesity and osteoarthritis has been evident for many years, but whether obesity was a cause or a consequence of the disease was unclear. It now appears that obesity not only predates osteoarthritis, but also increases the rate of disease progression, especially in women and in those with osteoarthritis of the knee.[26,27]

Another feature of osteoarthritis that appears to differ between men and women is the degree of joint stiffness, especially stiffness of the joint cartilage. A reduction in cartilage compressive stiffness is one of the first manifestations of osteoarthritis, preceding cartilage erosion.[9] Abnormal mechanical stress on joint cartilage appears to increase the risk of cartilage erosion. The development of osteoarthritis subsequent to joint trauma is well established, although the mechanisms are unclear. Risk factors for posttraumatic osteoarthritis include joint biomechanical factors such as residual joint instability and malalignment, personal factors such as obesity, and lifestyle factors such as a very high (or perhaps a very low) level of physical activity (recreational or occupational).

The fact that physical activity is both a risk factor and a treatment for osteoarthritis is testament to the complex nature of the interactions among the disorder, physical activity, and lifestyle. Occupational or recreational activities associated with excessive, repetitive, or high-impact joint loads are risk factors for osteoarthritis. In contrast, moderate physical activity such as running decreases the risk for osteoarthritis, at least in men.[28] Muscle weakness is associated with osteoarthritis, but it remains unclear whether it is a contributor to or a consequence of the condition. Muscle strength or weakness is related to the level of habitual physical activity and lifestyle, but weakness of the quadriceps may itself be a risk factor for structural damage to the knee joint.[29] The risk of osteoarthritis due to muscle weakness seems greater in women than in men, but this may be due in part to their relative weakness and to corresponding differences of lean body mass between women and men.

In sum, osteoarthritis is a complex disease, or series of diseases, with risk factors in multiple domains. The relative contribution of each of these factors is unclear, but it is likely that the occurrence, progression, and effect of osteoarthritis on disability are based on interplay, interaction, and linkages among these multiple factors. Some of the factors associated with the occurrence of specific diseases such as arthritis cannot be modified. They include genetic influences, age and gender, and some anthropometric characteristics such as height and body build. Other factors such as overweight/obesity, physical fitness, and smoking habits are modifiable, albeit with difficulty and with mixed success. Exercise has played a changing role in the management of arthritis. Historically, rest and avoidance of physical activity were the mainstays of treatment; however, it is now apparent that inactivity causes many of the same problems originally attributed to arthritis (e.g., muscle weakness, decreased flexibility) and obesity.

Rheumatoid arthritis is a systemic inflammatory disorder arising from a pathological reaction of the immune system against joint tissues and involving multiple joints. A chronic disease that affects primarily synovial joints, it is also a systemic disease, so manifestations such as fever, weight loss, skin thinning, corneal ulcers, and formation of subperiosteal nodules may develop. The etiology is unknown; it may be multifactorial, including immune reactions to viral, bacterial, and/or environmental events. Release of cytokines, proinflammatory mediators, and proteinases participates in the ultimate destruction of the joint.

The disease begins with an inflammatory reaction in the synovium. Monocytes and macrophages are activated by an autoimmune process. They interact with and present antigen to the T cells. The inflammatory biochemical cascade results in further activation of monocytes, macrophages, T and B cell activation, and increased endothelial cell activity. Polymorphonuclear cells are attracted to the inflamed joint by the elaboration of multiple cytokines, some of which may further enhance the inflammatory process. Several cytokines, including IL-1 α or β, IL-8, TNF-α, platelet-derived growth factor and heparin-binding growth factor, IFN-γ, TGF-α, IL-2, and IL-6 lead to increased activation of fibroblast-like cells in the synovium. This activates the release of prostaglandins, and proteinases such as collagenase, with the recruitment of osteoclast precursors culminating in destruction of bone and cartilage by the invasive proliferative synovium. The progression of rheumatoid arthritis is variable. Some individuals have a very mild form of the disease with spontaneous remission, but for others rheumatoid arthritis progresses in a series of acute exacerbations and remissions, with ultimate destruction of the joints involved. Elderly-onset rheumatoid arthritis is characterized by a higher frequency of acute systemic manifestations, involvement of the shoulder, greater radiographic damage, and greater functional decline.[10] This may be because degenerative joint changes predated the elderly-onset rheumatoid arthritis.

The diagnosis of rheumatoid arthritis is based on history, physical examination, and laboratory tests. Individuals usually present with symmetrical involvement of small and large joints. They may complain of weight loss and fatigue. Depending on the duration, activity, and acuity of the disease, individuals may present with red, warm, swollen, and painful joints and uncontrolled systemic disease, or with subacute or chronic joint symptoms and no signs of active inflammation. Laboratory tests reveal the presence of rheumatoid factor in more than 90% of affected individuals. The radiographic abnormalities may include evidence of juxta-articular osteoporosis, marginal joint erosions, and joint space narrowing due to cartilage erosion. Women with rheumatoid arthritis have been found to have decreased bone mineral density in both the axial and appendicular skeleton when compared to cohorts of similar age.[30] Both steroid use and the level of physical function appear to contribute to the relatively low levels of BMD and the risk of osteoporotic fractures. Thus management of rheumatoid arthritis to prevent physical dysfunction and avoidance of long-term steroid use when possible should decrease the risk of osteoporotic fracture.

9.3.2 Osteoporosis

Osteoporosis is a complex dynamic process where genetic factors act alone or in concert with physical, hormonal, nutritional, and pharmacological influences to diminish skeletal integrity.[13] These factors not only impact adult bone mass, but also modify the acquisition of peak bone mass. Bone mass at any time in adult life reflects the difference between the peak amount attained at skeletal maturity and subsequent losses.[13] Thus, the two major risk factors for developing osteoporosis are a low peak bone mass and the magnitude of subsequent bone loss. Knowledge of both these variables and their interaction is necessary in order to understand the pathogenesis of osteoporosis.

The three major functions of bone are (1) mechanical support, (2) homeostasis of calcium and other ions, and (3) hemopoiesis.[13,31] Changes in bone are the result of continual processes of bone resorption and bone formation, together known as bone remodeling. Remodeling is initiated by stimuli generated to meet the three functions of bone;[31] the process occurs throughout the life span. Once peak bone mass has been achieved, bone formation generally equals bone resorption, so the density of the bone remains unchanged. Peak bone density (or peak bone mass) is defined for most purposes as the highest amount of bone mass attained during life. Bone loss begins when bone resorption exceeds formation, whether through an increase in resorption, a decrease in formation, or a combination of the two processes.

Peak bone mass appears to be achieved between the ages of 16 and 40 years, depending on the type of bone tissue (whether cortical or trabecular) and the site examined.[32,33] Spinal bone density has been reported to increase significantly during the 20s, peaking in the mid-30s; bone loss then begins at a rate of about 1% per year.[34] However, it has also been estimated that spinal bone density peaks around the time of epiphyseal plate closure, when longitudinal growth ceases, or that trabecular bone mass reaches its peak prior to the age of 20, but that cortical bone mass does not peak until the mid-30s.[34] Other researchers indicate that most of the skeletal mass has accumulated in both cortical and trabecular bone by the average age of 18.[32] Bone mass peaks earlier in women than in men. The greater bone mass in men compared to women reflects the prolonged duration of pubertal maturation rather than a greater rate of bone accretion.[35] Although the age at which peak bone density is achieved is debated, genetics appear to have a major influence on when and how much peak bone mass is attained, particuarly at sites with a high proportion of trabecular bone, such as the lumbar vertebrae and Ward's triangle in the femur.[36] Although genetics are a significant determinant of bone density in the young, a genetic component is less often seen in adults.[37] This suggests the important influence of other factors, such as exercise, nutrition, or estrogen, on the amount of bone mass found in the adult.[37]

The total magnitude of bone loss as an adult is influenced by duration and rate of loss. In normal remodeling, the bone removed by the resorbing cells (osteoclasts) is replaced by an equal amount of bone formed by the osteoblasts. Bone loss results if either the amount of bone removed by the osteoclasts is more than the amount deposited by the osteoblasts, or the amount of bone deposited is less than that removed. The former is osteoclast-mediated bone loss and is the remodeling abnormality observed in type I or postmenopausal osteoporosis. The latter is osteoblast-mediated, and is responsible for type II or age-related bone loss.[14]

Type I osteoporosis typically impacts postmenopausal women within 15 to 20 years of menopause. The accelerated bone loss observed around menopause is predominantly due to estrogen deficiency. The phase of rapid bone loss normally lasts 4 to 8 years; however, in 10 to 20% of postmenopausal women who develop type I osteoporosis, the phase of rapid bone loss is prolonged for 15 to 20 years. At present, it is unclear what factors other than estrogen deficiency contribute to the increased bone resorption in postmenopausal osteoporosis.[14] Recent findings suggest that cytokines, a potent inducer of bone resorption, may play a role in type I osteoporosis.[14]

Type II osteoporosis occurs in men and women over the age of 70 years; it is twice as common in women as in men.[14] Even though the rates of bone loss are similar in elderly men and women, the accelerated bone loss at menopause, along with environmental factors, explains the twofold gender disparity in the incidence of hip fractures. The major causes for age-related slow bone loss in the entire population of men and women are secondary hyperparathyroidism (PTH), impaired osteoblast function, vitamin D deficiency (especially among house-bound elderly), and estrogen deficiency. A decrease in intestinal calcium absorption causes a rise in PTH resulting in an increased bone turnover. The impaired osteoblast function results in a remodeling imbalance; it may reflect a decrease in the number and/or sensitivity of the osteoblasts. The level of parathyroid function distinguishes type I from type II osteoporosis. In type I osteoporosis, PTH may be normal or decreased as a response to increased bone loss. The opposite is observed in type II osteoporosis: PTH concentrations increase with age, and are higher among osteoporotic hip-fracture patients than in age-matched controls.

There are also differences in the fracture site and the type of bone lost between the two categories of osteoporosis. The two main forms of bone tissue are cortical and trabecular. The proportions of the two types of bone differ throughout the body. Cortical or compact bone forms the dense outer wall of bone; it comprises almost 80% of the total skeleton, and trabecular bone makes up the remaining 20%. Trabecular bone, also known as cancellous or spongy bone, is found at the ends of long bones within the central core of their shafts, and is the primary component of the vertebrae. Trabecular bone has a much higher surface to volume ratio than cortical bone, making it much more active metabolically. Cortical bone may be more responsive to weight bearing or mechanical stress than is trabecular bone. Trabecular bone seems to be influenced more by hormonal or metabolic factors and is susceptible to fracture. The predominant location of fractures in the two osteoporotic syndromes is determined by the respective proportions of trabecular or cancellous bone. In the type I condition, fractures occur at sites that contain 50 to 75% trabecular bone — for instance, the distal radius (Colles' fractures) and vertebral crush fractures. Fractures in the type II condition typically occur at the hip (femoral neck), which contains only 25 to 50% of trabecular bone.[14]

9.4 Role of Physical Activity

9.4.1 Rheumatoid/Osteoarthritis

Arthritis is a simple label for a complex multidimensional (biopsychosocial) problem that is managed rather than cured. Exercise plays an important role in that management. Most individuals with arthritis adapt to and cope with persistent and recurrent symptoms of pain and limitation of physical activity. General exercise and physical activities are not harmful to the arthritic process, as was once thought. This is an important conceptual shift that may not yet be fully recognized and practiced. Although vigorous exercise is contraindicated in the presence of acute inflammation (hot, swollen, and painful joints) or uncontrolled systemic disease,[38] it is otherwise recommended. Unfortunately, prolonged physical inactivity can put individuals at risk for a variety of inactivity-related health problems such as cardiovascular disease and obesity. Philbin et al.[39] reported that individuals with severe osteoarthritis were not only severely deconditioned ($\dot{V}O_{2\,peak}$ 12.8 and 14.9 ml/[kg·min] for individuals with osteoarthritic knees and hips, respectively), but also had more frequent manifestations of coronary heart disease compared to an age- and gender-matched cohort. Likewise, physical inactivity can have deleterious effects on muscle strength and joint range of motion, further aggravating the arthritic process. Weak muscles are less able either to attenuate impact loads on the joints or to provide for joint stability. Decreased joint motion and elasticity of the periarticular tissues hinder cartilage nutrition and repair.[40] The beneficial effects of exercise on local joint structures, physical function, and psychological mood are all well established. Clinical guidelines now recommend that management of arthritis should be based on a combination of exercise/activity and education. Unfortunately, adherence to the recommended exercise and physical activity remains problematic. A variety of factors account for this including, it seems, basic human nature.

Castaneda and colleagues[41] characterized the activity behavior of 70 men and 126 women with osteoarthritis who were aged 60 years or older. Walking was the most common form of exercise for both men and women in this group. However, fewer women than men reported exercising regularly. There was no difference in health care utilization between men and women who exercised. However, exercise behavior was best predicted by differing factors in men and women. Quality of well-being was the best predictor of exercise participation in women, whereas extroversion was the best predictor in men. This indicates the strong influence of psychosocial rather than disease-related variables upon exercise habits. Current exercise behavior in the combined group (men and women) was also influenced by the perceived benefits of exercise. Individuals with longer disease durations appeared to perceive fewer benefits from exercise.[42] Whether the *perceived* benefit/cost ratio is matched by the *actual* benefit/cost ratio is unclear. Disease duration may or may not be matched with the level of joint destruction. However, individuals with longer disease durations may have been inactive for longer and they may thus have experienced pain associated with inadequately managed movement. They may have avoided activity that aggravates pain, in the mistaken belief that pain and ongoing tissue injury are closely related. Although this is a reasonable assumption in the case of acute pain, it is not so for chronic ongoing pain. A variety of neural and biochemical mechanisms contribute to persistent pain, and these do not indicate ongoing tissue damage.

Regardless of the reasons for physical inactivity, the consequences are clear: prolonged inactivity influences the physical characteristics of the arthritic joint, decreasing muscle strength and joint range of motion. Physiological fitness (for example, $\dot{V}O_{2\,max}$) is also diminished, and the sense of psychological well-being may be reduced. Psychosocial distress and depression can be a consequence of physical dysfunction and inactivity. Given the cumulative physical and psychological consequences of prolonged inactivity, individuals with arthritis may perceive the ratio of the anticipated effort associated with an increase of physical activity and the potentially modest immediate gains in condition too great to change their level of habitual activity.

It is ironic that the anticipated effort of exercise participation may preclude exercise adoption, when in fact regular participation in aerobic type exercise would decrease perceived fatigue.[43] Fatigue can be particularly problematic in rheumatoid arthritis because of its systemic nature; however, aerobic exercise can reduce fatigue. Twenty-five individuals (14 women and 11 men) with rheumatoid arthritis completed a low impact aerobic exercise for 1 hour, 2 times a week for 12 weeks.[43] Fatigue increased initially and then decreased to its lowest point at the 12-week period. Unfortunately, the persistence of the decrease in fatigue and adherence of subjects to the exercise program remains unclear, and so warrants further study. The effects of age and gender on fatigue and other outcomes were not explored specifically in this small sample of patients.[43]

A variety of exercise regimens have been tested in individuals with osteoarthritis and rheumatoid arthritis, but data are very limited in regard to the specific influences of gender and age. The literature is characterized by heterogeneity. Studies differ in regard to the subjects sampled and the stage of their disease, the types of exercise regimen (intensity, type, and duration), the location of exercise (community or clinic) and the extent of supervision, the methods of measuring outcomes, and the length of follow-up. Despite many interstudy differences of methodology, there is consistent support for the notion that exercise and physical activity can and should play a role in both prevention and rehabilitation. Nevertheless, activities associated with excessive, repetitive, or high-impact joint loads are risk factors for arthritis and should be avoided.

Muscle weakness is both a risk factor for and a consequence of arthritis; women appear to be at greater risk than men.[29] Sarcopenia, loss of muscle mass and strength, is a normal part of aging, but it is accelerated by physical inactivity and may be aggravated further by arthritis. Toda et al.[44] assessed lean body mass in 235 Japanese women aged between 45 and 69 years. The sample included 117 women who had suffered from osteoarthritis of the knee for less than 5 years, and 118 age- and gender-matched controls. The lean body mass in the legs (but not in the arms or trunk) was significantly lower in the osteoarthritic group than in the controls. No correlation was seen between lean body mass and disease duration or disease severity; the correlation between lean body mass and level of physical activity was not reported.

Komatireddy and associates[45] evaluated the effects of a 12-week resistance exercise regimen on functional impairment and physiological outcomes. Individuals participated in low load resistance circuit training 3 times a week for 12 weeks. There were significant improvements in grip strength, sit-to-stand time, and treadmill time, but no change in $\dot{V}O_{2\,peak}$ at reassessment. Individuals improved in function but not fitness; more importantly, the number of painful joints decreased. The mechanism of this change is not clear. It may include such physiological and psychological factors as improvements in joint circulation and mobility, decreased anxiety, or an exercise-induced improvement in well-being that enhanced the individual's ability to cope with pain.

Walking is the most frequently adopted recreational activity. Its effectiveness has been investigated in arthritis. Although walking improves both postural stability and function, adherence is a problem.[46,47] Measurable improvements in function can be achieved in the short term (8 weeks), but they are not maintained (at 1 year) at least in part because adherence to walking programs is poor.[47]

Exercise compliance in older participants with knee osteoarthritis was examined by Rejeski et al.[48] Study participants (n = 439) were randomly assigned to a 3-week center phase, followed by a 15-month home phase of aerobic exercise, resistance exercise, or health education. Prior exercise behavior was the single best predictor of time spent exercising. Factors such as demographics, psychosocial characteristics, fitness level, and extent of disability did not contribute to description of the time spent exercising at any phase of the trial, supporting the notion that a complex and poorly understood multiplicity of factors influences exercise participation.

The one fairly robust finding across studies of exercise adherence is past exercise behavior. Enjoyment of exercise and attitudes towards exercise probably influence perceptual judgments of the benefits of exercise, especially in those with arthritis. Optimistic judgments about the benefits of exercise may be due in part to exercise-induced mood improvements. However, it is also plausible that individuals engaging in regular physical activity have accrued less joint damage than their sedentary counterparts, despite a prolonged duration of joint disease. The fact that current exercise behavior appears to be best predicted by past exercise behavior is not surprising, but it is disconcerting, given that those individuals who most need to exercise are also those who are least likely to exercise. Further research must focus on the barriers to exercise and methods of encouraging and maintaining an active lifestyle across the life span.

9.4.2 Osteoporosis

Physical activity and exercise have important roles in allowing individuals to attain peak bone mass, reducing subsequent rates of bone loss, and modifying the risk of muscle weakness-related falls. However, the extent of benefit remains controversial, and optimal training programs for maximizing peak bone mass and maintaining skeletal integrity have yet to be defined.[49,50] Data on the effects of physical activity and exercise on bone density are conflicting. It is not surprising that disparities exist, given the complex interactions of bone metabolism with diet, hormones, genetics, and aging. Conflicts in the results may also be a function of differences in study design, types of exercise intervention, and techniques of determining bone density and the sites measured.

Based on current experimental knowledge, it has been proposed that an osteogenic exercise regime should include load-bearing activities at high magnitude with few repetitions, creating versatile strain distributions throughout the bone structure (i.e., loading the bone in directions to which it is unaccustomed); it should also be long term and progressive in nature.[51,52] Difficulty arises when trying to determine whether specific physical activities, sports, or exercises meet these osteogenic criteria. The variety of terms used to describe exercise adds to the confusion: weight-bearing or non-weight-bearing; impact or nonimpact; strength, resistance or endurance, aerobic; loading or nonloading. For example, walking is a weight-bearing exercise when compared to swimming; however, whether the bone is sufficiently loaded depends on the initial fitness level and the bone mineral density of the individual.[49]

Critical interpretation of the literature involves evaluating the exercise program on the five basic principles of physical training: (1) specificity, (2) overload, (3) reversibility, (4) initial values, and (5) diminishing returns.[49] Physical exercise creates an osteogenic response in the elderly if the mechanical stress is indeed an overload. In a classic early study, Dalsky and her associates[53] examined the impact of weight-bearing exercises, including walking, jogging, and stair climbing, in postmenopausal women between 55 and 70 years of age. After 9 months, the exercise group showed a significant gain in bone mineral density (5.2%) compared to the 1.4% decrease in the controls ($n = 18$). Despite the expected increase in aerobic power (17%) of the exercise group, there was no correlation between aerobic power ($\dot{V}O_{2\,max}$) and bone mineral content. Eleven of the 17 original individuals from the exercise group continued the exercise regimen for an additional 13 months; however, the lumbar bone mineral density did not show any appreciable further increase (+1.6%). Nevertheless, a greater change in bone mass might have been observed during the additional year of training if exercise intensity had been increased. Stopping the exercise program or training less than three days per week caused the lumbar bone mineral density to return to baseline values. These findings support the first three of the five principles of training: bone adaptation occurs from a *specific* exercise *overload* to the skeletal system, which may involve different exercises from those prescribed for cardiovascular fitness. Also, bone modeling is a dynamic process coupled to a continuing load stimulus, as evidenced in the *reversing* of bone mass gain in the detrained individuals.

Whether an exercise intervention increases bone mass or not depends on the initial bone mineral density (principle of initial values). Individuals with a low bone mass at the start of a training program would be expected to show a greater increase in bone mass than those with a higher bone mass.[49] Further, gains in bone mineral density would be expected to be small if an individual were approaching his or her biological ceiling (principle of diminishing returns).[49] The impact of these principles on the interpretation of findings is illustrated in a study conducted by Nichols et al.[54] The authors examined the impact of a high-intensity resistance program on elderly women. The resistance exercise program comprised 8 exercises, 3 sets of 3 exercises with 10 to 12 repetitions per set, conducted 3 times per week for 1 year. No significant increases in bone mineral density were found. These findings would appear to contradict other studies which found significant increases with a similar program in premenopausal women[55,56] and in postmenopausal women who performed fewer sets and repetitions.[57] However, in the study of Nichols et al., the women were very active prior to recruitment, and they had a high baseline bone mineral density. Thus, the exercise program was unlikely to yield any gains.[58]

Another explanation for inconsistency in the literature on exercise and bone mass stems from study design. Most reviews do not distinguish among epidemiological studies, longitudinal observational studies, and randomized vs. nonrandomized intervention studies.[50,59] The best studies to generate causal inferences are randomized intervention trials; epidemiological and observational studies are subject to selection bias.[50,59] Meta-analysis allows a systematic pooling of results from interventional studies examining the overall relative effect of exercise on bone mass.

Wolff and colleagues[59] conducted such a meta-analysis of published randomized and nonrandomized controlled trials in pre-and postmenopausal women. Sixty-two articles were found between 1966 and 1996; however, only 16 randomized control trials and nine nonrandomized control trials met the inclusion criteria of being human prospective studies with two or more interventions. Overall, the exercise training programs prevented or reversed bone loss by almost 1% per year relative to controls, regardless of menopausal status, compared with the controls. The exercise training programs varied in type, intensity, frequency, and duration; therefore, specific exercise recommendations could not be developed. In the nonrandomized controlled trials, the overall treatment effect was twice as high, illustrating the confounding impact of nonrandomization in clinical trials. The length of the training programs ranged from 6 to 24 months; therefore, the impact of longer duration exercise programs remains unknown.

Wallace and Cumming[50] conducted a similar meta-analysis, but limited their literature search to randomized trials conducted between 1977 and 1998. They examined the types of exercise programs, classifying them as either impact or nonimpact, based on typical ground reaction forces for the activities specified. They did not explore the effects of intensity and duration of the exercise program. Impact exercises included walking, running, aerobics, and "heel drops" (raising the body weight onto the toes and dropping the heels to the floor with knees and hips extended). Nonimpact exercises included studies that involved strength training through weight lifting (free weights, weight machines, or weighted backpacks). The nonimpact studies were labeled by several different terms (resistance training, strength training, and weightlifting), although they all involved similar weight lifting exercise programs differing only in the number of sets and repetitions. This illustrates the need to adopt a standard nomenclature for this area of research. Overall, weight-bearing exercises that loaded the skeleton through ground-reaction forces yielded a positive effect in both pre- and postmenopausal women of approximately 1.5% at the lumbar spine and 1% at the femoral neck. Non-impact exercise (strength training through weight lifting) had a positive effect at the lumbar spine (approximately 1.0%) in pre-and postmenopausal women, but studies were too few to draw conclusions on the femoral neck. Based upon these systematic reviews of randomized investigations, the effect of exercise on bone mass appears to be a gain of approximately 1% per year, regardless of menopausal status. Data comparing male and female subjects are limited, and essentially nonexistent when examining interaction between age- and gender-specific exercise responses.[60] It appears that men and women respond similarly to high-impact aerobics.[60,61]

Data on the role of exercise in combination with calcium intake are conflicting. Uncertainty may stem from the fact that, although calcium is crucial to skeletal integrity, its role in the development of osteoporosis is more permissive than causal.[62] In a critical review of the literature, Specker[63] found indirect evidence that the beneficial effects of exercise on bone may only occur with calcium intakes greater than 1000 mg/day. Conversely, the beneficial effect of calcium may only be present when physical activity is adequate. The additive effects of exercise, calcium supplementation, and hormone-replacement therapy have been examined in postmenopausal women.[64-66] The efficacy of estrogen therapy was enhanced by combining it with weight-bearing exercises,[66] weight training,[64] and weight-bearing plus calcium supplementation.[65]

The most important benefit of physical activity and exercise for the frail elderly may not be an increase in bone mass per se, but a reduced risk of falling. The most common cause of osteoporotic hip fractures is falling.[67-69] Poor balance and muscle weakness play an essential role in increasing the propensity to fall. Strength training programs in older men and women, even during the ninth decade,[70] have resulted in substantial increases in muscle strength and neuromuscular performance (see Chapter 6). An optimal exercise prescription for decreasing the incidence of fractures should thus target an increase in muscle strength, balance, and agility, as well as the loading bone in a weight-bearing manner.

9.5 Conclusions

Osteoarthritis, rheumatoid arthritis, and osteoporosis are common yet complex diseases that are the most frequent causes of pain, limitation of physical activity, and decreased quality of life in the elderly. The prevalence of osteoarthritis increases with age, and after the age of 50 years it is more common in women than in men. Osteoporosis has been viewed as primarily a problem of older white women, although osteoporotic fractures are an important and growing problem among men and women of all races. There appears to be an inverse relationship between the development of osteoarthritis and the risk of osteoporosis. Women with knee and hip osteoarthritis and osteophyte formation have greater bone densities and lose bone more slowly around menopause than do their nonosteoarthritic peers. Rheumatoid arthritis is a systemic disease more common in women than in men, regardless of age. Physical inactivity due to arthritis places individuals at risk for other health problems, e.g., cardiovascular problems, obesity, and osteoporosis. Such inactivity also contributes to muscle weakness and joint stiffness, placing the joints at risk of further recurrent injury. Although arthritis can be disabling across the life span, the impact is greatest in elders if and when there is a low reserve capacity due to overall functional decline. Exercise and physical activity can reduce joint pain and stiffness, strengthening the supporting muscles and improving physical function without aggravating joint disease. However, exercise adherence remains problematic. Finally, physical activity and exercise programs can have not only direct osteogenic effects, but can also yield indirect benefits such as decreasing the propensity to fall and improving overall muscular strength.

Acknowledgments

The authors wish to express their gratitude to Ms. Juanita Hernandez for her help in researching material and to Dr. David Nichols for his critical review of the manuscript.

References

1. Melton, L.J., Who has osteoporosis? A conflict between clinical and public health perspectives, *J. Bone Miner. Res.*, 15, 2309–2314, 2000.
2. National Institutes of Health, Consensus Development Conference Statement, 1-36, National Institutes of Health, Bethesda, MD, 2000.
3. Lavsky-Shulen, M.R. et al., Prevalence and functional correlates of low back pain in the elderly. The Iowa 65+ rural study, *J. Am. Geriatr. Soc.*, 33, 23–28, 1985.
4. Brattburg, G., Thorslund, M., and Wikman, A., The prevalence of pain in a general population. The results of a postal survey in a county of Sweden, *Pain*, 37, 215–222, 1989.
5. Brochet, B. et al., Pain in the elderly: an epidemiological study in southwestern France, *Pain Clin.*, 5, 73–79, 1991.

6. McAlindon, T. et al., Knee pain and disability in the community, *Br. J. Rheumatol.*, 189–192, 1992.
7. Jette, A. and Branch, L., The Framingham disability study: II. Physical disability among the aging, *Am. J. Publ. Health,* 71, 1211–1216, 1981.
8. Canada and Health and Welfare, Aging and independence: overview of a national survey, Minister of Supply and Services, Ottawa, 1993.
9. Jordan, J. et al., Systemic risk factors for osteoarthritis, *Ann. Intern. Med.*, 133, 637–639, 2000.
10. van Schaardenburg, D., Rheumatoid arthritis in the elderly. Prevalence and optimal management, *Drugs Aging*, 7, 30–37, 1995.
11. Guccione, A. et al., The effects of specific medical conditions on functional limitations of elders in the Framingham study, *Am. J. Publ. Health,* 84, 351–358, 1994.
12. Marwick, C., Treat arthritis earlier, better, *JAMA,* 281, 2174, 1999.
13. Marcus, R., The nature of osteoporosis, in *Osteoporosis,* Marcus, R., Feldman, D., and Kelsey, J., Eds., Academic Press, San Diego, 1996, 647–659.
14. Kassem, M., Melton, L.J., and Riggs, B.L., The type I/type II model for involutional osteoporosis, in *Osteoporosis,* Marcus, R., Feldman, D., and Kelsey, J., Eds., Academic Press, San Diego, 1996, 691–702.
15. Kanis, J.A. et al., The diagnosis of osteoporosis, *J. Bone Miner. Res.*, 9, 1137–1141, 1994.
16. McCreadie, B.R. and Goldstein, S.A., Biomechanics of fracture: is bone mineral density sufficient to assess risk? *J. Bone Miner. Res.*, 15, 2305–2308, 2000.
17. Cooper, C. and Melton, L.J., Magnitude and impact of osteoporosis and fractures, in *Osteoporosis,* Marcus R., Feldman, D., and Kelsey, J., Eds., Academic Press, San Diego, 1996, 419–434.
18. Looker, A.C., et al., Prevalence of low femoral bone density in older U.S. women from NHANES III, *J. Bone Miner. Res.*, 10, 796–802, 1995.
19. Brandt, K., Osteoarthritis, in *Primer on the Rheumatoid Disease,* Schumacher, R., Klippel, J.H., and Koopman, J.S., Eds., Arthritis Foundation, Atlanta, 1993, 184–187.
20. Anderson, J. and Felson, D., Factors associated with osteoarthritis of the knee in the first national health and nutrition examination survey (HANES I). Evidence for an association with overweight, race, and physical demands of work, *Am. J. Epidemiol.*, 128, 179–189, 1988.
21. Tepper, S. and Hochberg, M., Factors associated with hip osteoarthritis: data from the first national health and nutrition examination survey (NHANES-I), *Am. J. Epidemiol.*, 137, 1081–1088, 1993.
22. Jordan, J. et al., The impact of arthritis in rural populations, *Arthritis Care Res.*, 8, 242–250, 1995.
23. Specter, T. et al., Genetic influences on osteoarthritis in women: a twin study, *Br. Med. J.*, 312, 940–943, 1996.
24. Nevitt, M. et al., Radiographic osteoarthritis of the hip and bone mineral density. The study of osteoporotic fractures research group, *Arthritis Rheum.*, 38, 907–916, 1995.
25. Hannon, M. et al., Bone mineral density and knee osteoarthritis in elderly men and women. The Framingham study, *Arthritis Rheum.*, 36, 1671–1680, 1993.
26. Manninen, P. et al., Overweight, gender and knee osteoarthritis, *Int. J. Obes. Relat. Metab. Disord.*, 20, 595–597, 1996.

27. Dougados, M. et al., Longitudinal radiologic evaluation of osteoarthritis of the knee, *J. Rheumatol.*, 19, 378–383, 1992.
28. Lane, N. et al., The risk of osteoarthritis with running and aging: a 5-year longitudinal study, *J. Rheumatol.*, 20, 461–468, 1993.
29. Slemenda, C. et al., Reduced quadriceps strength relative to body weight: a risk factor for knee osteoarthritis in women? *Arthritis Rheum.*, 41, 1951–1959, 1998.
30. Lane N. et al., Rheumatoid arthritis and bone mineral density in elderly women, *J. Bone Miner. Res.*, 1995, 10, 57–63.
31. Rodan, G.A., Coupling of bone resorption and formation during bone remodeling, in *Osteoporosis*, Marcus, R., Feldman, D., and Kelsey, J., Eds., Academic Press, San Diego, 1996, 289–299.
32. Matkovic, V. et al., Timing of peak bone mass in Caucasian females and its implication for the prevention of osteoporosis. Inference from a cross-sectional model, *J. Clin. Invest.*, 93, 799–808, 1994.
33. Theintz, G.B. et al., Longitudinal monitoring of bone mass accumulation in healthy adolescents: evidence for a marked reduction after 16 years of age at the levels of lumbar spine and femoral neck in female subjects, *J. Clin. Endocrinol. Metab.*, 75, 1060–1065, 1992.
34. Rodin, A. et al., Premenopausal bone loss in the lumbar spine and neck of femur: a study of 225 Caucasian women, *Bone*, 11, 1–5, 1990.
35. Bongour, J. and Rizzoli, R., Bone acquisition in adolescence, in *Osteoporosis*, Marcus, R., Feldman, D., and Kelsey, J., Eds., Academic Press, San Diego, 1996, 465–476.
36. Pocock, N.A. et al., Genetic determinants of bone mass in adults. A twin study, *J. Clin. Invest.*, 80, 706–710, 1987.
37. Dequeker, J. et al., Genetic determinants of bone mineral content at the spine and radius: a twin study, *Bone*, 8, 207–209, 1987.
38. Minor, M.A. and Kay, D.R., Arthritis, in *Exercise Management for Persons with Chronic Diseases and Disabilities*, Durstine, J.L., Ed., Human Kinetics, Champaign, IL, 1997, 149–154.
39. Philbin, E. et al., Cardiovascular fitness and health in patients with end-stage osteoarthritis, *Arthritis Rheumat.*, 38, 799–805, 1995.
40. Hochberg, M., McAlindon, T., and Felson, D., Systemic and topical treatments, *Ann. Intern. Med.*, 133, 726–729, 2000.
41. Castaneda, D., Bigatti, S., and Cronan, T., Gender and exercise behavior among women and men with osteoarthritis, *Women Health*, 27, 33–53, 1998.
42. Neuberger, G. et al., Determinants of exercise and aerobic fitness in outpatients with arthritis, *Nurs. Res.*, 43, 11–17, 1994.
43. Neuberger, G. et al., Effects of exercise on fatigue, aerobic fitness, and disease activity measures in persons with rheumatoid arthritis, *Res. Nurs. Health*, 20, 195–204, 1997.
44. Toda, Y. et al., Decline in lower extremity lean body mass per body weight is characteristic of women with early phase osteoarthritis of the knee, *J. Rheumatol.*, 27, 2449–2454, 2000.
45. Komaitireddy, G.R. et al., Efficacy of low load resistive muscle training in patients with rheumatoid arthritis functional class II and III, *J. Rheumatol.*, 24, 1531–1539, 1997.

46. Messier, S. et al., Long-term exercise and its effect on balance in older, osteoarthritic adults: results from the fitness, arthritis, and seniors trial (FAST), *J. Am. Geriatr. Soc.*, 48, 131–138, 2000.
47. Sullivan, T. et al., One-year follow-up of patients with osteoarthritis of the knee who participated in a program of supervised fitness walking and supportive patient education, *Arthritis Care Res.*, 11, 228–233, 1998.
48. Rejeski, W. et al., Compliance to exercise therapy in older participants with knee osteoarthritis: implications for treating disability, *Med. Sci. Sports Exerc.*, 29, 977–985, 1997.
49. Drinkwater, B.L. et al., ACSM position stand on osteoporosis and exercise, *Med. Sci. Sports Exerc.*, 27, i-vii, 1995.
50. Wallace, B.A. and Cumming, R.G., Systematic review of randomized trials of the effect of exercise on bone mass in pre- and postmenopausal women, *Calcif. Tissue Int.*, 67, 10–18, 2000.
51. Lanyon, L.E. and Rubin, C.T., Regulation of bone mass in response to physical activity, in *Osteoporosis, A Multidisciplinary Problem*. Dixon, A.J., Russell, R.G.G., and Stamp, T.B.C., Eds., Royal Society of Medicine, London, 1983, 51–61.
52. Skerry, T.M., Mechanical loading and bone: what sort of exercise is beneficial to the skeleton? *Bone*, 20, 179–181, 1997.
53. Dalsky, G.P. et al., Weight-bearing exercise training and lumbar bone mineral content in postmenopausal women, *Ann. Intern. Med.*, 108, 824–828, 1988.
54. Nichols, J.F. et al., Bone mineral density responses to high-intensity strength training in active older women, *J. Aging Phys. Act.*, 3, 26–38, 1995.
55. Lohman, T.G. et al., Effects of resistance training on regional and total bone mineral density in premenopausal women: a randomized prospective study, *J. Bone Min. Res.*, 10, 1015–1024, 1995.
56. Snow-Harter, C. et al., Effects of resistance and endurance exercise on bone mineral status of young women: a randomized exercise intervention trial, *J. Bone Min. Res.*, 7, 761–769, 1992.
57. Pruitt, L.A., Jackson, R.D., and Bartels, R.L., Weight-training effects on bone mineral density in early postmenopausal women, *J. Bone Min. Res.*, 7, 179–185, 1992.
58. Layne, J.E. and Nelson, M.E., The effects of progressive resistance training on bone density: a review, *Med. Sci. Sports Exerc.*, 31, 25–30, 1999.
59. Wolff, I. et al., The effect of exercise training programs on bone mass: a meta-analysis of published controlled trials in pre- and postmenopausal women, *Osteopor. Internat.*, 9, 1–12, 1999.
60. Beck, B. and Marcus, R., Impact of physical activity on age-related bone loss, in *The Aging Skeleton*, Rosen, C.J. and Glowacki, J., Eds., Academic Press, San Diego, 1999, 467–478.
61. Welsh, L. and Rutherford, O.M., Hip bone mineral density is improved by high-impact aerobic exercise in postmenopausal women and men over 50 years, *Eur. J. Appl. Physiol.*, 74, 511–517, 1996.
62. Heaney, R.P., The role of nutrition in prevention and management of osteoporosis, *Clin. Obstetr. Gynecol.*, 50, 833–846, 1987.
63. Specker, B.L., Evidence for an interaction between calcium intake and physical activity on changes in bone mineral density, *J. Bone Min. Res.*, 11, 1539–1544, 1996.

64. Notelovitz, M. et al., Estrogen therapy and variable-resistance weight training increase bone mineral in surgically menopausal women, *J. Bone Min. Res.*, 6, 583–590, 1991.
65. Prince, R.L., et al., Prevention of postmenopausal osteoporosis: a comparative study of exercise, calcium supplementation, and hormone-replacement therapy, *N. Engl. J. Med.*, 325, 1189–1195, 1991.
66. Kohrt, W.M. et al., Additive effects of weight-bearing exercise and estrogen on bone mineral density in older women, *J. Bone Min. Res.*, 10, 1303–1311, 1995.
67. Cummings, S.R. et al., Risk factors for hip fracture in white women, *N. Engl. J. Med.*, 332, 767–773, 1995.
68. Kannus, P., Preventing osteoporosis, falls, and fractures among elderly people. Promotion of lifelong physical activity is essential, *Br. Med. J.*, 318, 205–206, 1999.
69. Hayes, W.C. et al., Etiology and prevention of age-related hip fractures, *Bone*, 18, 77S-86S, 1996.
70. Fiatarone, M.A. et al., High-intensity strength training in nonagenarians: effects on skeletal muscle, *JAMA*, 263, 3029–3034, 1990.

10

Aging, Obesity, and Metabolic Regulation: Influence of Gender and Physical Activity

Wendy M. Kohrt

CONTENTS

0-8493-1027-X/02/$0.00+$1.50

10.1 Introduction

A comprehensive review of the effects of aging, obesity, gender, and physical activity on the regulation of metabolism would exceed the limits imposed for this topic. Therefore, the discussion of the effects of these factors on metabolic regulation will focus primarily on resistance to the glucoregulatory actions of insulin. The effects of aging and obesity will be reviewed briefly, with more attention paid to the effects of gender and physical activity. Although it is recognized that the relative strength of these factors as determinants of insulin action may vary by ethnicity, this factor is not considered in the present chapter.

10.2 Aging and Insulin Resistance

The effectiveness of insulin in regulating blood glucose levels declines with advancing age, particularly in individuals who live in technologically advanced societies, leading to an increased risk of impaired glucose tolerance and type 2 diabetes mellitus.[1-4] The progression from normal glucose tolerance to glucose intolerance in aging is characterized by defects in both insulin secretion and action.[5-7] It is likely that reduced insulin action (i.e., insulin resistance) is an early impairment; initially, this is compensated effectively by increased insulin secretion, thereby maintaining blood glucose levels within the broad range considered normal. As insulin resistance progresses and the ability to hypersecrete insulin becomes impaired, glucose intolerance develops and can lead to type 2 diabetes mellitus. Thus, insulin resistance is viewed as an early, subclinical marker of risk for glucose intolerance.

Although a component of the decline in insulin action and glucose tolerance may, indeed, be attributable to the aging process, secondary characteristics of aging also play a significant role. The decrease in physical activity and increase in adiposity, particularly in the abdominal region, that typically occur with aging are both associated with insulin resistance. Among healthy individuals who stay relatively lean and physically active, it is not unusual for glucose tolerance to remain normal well into old age.[8,9] This suggests that secondary correlates of aging are more important determinants of insulin resistance and glucose intolerance than aging per se.

10.3 Aging, Obesity, and Insulin Resistance

The potent effect of adiposity, and specifically abdominal adiposity, on insulin resistance across the age spectrum is well documented.[6,10-13] A disproportionate accumulation of abdominal fat, even in normal-weight individuals, is associated with metabolic dysfunction, including insulin resistance, glucose intolerance, dyslipidemia (primarily decreased high-density lipoprotein cholesterol and increased triglycerides), and hypertension. The specific role of intraabdominal, or visceral, fat in the development of insulin resistance and glucose intolerance was clearly demonstrated by Ronnemaa et al.[14] in a study of monozygotic twin pairs who were discordant for body mass. Although the average interpair difference in body mass was 18 kg, differences in insulin action and glucose tolerance were apparent only in those twin pairs that differed in the degree of visceral adiposity.

Several studies have evaluated specifically whether the age-associated increase in abdominal obesity accounts for insulin resistance in aging.[2,6,10,11] Kohrt and colleagues[6] assessed insulin action during hyperinsulinemic, euglycemic clamp procedures in 84 young (21 to 33 years) and older (60 to 72 years) women and men. Both age ($r = -0.45$) and waist circumference ($r = -0.72$) were significant determinants of insulin-stimulated glucose uptake, but age explained less than 2% of the variance in insulin action independently of waist size. Similarly, Weidner et al.[10] found that several anthropometric measures of central body adiposity were more strongly associated with insulin sensitivity than age in 84 women and men aged 18 to 80 years. The minimal waist girth was the strongest determinant of insulin action in both sexes, accounting for about 37% of the variance.

The finding that waist circumference, a simple but robust anthropometric measure of abdominal obesity,[15,16] accounted for nearly all of the age-associated increase in insulin resistance[6,10] was subsequently extended by Cefalu and colleagues.[11] They quantified abdominal subcutaneous and intra-abdominal fat depots by magnetic resonance imaging (MRI) in 60 healthy women and men aged 23 to 83 years. In multivariate regression analyses, intra-abdominal fat area accounted for 51% of the variance in insulin sensitivity, whereas the independent contribution of age was <1%. The multicenter European Group for the Study of Insulin Resistance conducted hyperglycemic, euglycemic clamp procedures to evaluate insulin action in 1146 women and men aged 18 to 85 years.[2] Those investigators also concluded that the effect of age on insulin action could be explained by age-related differences in body composition and substrate competition. Collectively, these studies[2,6,10,11,15,16] provide compelling evidence that insulin resistance in aging develops largely as a result of increasing adiposity and, therefore, is likely an avoidable consequence of aging.

10.4 Gender and Insulin Resistance

10.4.1 Gender Differences in Muscle Mass

Under hyperinsulinemic conditions, the majority of glucose is directed to skeletal muscle for storage.[17] It has therefore been suggested that the increased incidence of glucose intolerance in old age is due, in part, to a decline in muscle mass (i.e., sarcopenia) and that women are at higher risk than men simply because they have less muscle mass. To evaluate this, a standard 75-g oral glucose challenge was administered to healthy young and old women and men. Averages for lean body mass and, presumably, muscle mass varied widely among groups, with lean mass more than two times greater in young men than in older women.[18] Despite the large differences in lean mass, the glucose and insulin responses to the oral challenge did not differ (Figure 10.1). Thus, muscle mass does not appear to play a major role in determining glucose tolerance, and the decline in muscle mass with aging is unlikely to increase the risk of glucose intolerance.

10.4.2 Gender Differences in Prevalence of Glucose Intolerance

The Third National Health and Nutrition Examination Survey, conducted in the U.S. between 1988 and 1994, provided evidence that the prevalence of abnormal glucose tolerance is less in women than in men (Figure 10.2).[3] Among individuals between the ages of 20 and 49 years, the prevalence of undiagnosed diabetes and impaired fasting glucose was more than two times higher in men than in women. Gender differences in the prevalence of glucose intolerance were reduced in older individuals. In fact, when the diagnosis of diabetes or impaired glucose tolerance was based on the serum glucose response to an oral challenge, rather than on fasted glucose levels, the incidence was somewhat lower in 40- to 49-year-old women than men (13.0% vs. 15.5%, respectively), but was essentially identical in 50- to 59-year-old women and men (21.3% vs. 20.1%, respectively) and in 60- to 74-year-olds (31.4% vs. 31.6%, respectively);[3] these tests were not administered to younger individuals.

10.4.3 Gender Differences in Abdominal Obesity

The strong association between the glucoregulatory action of insulin and abdominal obesity suggests that the lower prevalence of glucose intolerance in women, particularly before the age of 50, is related to the conspicuous sex dimorphism in regional fat deposition. Whereas men preferentially accumulate adipose tissue in the abdominal region, women typically store excess fat in the gluteal-femoral region. However, evidence is accumulating that the menopausal transition diminishes or possibly eliminates the protection women are afforded from abdominal obesity prior to menopause. Cross-sectional data from 1179 participants in the Baltimore Longitudinal Study on Aging (BLSA) suggest that waist girth begins to increase at a relatively young age in men, but does not increase markedly in women until after the age of 50 years (Figure 10.3).[19] In the BLSA, the difference in average waist size between 20- and 50-year-olds was 12 cm in men compared with only 4 cm in women. In contrast, the difference in average waist size between 50- and

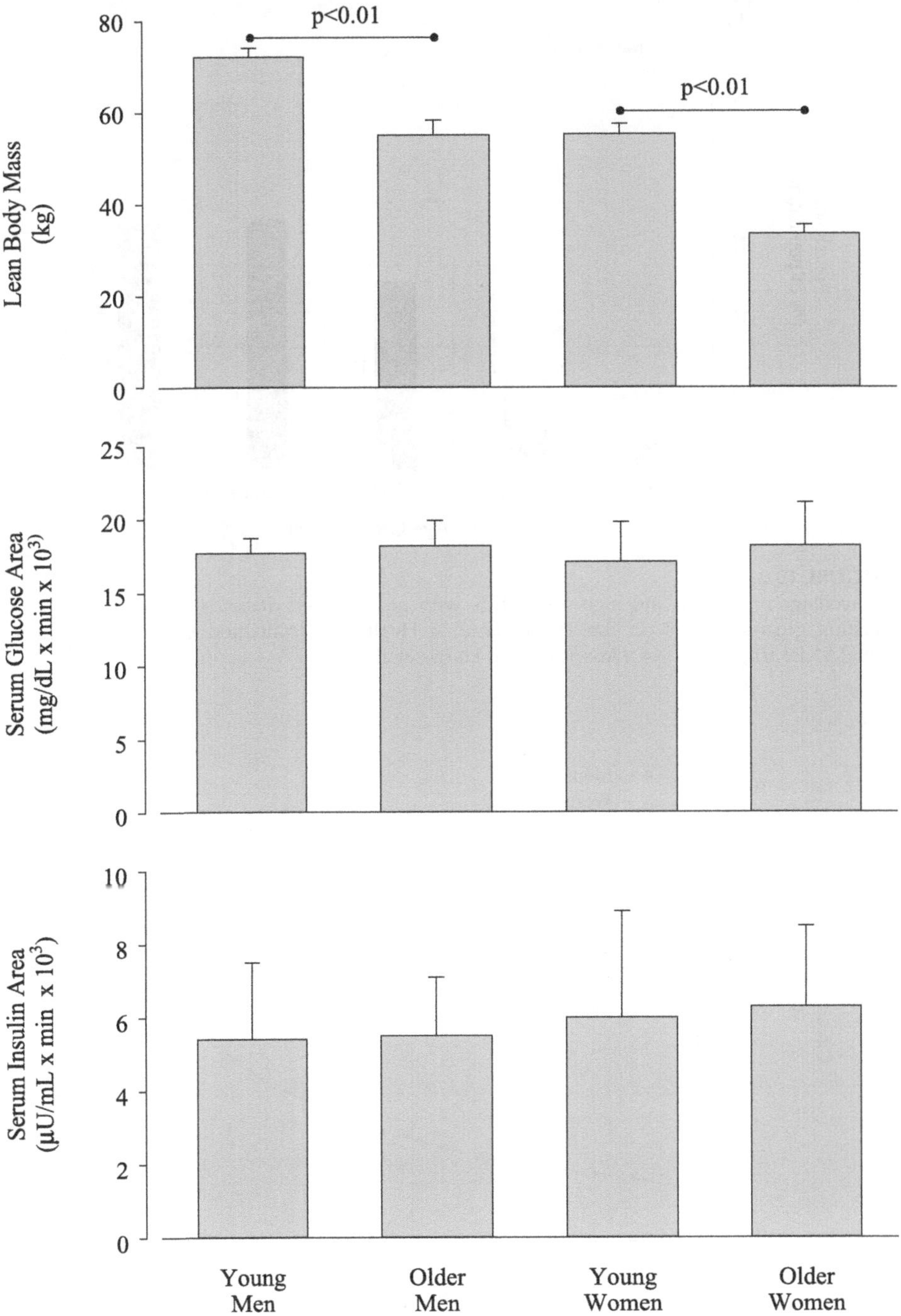

FIGURE 10.1
Lean body mass (top panel), serum glucose (middle panel), and insulin (bottom panel) responses to an oral glucose tolerance test (OGTT) in young and older women and men. Glucose and insulin responses are the integrated areas under the OGTT curve. (Adapted from Kohrt and Holloszy.[18])

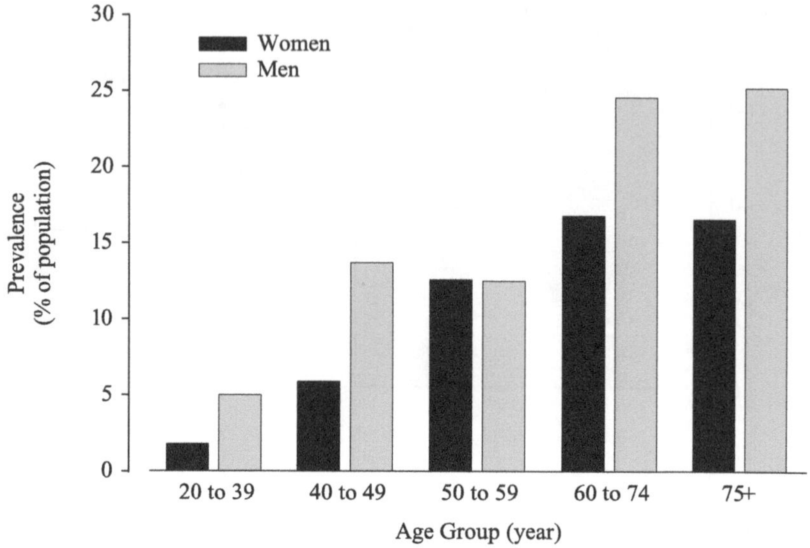

FIGURE 10.2
Percentage of women and men in the U.S. with undiagnosed diabetes mellitus or impaired fasting glucose, based on the Third National Health and Nutrition Examination Survey (NHANES III), 1988–1994. (Adapted from Harris et al.[3])

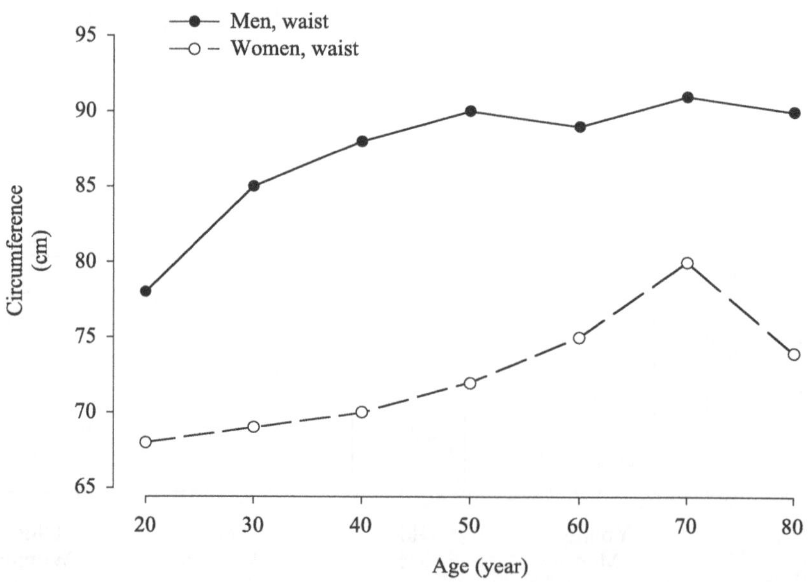

FIGURE 10.3
Cross-sectional average values for waist circumference by decade of age for women and men in the Baltimore Longitudinal Study on Aging. (Adapted from Shimokata et al.[19])

70-year-olds was only 1 cm in men but 8 cm in women. Cross-sectional evaluations of the effects of age and gender on abdominal subcutaneous and visceral adiposity as measured by computed tomography also indicate that the accumulation of abdominal fat, particularly in the visceral region, is increased at an older age in women than in men.[20,21]

10.4.3.1 Effects of Menopause

There is evidence that the increase in abdominal adiposity in women is not a general aging phenomenon, but rather is triggered by menopause, and specifically by the withdrawal of estrogens. Poehlman and colleagues[22] studied a group of age-matched women prospectively over six years; all were initially premenopausal. There were no significant changes in body composition in women who remained premenopausal over the 6-year period. However, women who went through the menopausal transition over the course of the study lost an average of 3 kg of lean mass and gained 2.5 kg of fat mass. There was an increase in the waist-to-hip circumference ratio only in the postmenopausal women, indicating they had developed a disproportionate increase in abdominal adiposity.

10.4.3.2 Effects of Estrogen Replacement

Further evidence that changes in body composition and fat distribution at menopause are related to the withdrawal of sex hormones came from the Postmenopausal Estrogen-Progestin Interventions (PEPI) study. In this investigation, 875 postmenopausal women were randomly assigned to receive conjugated estrogen replacement (either alone or in combination with progestins) or placebo treatment.[23] After 3 years, the women receiving hormone replacement therapy (HRT) gained significantly less body mass and had a lesser increase in waist size than women in the placebo group. The smallest increases in body mass and waist size occurred in the women treated with estrogens only, but changes in this group did not differ significantly from those that occurred in the groups treated with estrogens and progestins. These observations suggest that changes in body composition and fat distribution are mediated by an estrogen-dependent mechanism. The attenuating effect of HRT on weight gain in postmenopausal women was also observed by Kohrt et al.[24] Women using HRT who lost weight and reduced waist size as a result of participating in a 9-month exercise training program had less regain of weight and less increase in waist girth over the next 6 months than women not receiving HRT.

To date, there have been no studies of the specific effects of HRT on visceral fat accumulation in women. However, in light of the cross-sectional observations that visceral fat mass is increased at an older age in women than in men,[20,21] despite similar age-related increases in total adiposity,[25] and the prospective evidence that HRT attenuates the increase in waist size, it seems likely that menopausal withdrawal of sex hormones accelerates visceral fat accumulation in women. The mechanisms by which estrogens regulate visceral fat metabolism are unknown. The low density of estrogen receptors in adipocytes[26] suggests that the action may be through indirect rather than direct, receptor-mediated mechanisms. As one possible indirect mechanism of action, hyperactivity of the hypothalamic–pituitary-adrenal axis has been shown to be associated with increased intra-abdominal fat accumulation.[27,28] Interleukin-6 (IL-6), which increases after menopause and is suppressed in response to HRT,[29] is a potent stimulator of the HPA axis.[30] Thus, it seems plausible that estrogens could modulate cortisol-mediated regulation of visceral fat metabolism.

The effect of HRT in attenuating abdominal fat accumulation is not generally considered one of the mechanisms for the purported cardioprotective effects of HRT reported in observational studies of postmenopausal women.[31] However, given the firm associations of abdominal adiposity with insulin resistance and risk factors for coronary artery disease in both women and men,[6,10-13] it seems likely that a diminution of abdominal fat accumulation by estrogens would be cardioprotective. This conjecture may seem to contrast with findings from the first randomized clinical trial of HRT to include cardiovascular events as outcome measures — the Heart Estrogen Replacement Study (HERS).[32] This secondary prevention trial found a trend for increased cardiovascular events in the first year of HRT use in women with coronary artery disease. However, there was also a trend for reduction in cardiovascular events after 4 years of HRT use. This "early harm, late benefit" paradigm of HRT is compatible with the notion that the late benefit is attributable to an action of estrogen, that brings about changes slowly over time, such as the attenuation of abdominal fat accumulation. Studies by the author and others to evaluate such potential effects of HRT are in progress, but results may not be available for several years.

10.4.4 Gender Differences in Insulin Resistance

The increase in abdominal adiposity in women after menopause probably contributes to the increased prevalence of insulin resistance and glucose intolerance observed in women over the age of 50 years.[3] In support of this, the relationship between waist circumference and glucose disposal rate at a physiologic level of hyperinsulinemia is illustrated in Figure 10.4.[6] In both women (top panel) and men (bottom panel), waist size explained nearly 50% of the variance in insulin action; this measure was a better predictor of insulin resistance than age, physical fitness level, or total degree of adiposity. Moreover, regression equations describing the associations between waist size and insulin resistance were essentially identical in women and men. Cefalu and colleagues[11] evaluated the relationship between insulin sensitivity and intra-abdominal fat levels separately in women and men; they also found that the regression lines were essentially superimposable. These observations are compatible with the findings of Pouliot et al.[16] that the degree of visceral adiposity for a certain waist size is similar in women and men and that,

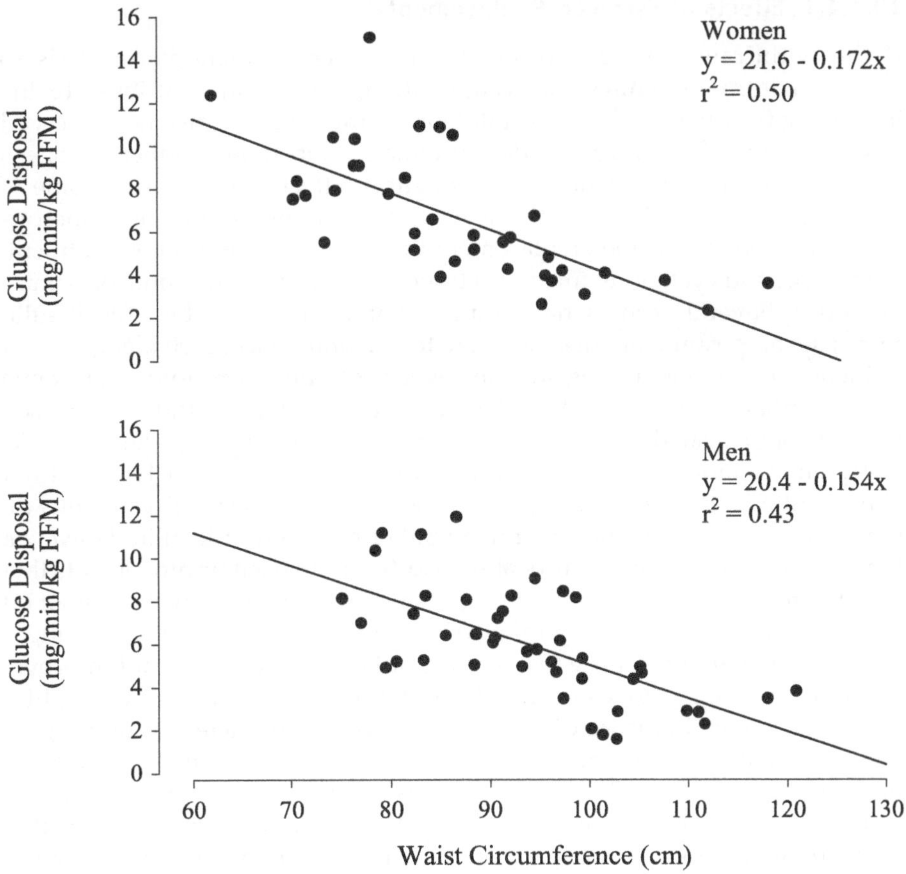

FIGURE 10.4
Relation between insulin sensitivity, assessed as glucose disposal rate per kilogram of fat-free mass during a hyperinsulinemic, euglycemic clamp procedure, and waist circumference in women (top panel) and men (bottom panel) aged 21 to 72 years. (Adapted from Kohrt et al.[6])

regardless of gender, a waist circumference in excess of 100 cm is likely to be associated with insulin resistance. However, the clinical standards of waist size for women and men gaining acceptance[4,33,34] adhere to the concept that there is a sexual dimorphism in the degree of disease risk associated with waist circumference. It has been recommended that there be two sex-specific thresholds for waist size to designate moderate and high risk for coronary artery disease: 80 and 88 cm for women and 94 and 102 cm for men. Certainly, the evidence for an increase in disease risk with abdominal fat accumulation is sufficiently strong that it is prudent to recommend that increases in waist size with aging be held to a minimum. However, it seems premature to recommend specific cut-points of waist size for degree of risk, particularly in women, since so little is known about the effects of menopause and sex hormones on abdominal fat metabolism.

10.4.4.1 Effects of Estrogen Replacement

If the withdrawal of sex hormones in women at menopause leads to increased intra-abdominal fat accumulation, this could contribute to the increasing prevalence of glucose intolerance and insulin resistance observed in women aged 50 years and older.[3] It remains uncertain whether estrogens have effects on insulin action independent of effects on adiposity. Some of the uncertainty is related to the incongruity among studies of numerous factors related to hormone replacement therapy (e.g., duration of treatment; dose, type, and cycling regimen of estrogens and progestins; route of administration). Several studies have found that HRT diminished the insulin response of postmenopausal women to an oral glucose challenge.[35-39] A reduction in the circulating insulin level necessary to restore euglycemia reflects enhanced insulin action. However, among recent studies that used a more sophisticated measure of insulin action (i.e., the hyperinsulinemic, euglycemic clamp), the majority found that 6 to 12 weeks of HRT did not alter insulin action significantly.[40-43] These results suggest that estrogens do not have a direct effect on the glucoregulatory action of insulin. However, the period of treatment was probably insufficient to elicit improvements that could potentially be mediated through effects of estrogens on abdominal fat metabolism. One study that employed the clamp procedure to assess changes in insulin action in response to 6 months of HRT found significant improvements in women who were initially hyperinsulinemic and overweight.[44] Insulin-stimulated glucose disposal during the clamp increased by roughly 50% in that study, and there was a 30% reduction in insulin response to an oral glucose challenge. The improvements in insulin action did not appear to be related to changes in the waist-to-hip circumference ratio, but that measurement is not a sensitive index of change in abdominal obesity.[45] Values for waist circumference only, a more sensitive index of change, were not reported.

The results of the multicenter Menopause Study Group trial could be interpreted as supporting the contention that effects of estrogens on insulin action are mediated through changes in fat metabolism.[37] Women were randomly assigned to receive conjugated estrogens alone or with various combinations of medroxyprogesterone acetate (low vs. high dose, continuous vs. cyclic) and were followed through thirteen 28-day cycles of HRT. Oral glucose tolerance tests were administered at baseline and after cycles 3, 6, and 13. There were significant decreases of 20 to 40% in the insulin response to glucose in all of the treatment groups except the one treated with continuous low-dose medroxyprogesterone acetate. Moreover, the decreases in insulin response to glucose in each group were progressively larger with increasing duration of HRT. It seems plausible that progressive reduction in hyperinsulinemia with increasing duration of HRT resulted from a slow, steady decline in visceral adiposity. Further research is necessary to elucidate the effects of estrogens on abdominal obesity and insulin resistance.

10.5 Physical Activity and Insulin Resistance

10.5.1 Physical Activity and Risk of Glucose Intolerance

As reviewed in the U.S. Surgeon General's report on physical activity and health, epidemiological studies provide convincing evidence that lack of physical activity is a risk factor for insulin resistance, glucose intolerance, and type 2 diabetes mellitus.[46] For example, the multicultural Insulin Resistance Atherosclerosis Study of 1467 women and men, aged 40 to 69 years, found that increased levels of physical activity, either vigorous or nonvigorous, were associated with increased insulin sensitivity.[47] Positive associations between physical activity and insulin sensitivity remained apparent in subgroup analyses by diabetes status, ethnicity, and gender.

Prospective cohort studies also provide evidence that habitual physical activity confers protection against development of diabetes independently of the effects of age, body mass index, and other risk factors for coronary artery disease.[48,49] The results of these studies suggest that the relative risk for diabetes is reduced by as much as 50% in women and men who exercise regularly. They suggest further that even modest levels of physical activity are associated with significant benefit in this regard.

The most rigorous evidence for the important role of physical activity in preventing insulin resistance in aging comes from studies involving exercise interventions. Both short-term exercise interventions, involving only 7 to 10 days of exercise,[50,51] and interventions carried out over several months involving endurance or resistive exercise training,[52-62] demonstrate the insulin-enhancing effects of exercise in women and men up to the age of 80 years. Benefits are apparent in healthy individuals and in those with abnormal glucose tolerance. In studies that included women,[51,52,55,56,60-62] there was no indication that the response to exercise was gender dependent.

10.5.2 Older Athletes as a Model of Primary Effects of Aging

The primary effects of aging on physiological measures are always difficult to evaluate independently of secondary characteristics of aging that seem to accelerate the aging process (e.g., physical inactivity and obesity). However, it is important to try to distinguish these effects because changes consequent to primary aging factors are often viewed as inevitable, whereas changes associated with secondary characteristics of aging may be avoidable. In this respect, physiological changes that occur with advancing age in people maintaining relatively high levels of vigorous physical activity and low levels of body fat over much of their lifetime, i.e., older athletes, are thought to reflect changes due to the aging process per se. It has been argued that the superiority of older athletes in certain physiological, and possibly inherited, characteristics makes them a poor model of aging, in that they are not representative of the general population. However, results from long-term (i.e., 20+ years) follow-up studies of former athletes who did not maintain their exercise habits indicate few residual benefits of previous athletic status in those who become sedentary, and that these individuals are physiologically similar to their age-matched, nonathletic peers.[63-66] This suggests that the aged athlete is a useful model from which to glean information regarding the primary physiological effects of aging.

10.5.3 Glucose Tolerance and Insulin Action of Older Athletes

Studies of older endurance athletes and age-matched controls with normal glucose tolerance indicate that athletes had less excursion in blood glucose levels in response to an oral challenge; [67-69] the glucose response of older athletes also did not differ from that of young athletes.[69] Moreover, the insulin responses of athletes to an oral glucose challenge were less than half as great as those of controls, and did not differ from those of young athletes. These studies indicate that the glucose tolerance of older athletes is indistinguishable from that of healthy young people. Studies that utilized the hyperinsulinemic, euglycemic clamp procedure to assess older athletes and age-matched sedentary controls[67,70] found that insulin sensitivity was about 40% greater in the athletes. Insulin sensitivity was also about 20% higher in older athletes than in young, sedentary controls.[70]

The maintenance of normal glucose tolerance and enhanced insulin action with aging in people who exercise habitually is likely due to the physical activity per se, and to the maintenance of normal body mass. Importantly regarding the latter, modest changes in body composition and fat distribution with aging, when accompanied by regular exercise, do not appear to have a deleterious effect on these measures. Endurance athletes who continued to train vigorously for 20 years or more maintained their body mass, but increased their body fat content by 3 to 5% and their waist size by 5 cm.[64,65] These changes were larger in former athletes who continued to exercise, though not as vigorously, and larger still in former athletes who reduced their physical activity levels markedly. The importance of physical activity per se to the maintenance of normal glucose tolerance and insulin action was demonstrated by Rogers et al.,[71] who performed oral glucose tolerance tests in 14 older endurance athletes in their usual physical activity state and after 10 days without exercise. The insulin response to the oral challenge was nearly two times larger after this short period without exercise but, despite this, the glucose response was also increased, indicating a marked increase in insulin resistance.

The studies of older athletes discussed here included only men. There have been fewer characterizations of older females athletes and, apparently, no longitudinal studies. Body mass, body fat content, and abdominal obesity are significantly less in older female athletes than in age-matched sedentary women.[72-75] Thus, it seems likely that habitual exercise would be effective in maintaining normal glucose tolerance and enhanced insulin action with aging in women. However, it is not known whether the withdrawal of estrogens at menopause compromises the benefits of regular exercise in women. For example, if estrogen deficiency triggers an accumulation of abdominal fat, insulin action may be affected negatively despite maintenance of high levels of physical activity.

10.5.4 Physiological Mechanisms for the Enhancing Effects of Exercise on Insulin Action

10.5.4.1 Acute Effects of Exercise

The potent insulin-lowering effect of exercise occurs in both young and older individuals.[50,52,67-69,76] The decline in insulin secretion in response to exercise counters the enhancing effect of exercise on insulin-stimulated glucose uptake by skeletal muscle, thereby preventing hypoglycemia.

As reviewed recently by Holloszy and Hansen,[77] there are at least three mechanisms by which exercise enhances the passage of glucose from the blood into skeletal muscle. During and immediately after exercise, there is an increase in insulin-independent glucose transport into muscle. When measured under *in vitro* conditions, this effect persists less than 1 hour after cessation of muscle contractile activity.[78] An insulin-dependent increase in glucose transport also occurs after exercise. This increased insulin sensitivity persists until the exercise-induced decrease in muscle glycogen stores is reversed,[79] typically 1 to 2 days after a strenuous or prolonged exercise bout for an individual on a normal or high-carbohydrate diet. The third mechanism by which glucose uptake into muscle is enhanced after exercise is through an increase in the protein that facilitates the entry of glucose into muscle, GLUT4. Because this protein has a half-life of only a few days, significant increases can occur within 48 hours of exercise,[80] but the adaptation is also completely reversed within 48 hours, even when exercise has been performed regularly for several weeks.[81] Thus, under normal dietary conditions, all of these exercise-induced adaptations in muscle glucose uptake are short-lived, lasting only 1 to 2 days unless repeated bouts of exercise are performed.

10.5.4.2 Chronic Effects of Exercise Training

Even when exercise training is carried out over several months, the adaptive increase in insulin action is completely lost within a few days if energy balance is maintained, so that there is no weight loss during the training program.[82] More persistent improvements in insulin action in response to exercise training are likely mediated through a reduction in total body and abdominal fat stores. Indeed, there is evidence in older women and men that improvements in insulin action and glucose tolerance in response to exercise training are independently enhanced by reductions in waist circumference and body fat content.[52,58]

GLUT4 protein levels are lower in sedentary older individuals than in young individuals,[83] but the ability to adapt to exercise with increased GLUT4 appears to be retained with aging.[51,84] Houmard and colleagues[51] found that insulin sensitivity and GLUT4 protein levels increased similarly in young and older women and men in response to 7 days of exercise training. The lower GLUT4 protein levels in sedentary older people suggest that a decline in physical activity levels could account for a portion of insulin resistance and glucose intolerance in aging, even among those who remain relatively lean. Increases in total and abdominal adiposity with aging would be expected to have further detrimental effects on insulin resistance.

10.5.4.3 Effects of Negative Energy Balance — Diet vs. Exercise

Physical activity can enhance insulin action both acutely, through effects of muscle contractile activity on GLUT4 protein and other cellular mechanisms, and chronically, by reducing adiposity. This suggests that weight loss induced through exercise should result in larger improvements in insulin action (via both acute and chronic effects) than weight loss induced through diet (chronic effects only). Arciero et al.[50] evaluated this contention by having overweight, middle-aged and older women and men with glucose intolerance undergo either 10 days of a low-energy diet or 10 days of exercise training. Insulin action was evaluated before and after the intervention, using a modified hyperglycemic clamp procedure. Prior to the intervention, insulin action was similar in both groups of subjects (Figure 10.5). The estimated energy deficit during the 10-day intervention was more than 2.5 times greater in the diet group (–4.80 MJ/d) than in the exercise group (–1.76 MJ/d). Despite this, the increase in insulin action in response to exercise was significantly greater than the increase that occurred in the diet group.

10.6 Conclusions

Aging, per se, appears to have only a small effect on glucose intolerance and insulin resistance. The majority of insulin resistance that develops in older women and men is explained by increased adiposity, particularly in the abdominal region. However, there have been few studies of women and men aged 80+ years of age; it will be important to evaluate further the effects of aging on glucose tolerance and insulin action in the elderly.

The prevalence of glucose intolerance appears to be less in women than men before the age of 40 years, but gender differences in the prevalence of glucose intolerance diminish with aging. The independent effects of menopausal withdrawal of sex hormones on insulin action are largely unknown.

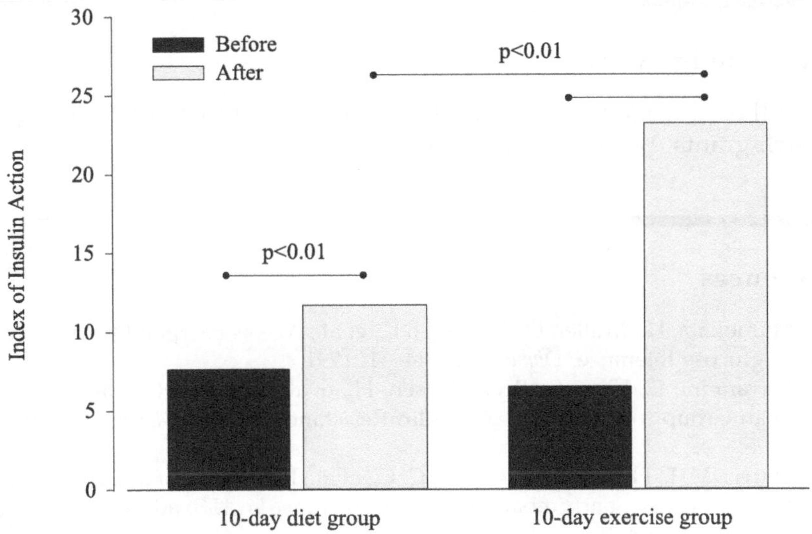

FIGURE 10.5
Effects of 10 days of either a low-energy diet or exercise on insulin action. The index of insulin action is the slope of the regression line describing the relation between glucose disposal rate and serum insulin concentration during a modified hyperglycemic procedure. (Adapted from Arciero et al.[50])

Results of studies of the effects of estrogen replacement on glucose tolerance and insulin action are not uniform, although generally demonstrating either beneficial or neutral effects. There is emerging evidence that the potential effect of menopause in inducing insulin resistance could be mediated through an accumulation of abdominal fat. The menopausal withdrawal of sex hormones appears to trigger an increase in abdominal adiposity in women, thereby diminishing the benefit of female gender in the risk profile for cardiovascular disease. An attenuation of abdominal fat accumulation by HRT may contribute to the purported cardioprotective effects of HRT in women.

Exercise has a potent enhancing effect on insulin action, independent of gender. This is mediated acutely by cellular adaptations to exercise and chronically by the beneficial effects of exercise on body composition and fat distribution. A decline in physical activity likely contributes to insulin resistance in aging, even in the absence of weight gain.

In summary, secondary characteristics of aging, specifically increased physical inactivity and adiposity, account for a large portion of the insulin resistance and glucose intolerance common in older women and men. The contribution of menopause, considered a primary aging factor in women, is unknown. The prevalence and determinants of glucose intolerance in the oldest old remain to be determined. At least through the eighth decade, life style appears to be a much stronger determinant of insulin resistance than aging per se.

Acknowledgments

The author's work is supported by National Institutes of Health (NIH) research grants AG18198 and AG18857.

References

1. Shimokata, H., Muller, D. C., Fleg, J. L., et al., Age as independent determinant of glucose tolerance, *Diabetes,* 40, 44–51, 1991.
2. Ferrannini, E., Vichi, S., Beck-Nielsen, H., et al., Insulin action and age. European Group for the Study of Insulin Resistance (EGIR), *Diabetes,* 45, 947–953, 1996.
3. Harris, M. I., Flegal, K. M., Cowie, C. C., et al., Prevalence of diabetes, impaired fasting glucose, and impaired glucose tolerance in U.S. adults, *Diabetes Care,* 21, 518–524, 1998.
4. Iwao, S., Iwao, N., Muller, D. C., et al., Effect of aging on the relationship between multiple risk factors and waist circumference, *J. Am. Geriatr. Soc.,* 48, 788–794, 2000.
5. Reaven, G. M., Chen, N., Hollenbeck, C., et al., Effect of age on glucose tolerance and glucose uptake in healthy individuals, *J. Am. Geriatr. Soc.,* 37, 735–740, 1989.
6. Kohrt, W. M., Kirwan, J. P., Staten, M. A., et al., Insulin resistance in aging is related to abdominal obesity, *Diabetes,* 42, 273–281, 1993.
7. DeFronzo, R. A., Bonadonna, R., and Ferrannini, E., Pathogenesis of NIDDM: a balanced overview, *Diabetes Care,* 15, 318–368, 1992.
8. Zavaroni, I., Dall'Aglio, E., Bruschi, F., et al., Effect of age and environmental factors on glucose tolerance and insulin secretion in a worker population, *J. Am. Geriatr. Soc.,* 34, 271–275, 1986.
9. Paolisso, G., Gambardella, A., Ammendola, S., et al., Glucose tolerance and insulin action in healthy centenarians, *Am. J. Physiol.,* 270, E890–E894, 1996.
10. Weidner, M. D., Gavigan, K. E., Tyndall, G. L., et al., Which anthropometric indices of regional adiposity are related to the insulin resistance of aging? *Int. J. Obes. Relat. Metab. Disord.,* 19, 325–330, 1995.
11. Cefalu, W. T., Wang, Z. Q., Werbel, S., et al., Contribution of visceral fat mass to the insulin resistance of aging, *Metabolism,* 44, 954–959, 1995.
12. Després, J.-P., The insulin resistance-dyslipidemic syndrome of visceral obesity: effect on patients' risk, *Obes. Res.,* 6, 8S-17S, 1998.
13. Björntorp, P., Body fat distribution, insulin resistance, and metabolic diseases, *Nutrition,* 13, 795–803, 1997.
14. Ronnemaa, T., Koskenvuo, M., Marniemi, J., et al., Glucose metabolism in identical twins discordant for obesity. The critical role of visceral fat, *J. Clin. Endocrinol. Metab.,* 82, 383–387, 1997.
15. Han, T. S., Seidell, J. C., Currall, J. E., et al., The influences of height and age on waist circumference as an index of adiposity in adults, *Int. J. Obes. Relat. Metab. Disord.,* 21, 83–89, 1997.

16. Pouliot, M. C., Després, J.-P., Lemieux, S., et al., Waist circumference and abdominal sagittal diameter: best simple anthropometric indexes of abdominal visceral adipose tissue accumulation and related cardiovascular risk in men and women, *Am. J. Cardiol.*, 73, 460–468, 1994.
17. Shulman, G. I., Rothman, D. L., Jue, T., et al., Quantitation of muscle glycogen synthesis in normal subjects and subjects with noninsulin-dependent diabetes by ^{13}C nuclear magnetic resonance spectroscopy, *N. Engl. J. Med.*, 322, 223–228, 1990.
18. Kohrt, W. M. and Holloszy, J. O., Loss of skeletal muscle mass with aging: effect on glucose tolerance, *J. Gerontol. Biol. Sci. Med. Sci.*, 50, 68–72, 1995.
19. Shimokata, H., Tobin, J. D., Muller, D. C., et al., Studies in the distribution of body fat: I. Effects of age, sex, and obesity, *J. Gerontol.*, 44, M66–M73, 1989.
20. Enzi, G., Gasparo, M., Biondetti, P. R., et al., Subcutaneous and visceral fat distribution according to sex, age, and overweight, evaluated by computed tomography, *Am. J. Clin. Nutr.*, 44, 739–746, 1986.
21. Seidell, J. C., Oosterlee, A., Deurenberg, P., et al., Abdominal fat depots measured with computed tomography: effects of degree of obesity, sex, and age, *Eur. J. Clin. Invest.*, 42, 805–815, 1988.
22. Poehlman, E. T., Toth, M. J., and Gardner, A. W., Changes in energy balance and body composition at menopause: a controlled longitudinal study, *Ann. Int. Med.*, 123, 673–675, 1995.
23. Espeland, M. A., Stefanick, M. L., Kritz-Silverstein, D., et al., Effect of postmenopausal hormone therapy on body weight and waist and hip girths, *J. Clin. Endocrinol. Metab.*, 82, 1549–1556, 1997.
24. Kohrt, W. M., Ehsani, A. A., and Birge, S. J., HRT preserves increases in bone mineral density and reductions in body fat after a supervised exercise program, *J. Appl. Physiol.*, 84, 1506–1512, 1998.
25. Holloszy, J. O. and Kohrt, W. M., Exercise, in *Handbook of Physiology — Aging*, Masoro, E. J., Ed., University Press, Oxford, 1995, 633–666.
26. Pedersen, S. B., Fuglsig, S., Sjogren, P., et al., Identification of steroid receptors in human adipose tissue, *Eur. J. Clin. Invest.*, 26, 1051–1056, 1996.
27. Rosmond, R., Dallman, M. F., and Björntorp, P., Stress-related cortisol secretion in men: relationships with abdominal obesity and endocrine, metabolic, and hemodynamic abnormalities, *J. Clin. Endocrinol. Metab.*, 83, 1853–1859, 1998.
28. Pasquali, R., Anconetani, B., Chattat, R., et al., Hypothalamic-pituitary-adrenal axis activity and its relationship to the autonomic nervous system in women with visceral and subcutaneous obesity: effects of the corticotropin-releasing factor/arginine-vasopressin test and of stress, *Metabolism*, 45, 351–356, 1996.
29. Straub, R., Hense, H., Andus, T., et al., Hormone replacement therapy and interrelation between serum interleukin-6 and body mass index in postmenopausal women: a population-based study, *J. Clin. Endocrinol. Metab.*, 1340–1344, 2000.
30. Mastorakos, G., Chrousos, C., and Weber, J., Recombinant interleukin-6 activates the hypothalamic–pituitary-adrenal axis in humans, *J. Clin. Endocrinol. Metab.*, 77, 1690–1694, 1993.
31. Grodstein, F., Stampfer, M. J., Manson, J. E., et al., Postmenopausal estrogen and progestin use and the risk of cardiovascular disease, *N. Engl. J. Med.*, 335, 453–461, 1996.

32. Hulley, S., Grady, D., Bush, T., et al., Randomized trial of estrogen plus progestin for secondary prevention of coronary heart disease in postmenopausal women. Heart and estrogen/progestin replacement study (HERS) research group, *JAMA*, 280, 605–613, 1998.
33. NHLBI Obesity Education Initiative Expert Panel, Clinical guidelines on the identification, evaluation, and treatment of overweight and obesity in adults, *Obes. Res.*, 6, 209S-1998.
34. Lean, M. E. J., Han, T. S., and Morrison, C. E., Waist circumference as a measure for indicating need for weight management, *Br. Med. J.*, 311, 158–161, 1995.
35. Spencer, C. P., Godsland, I. F., Cooper, A. J., et al., Effects of oral and transdermal 17beta-estradiol with cyclical oral norethindrone acetate on insulin sensitivity, secretion, and elimination in postmenopausal women, *Metabolism*, 49, 742–747, 2000.
36. Crook, D., Godsland, I. F., Hull, J., et al., Hormone replacement therapy with dydrogesterone and 17 beta-oestradiol: effects on serum lipoproteins and glucose tolerance during 24 month follow-up, *Br. J. Obstetr. Gynaecol.*, 104, 298–304, 1997.
37. Lobo, R. A., Pickar, J. H., Wild, R. A., et al., Metabolic impact of adding medroxyprogesterone acetate to conjugated estrogen therapy in postmenopausal women. The menopause study group, *Obstetr. Gynecol.*, 84, 987–995, 1994.
38. Mendoza, S., Velazquez, E., Osona, A., et al., Postmenopausal cyclic estrogen–progestin therapy lowers lipoprotein, *J. Lab. Clin. Med.*, 123, 837–841, 1994.
39. Evans, E. M. et al., Effects of HRT and exercise training on body composition, glucose tolerance, and insulin action in older women, *J. Appl. Physiol.*, 2001.
40. Andersson, B., Mattsson, L. A., Hahn, L., et al., Estrogen replacement therapy decreases hyperandrogenicity and improves glucose homeostasis and plasma lipids in postmenopausal women with noninsulin-dependent diabetes mellitus, *J. Clin. Endocrinol. Metab.*, 82, 638–643, 1997.
41. Brussaard, H. E., Gevers Leuven, J. A., Frolich, M., et al., Short-term oestrogen replacement therapy improves insulin resistance, lipids and fibrinolysis in postmenopausal women with NIDDM, *Diabetologia*, 40, 843–849, 1997.
42. Duncan, A. C., Lyall, H., Roberts, R. N., et al., The effect of estradiol and a combined estradiol/progestagen preparation on insulin sensitivity in healthy postmenopausal women, *J. Clin. Endocrinol. Metab.*, 84, 2402–2407, 1999.
43. Kimmerle, R., Heinemann, L., Heise, T., et al., Influence of continuous combined estradiol-norethisterone acetate preparations on insulin sensitivity in postmenopausal nondiabetic women, *Menopause*, 6, 36–42, 1999.
44. Cucinelli, F., Paparella, P., Soranna, L., et al., Differential effect of transdermal estrogen plus progestagen replacement therapy on insulin metabolism in postmenopausal women: relation to their insulinemic secretion, *Eur. J. Endocrinol.*, 140, 215–223, 1999.
45. van der Kooy, K., Leenen, R., Seidell, J. C., et al., Waist-hip ratio is a poor predictor of changes in visceral fat, *Am. J. Clin. Nutr.*, 57, 327–333, 1993.
46. U.S. Department of Health and Human Services, Physical activity and health. A report of the Surgeon General, 1996.
47. Mayer-Davis, E. J., D'Agostino, R., Jr., Karter, A. J., et al., Intensity and amount of physical activity in relation to insulin sensitivity: the insulin resistance atherosclerosis study, *JAMA*, 279, 669–674, 1998.
48. Hu, F. B., Sigal, R. J., Rich-Edwards, J. W., et al., Walking compared with vigorous physical activity and risk of type 2 diabetes in women: a prospective study, *JAMA*, 282, 1433–1439, 1999.

49. Manson, J. E., Nathan, D. M., Krolewski, A. S., et al., A prospective study of exercise and incidence of diabetes among U.S. male physicians, *JAMA*, 268, 63–67, 1992.
50. Arciero, P. J., Vukovich, M. D., Holloszy, J. O., et al., Comparison of short-term diet and exercise on insulin action in individuals with abnormal glucose tolerance, *J. Appl. Physiol.*, 86, 1930–1935, 1999.
51. Cox, J. H., Cortright, R. N., Dohm, G. L., et al., Effect of aging on response to exercise training in humans: skeletal muscle GLUT-4 and insulin sensitivity, *J. Appl. Physiol.*, 86, 2019–2025, 1999.
52. Kirwan, J. P., Kohrt, W. M., Wojta, D. W., et al., Endurance exercise training reduces glucose-stimulated insulin levels in 60- to 70-yr-old men and women, *J. Gerontol.*, 48, M84–M90, 1993.
53. Dengel, D. R., Pratley, R. E., Hagberg, J. M., et al., Distinct effects of aerobic exercise training and weight loss on glucose homeostasis in obese sedentary men, *J. Appl. Physiol.*, 81, 318–325, 1996.
54. Hughes, V. A., Fiatarone, M. A., Fielding, R. A., et al., Long-term effects of a high-carbohydrate diet and exercise on insulin action in older subjects with impaired glucose tolerance, *Am. J. Clin. Nutr.*, 62, 426–433, 1995.
55. Hersey, W. C. 3., Graves, J. E., Pollock, M. L., et al., Endurance exercise training improves body composition and plasma insulin responses in 70- to 79-yr-old men and women, *Metabolism*, 43, 847–854, 1994.
56. Hughes, V. A., Fiatarone, M. A., Fielding, R. A., et al., Exercise increases muscle GLUT-4 levels and insulin action in subjects with impaired glucose tolerance, *Am. J. Physiol.*, 264, E855–E862, 1993.
57. Zachwieja, J. J., Toffolo, G., Cobelli, C., et al., Resistance exercise and growth hormone administration in older men: effects on insulin sensitivity and secretion during a stable-label IVGTT, *Metabolism*, 45, 254–260, 1996.
58. Pratley, R. E., Hagberg, J. M., Dengel, D. R., et al., Aerobic exercise training-induced reductions in abdominal fat and glucose-stimulated insulin responses in middle-aged and older men, *J. Am. Geriatr. Soc.*, 48, 1055–1061, 2000.
59. Dengel, D. R., Galecki, A. T., Hagberg, J. M., et al., The independent and combined effects of weight loss and aerobic exercise on blood pressure and oral glucose tolerance in older men, *Am. J. Hypertens.*, 11, 1405–1412, 1998.
60. Ryan, A. S., Pratley, R. E., Goldberg, A. P., et al., Resistive training increases insulin action in postmenopausal women, *J. Gerontol. Med. Sci.*, 51A, M199–M205, 1996.
61. DiPietro, L., Seeman, T. E., Stachenfeld, N. S., et al., Moderate-intensity aerobic training improves glucose tolerance in aging independent of abdominal obesity, *J. Am. Geriatr. Soc.*, 46, 875–879, 1998.
62. Ryan, A. S., Pratley, R. E., Elahi, D., et al., Changes in plasma leptin and insulin action with resistive training in postmenopausal women, *Int. J. Obes. Relat. Metab. Disord.*, 24, 27–32, 2000.
63. Robinson, S., Dill, D. B., Robinson, R. D., et al., Physiological aging of champion runners, *J. Appl. Physiol.*, 41, 46–51, 1976.
64. Trappe, S. W., Costill, D. L., Vukovich, M. D., et al., Aging among elite distance runners: a 22-yr longitudinal study, *J. Appl. Physiol.*, 80, 285–290, 1996.
65. Pollock, M. L., Mengelkoch, L. J., Graves, J. E., et al., Twenty-year follow-up of aerobic power and body composition of older track athletes, *J. Appl. Physiol.*, 82, 1508–1516, 1997.

66. Mengelkoch, L. J., Pollock, M. L., Limacher, M. C., et al., Effects of age, physical training, and physical fitness on coronary heart disease risk factors in older track athletes at twenty-year follow-up, *J. Am. Geriatr. Soc.*, 45, 1446–1453, 1997.
67. Pratley, R. E., Hagberg, J. M., Rogus, E. M., et al., Enhanced insulin sensitivity and lower waist-to-hip ratio in master athletes, *Am. J. Physiol.*, 268, E484–E490, 1995.
68. Larsson, B., Renstrom, P., Svardsudd, K., et al., Health and aging characteristics of highly physically active 65-yr-old men, *Eur. Heart J.*, 5, 31–35, 1984.
69. Seals, D. R., Hagberg, J. M., Allen, W. K., et al., Glucose tolerance in young and older athletes and sedentary men, *J. Appl. Physiol.*, 56, 1521–1525, 1984.
70. Yamanouchi, K., Nakajima, H., Shinozaki, A., et al., Effects of daily physical activity on insulin action in the elderly, *J. Appl. Physiol.*, 73, 2241–2245, 1992.
71. Rogers, M. A., King, D. S., Hagberg, J. M., et al., Effect of 10 days of inactivity on glucose tolerance in master athletes, *J. Appl. Physiol.*, 68, 1833–1837, 1990.
72. Kohrt, W. M., Malley, M. T., Dalsky, G. P., et al., Body composition of healthy sedentary and trained, young and older men and women, *Med. Sci. Sports Exerc.*, 24, 832–837, 1992.
73. Van Pelt, R. E., Davy, K. P., Stevenson, E. T., et al., Smaller differences in total and regional adiposity with age in women who regularly perform endurance exercise, *Am. J. Physiol.*, 275, E626–E634, 1998.
74. Stevenson, E. T., Davy, K. P., and Seals, D. R., Maximal aerobic capacity and total blood volume in highly trained middle-aged and older female endurance athletes, *J. Appl. Physiol.*, 77, 1691–1696, 1994.
75. Ryan, A. S., Nicklas, B. J., and Elahi, D., A cross-sectional study on body composition and energy expenditure in women athletes during aging, *Am. J. Physiol.*, 271, E916–E921, 1996.
76. King, D. S., Staten, M. A., Kohrt, W. M., et al., Insulin secretory capacity in endurance-trained and untrained young men, *Am. J. Physiol.*, 259, E155–E181, 1990.
77. Holloszy, J. O. and Hansen, P. A., Regulation of glucose transport into skeletal muscle, in *Reviews of Physiology, Biochemistry and Pharmacology*, Blaustein, M. P., et al., Eds., Springer-Verlag, Berlin, 1996, 99–193.
78. Gulve, E. A., Cartee, G. D., Zierath, J. R., et al., Reversal of enhanced muscle glucose transport after exercise: roles of insulin and glucose, *Am. J. Physiol.*, 259, E685–E691, 1990.
79. Cartee, G. D., Young, D. A., Sleeper, M. D., et al., Prolonged increase in insulin-stimulated glucose transport in muscle after exercise, *Am. J. Physiol.*, 256, E494–E499, 1989.
80. Ren, J. M., Semenkovich, C. F., Gulve, E. A., et al., Exercise induces rapid increases in GLUT4 expression, glucose transport capacity, and insulin-stimulated glycogen storage in muscle, *J. Biol. Chem.*, 269, 14396–14401, 1994.
81. Host, H. H., Hansen, P. A., Nolte, L. A., et al., Rapid reversal of adaptive increases in muscle GLUT4 and glucose transport capacity after training cessation, *J. Appl. Physiol.*, 84, 798–802, 1998.
82. Segal, K. R., Edano, A., Abalos, A., et al., Effect of exercise training on insulin sensitivity and glucose metabolism in lean, obese, and diabetic men, *J. Appl. Physiol.*, 71, 2402–2411, 1991.
83. Houmard, J. A., Weidner, M. D., Dolan, P. L., et al., Skeletal muscle GLUT4 protein concentration and aging in humans, *Diabetes*, 44, 555–560, 1995.
84. Gulve, E. A., Rodnick, K. J., Henriksen, E. J., et al., Effects of wheel running on glucose transporter (GLUT4) concentration in skeletal muscle of young adult and old rats, *Mech. Ageing Dev.*, 67, 187–200, 1993.

11

Aging of Immune and Hormonal Responses: Influences of Gender and Physical Activity

Shoji Shinkai

CONTENTS

0-8493-1027-X/02/$0.00+$1.50

11.1 Introduction

Human immune function undergoes adverse changes with aging,[1-3] potentially leading to an increased risk of infections,[4-6] a greater occurrence of autoantibodies and lymphoproliferative disorders,[7-9] and a greater morbidity and mortality[10-13] in the elderly. Immune function is apparently sexually dimorphic; women have more vigorous immunologic activity than do men, reducing the risks of infection in women.[14-17] However, the same mechanisms make women more susceptible to various autoimmune diseases. In old age, the gender difference in immune function does not seem to be predominant. In this context, a question arises whether regular physical activity can correct the detrimental effects of aging and gender on human immune function. This chapter first reviews how the human immune system ages, and then describes sexual dimorphism in the immune system and its possible causes. Following a brief review of exercise-induced immunomodulatory hormones, the latter part of the chapter is devoted to a review of cross-sectional and prospective data regarding the effects of regular physical activity on immune function in the elderly. The potential role of regular physical activity in correcting the aging of immune function is also discussed.

11.2 Aging of the Human Immune System

11.2.1 Thymus Involution

The thymus starts to involute at an early age, and in humans the process is completed by midlife.[18] Many age-related changes in the immune system follow the loss of thymic and T-lymphocyte function. The aged thymus has only a limited capacity to provide the circulation with "naïve" T cells.[19] In addition, the chronic antigenic load encountered over the course of aging causes a continuous attrition of circulating naïve T cells, so that there is a progressive shift from naïve T cells to "memory" T cells as a person ages.[19-22] Both positive and negative intrathymic T cell selections are compromised in the elderly; this leads to the appearance of anti-self-reactive T cells and T cells that do not express self-MHC-restricted antigen recognition.

11.2.2 Neuroendocrine System Associated with Immunosenescence

It is unclear why the thymus involutes with age. However, evidence is emerging which suggests that the neuroendocrine system plays a major role in this process.[23] Among the elements involved are the growth hormone insulin-like growth factor-I system,[24,25] adrenal dehydroepiandrosterone,[26,27]

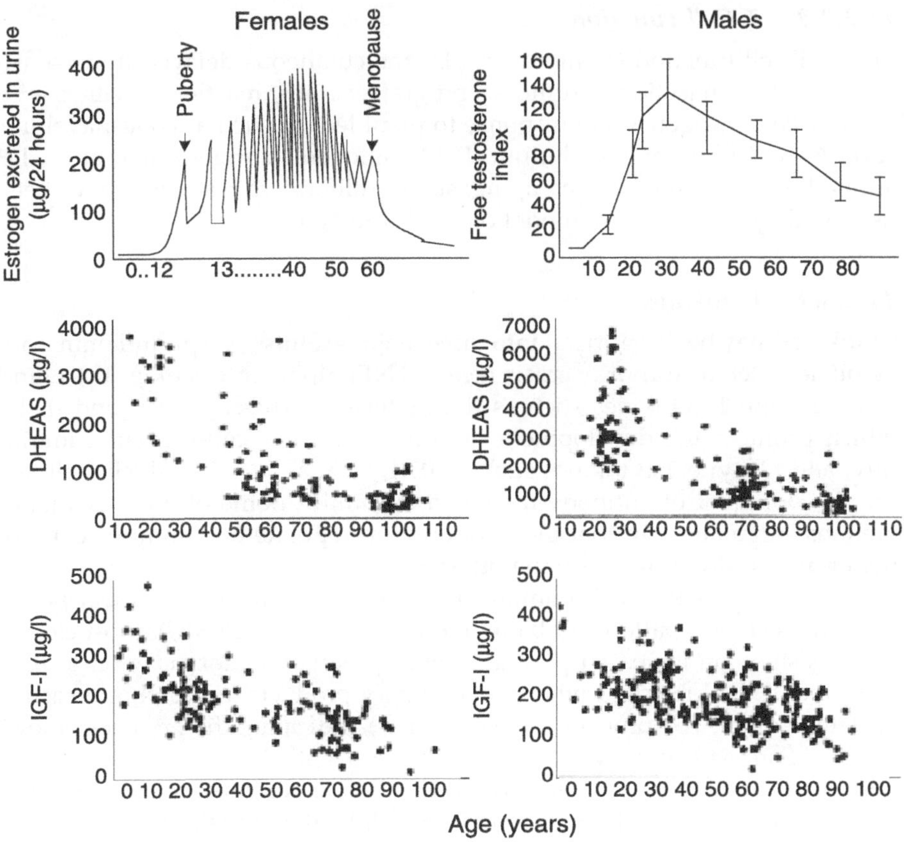

FIGURE 11.1
Changes occurring in the hormone levels of normal women (left) and men (right) during the aging process (Reprinted with permission from Lamberts, S.W.J. et al., The endocrinology of aging, *Science*, 278, 419–424, Copyright 1997, The American Association for the Advancement of Science.)

and the hypothalamic–pituitary–gonadal–thymic axis.[28] Changes occurring in the relevant hormone levels of normal women and men during the aging process are depicted in Figure 11.1.

11.2.3 Immune Senescence as Seen in Peripheral Blood

11.2.3.1 Cell Counts and Subsets

Age-related changes in cell counts and subsets include lower circulating numbers of $CD4^+$ and $CD8^+$ T cells, and B cells, although the proportion of activated T cells (cells expressing HLA-DR or IL-2R molecules) increases.[30-32] The number of circulating NK cells either remains unchanged or increases with age.[31-33] Aging also leads to a relative increase in the number of $CD45RO^+$ memory cells at the expense of $CD45RA^+$ naive cells, in both the $CD4^+$ and $CD8^+$ T cell populations.[30,34,35]

11.2.3.2 T Cell Function

In vivo T cell function (as monitored by the cutaneous delayed hypersensitivity reaction, rejection of tumors, and graft-vs.-host reaction) declines with age.[1,2] T cell mitogenesis in response to plant lectins such as concanavalin A (Con A) and phytohemagglutinin (PHA), allogenic antigens, and anti-CD3 antibodies diminishes during aging; such proliferative responses have been used widely as an *in vitro* model of T cell function.[36-40]

11.2.3.3 Cytokines

Cytokines may be categorized into three major groups:[41] (1) proinflammatory cytokines such as tumor necrosis factor (TNF)-alpha, interleukin (IL)-1, and IL-6; (2) type 1 cytokines such as IL-2, interferon (IFN)-gamma and IL-12, which promote the development of antigen-specific, cell-mediated immunity; and (3) type 2 cytokines such as IL-4, IL-5, and IL-10, which facilitate the development of antibody-mediated immunity. Some of these cytokines are cross-regulatory, in that they not only up-regulate one immune component but also down-regulate the other.[41,42]

Aging is associated with immune activation and changes in the balance of cytokine secretion patterns of blood mononuclear cells (PBMC). Most elderly subjects show an increased plasma level of proinflammatory cytokines (IL-1, IL-6, and TNF-alpha) and other inflammatory products (acute phase reactive proteins, soluble receptors of some cytokines), indicating the presence of low-grade inflammatory activity.[43] After induction with lipopolysaccharide, the peripheral blood mononuclear cells (PBMC) from elderly persons also produce larger amounts of IL-1, IL-6, IL-8, and TNF-alpha than the PBMC from young donors.[44] There is increasing evidence that high levels of inflammatory markers are associated with atherosclerosis, postmenopausal osteoporosis, and dementia, and can predict future disability in older persons.[45-50]

The PBMC from elderly donors show an increased capacity to produce type 2 cytokines (IL-4, IL-5, IL-6, IL-10), but a lower capacity to produce the type 1 cytokines (IFN-gamma, IL-2, IL-12) in comparison with those from young donors.[42,51,52] The shift of cytokine profile reflects in part a relative expansion of memory T cells at the expense of naïve T cells. The increased levels of type 2 cytokines correlate with the increased levels of serum antibodies and benign gammopathies in the elderly.[8,53,54]

Relatively little is known about changes in soluble receptors and other agonist/antagonists that may regulate cytokine actions in aging humans. Albright and Albright[55] recently reported that aging subjects (50 to 67 years) had significantly higher plasma levels of IL-1 receptor antagonist (IL-1ra) and significantly lower levels of soluble TNF receptor (TNFsRII) and soluble IL-6 receptor than young subjects (25 to 35 years), but no significant change in the level of soluble IL-1 receptor. There was less spontaneous output of IL-1ra and TNFsRII by the PBMC of aging subjects, but the output of both factors in response to PHA stimulation matched that of younger subjects, indicating that, although the basal output of these two factors had declined with age, the potential of stimulated PBMC to produce the factors remained unchanged.

11.2.3.4 B Cell Function

Some reports[56,57] have noted an age-dependent decline in the B-cell proliferative response to lipopolysaccharide, anti-Ig antibodies, or Fc fragments. An age-associated decline in the antibody response to tetanus toxoid, cholera toxin, and influenza vaccine has also been reported in humans.[4,58] An age-related increase of serum IgG (IgG_1, IgG_2, and IgG_3, but not IgG_4) and IgA, but not IgM levels, has been documented by several authors.[53,59]

11.2.3.5 Innate Immunity

Components of innate immunity such as neutrophils, macrophages, and natural killer cells retain their activity even in the aged.[60-62] There have been conflicting results concerning NK cell number and activity.[63-66] However, a recent study[67] demonstrating an age-related decline of perforin expression in human natural killer cells, as well as cytotoxic T lymphocytes supports a previous finding that NK cell activity expressed on a per-cell basis was decreased in the aged.[32,35]

11.3 Gender Difference in Immune Function

11.3.1 Premenopausal Women

When compared with their male peers, women have a lower incidence and mortality for several types of infection.[14,68] One proximate cause is a sexual dimorphism in immune function.[14-17] IgM levels are higher in adult women than in men,[69,70] and IgG responses to certain hepatitis B vaccine preparations are also three times higher in women.[71] However, the same mechanisms that reduce risks of infection in women also make them more susceptible to various autoimmune diseases.[14-17] The production of a variety of autoreactive antibodies is also more frequent in females than in males. Certain clinical conditions such as chlamydial and gonococcal infection rates are associated with specific phases of the menstrual cycle.[72,73] Urinary tract infections are less likely to recur if their initial onset is in the luteal phase.[74] Likewise, both the menstrual cycle and pregnancy have an impact on the severity of autoimmune diseases such as lupus erythematosus, Sjögren's syndrome, rheumatoid arthritis, and multiple sclerosis.[17,75]

Sex hormones, specifically estrogens in females and androgens in males, have direct immunological effects that impact the sexual dimorphism in immune function. Several experimental approaches have examined the underlying mechanisms:[4]

- Treating animals, or immune cells collected from animals, with sex steroids or nonsteroidal estrogenic compounds
- Gonadectomizing animals with or without hormone replacement therapy
- Observing immunological change during periods of altered hormonal status (human menstrual cycles, rodent estrus cycles, menopause, or pregnancy)

Available findings may be summarized as follows:[16,28]

- Estrogens increase B-cell response both *in vivo* and *in vitro*, whereas progesterone and androgens depress antibody production.
- T cell-mediated responses, such as transplant rejection and tumor-associated immunity, are depressed by androgens, progesterone, and, to a lesser extent, estrogens.
- Sex hormones modulate a large variety of mechanisms involved in immune responses, including thymocyte maturation and selection, cell trafficking, cytokine and monokine production, lymphocyte proliferation, expression of adhesion molecules, and HLA-class II receptors.

Taken together, estrogens enhance B cell-mediated diseases but suppress T cell-dependent conditions. Testosterone appears to suppress both B cell- and T cell-mediated responses and virtually always suppresses expression of disease.

Gender differences can be seen in resting peripheral blood samples. Circulating neutrophil counts are approximately 20% higher in women,[76] and the count varies in a cyclic fashion during the menstrual cycle, correlating with urinary estrogen measurements.[77] A greater respiratory burst reaction of monocytes has also been reported in women than in men.[78] Higher CD4:CD8 ratios are generally seen in females and hypogonadal males, due to relatively lower numbers of circulating CD8 T cells.[79,80] Using sensitive enzyme-linked immunospot assays, Verthelyi and Klinman[81] found that the physiological fluctuation in sex hormone levels influences the activity of peripheral blood cytokine-producing cells in premenopausal women; the number of PBMC able to secrete IL-4 in response to stimulation correlated significantly with plasma estrogen levels and fluctuated with the menstrual cycle, whereas the activity of IFN-gamma-secreting cells varied as a function of serum DHEA levels.

Overall, sexual dimorphism is apparent in sexually mature individuals.

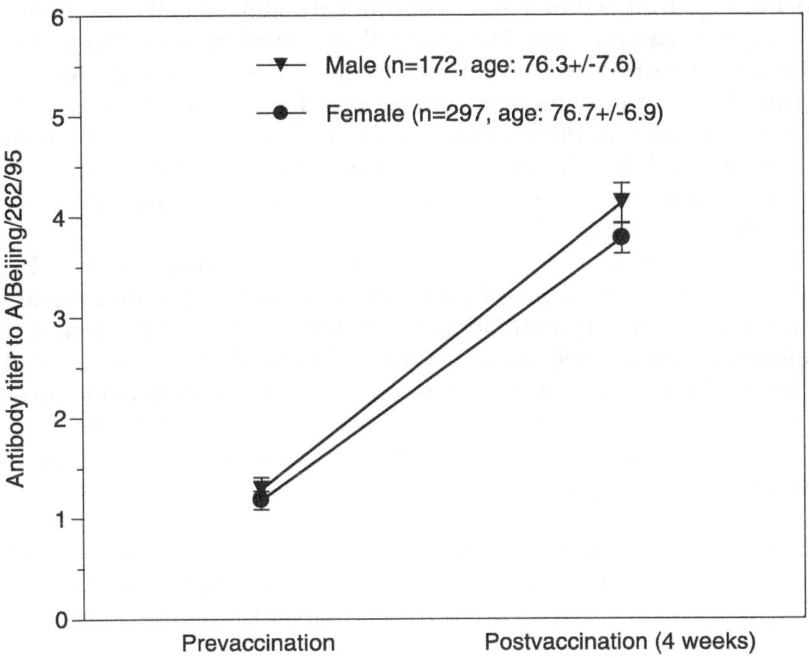

FIGURE 11.2
Comparison of antibody production in response to influenza vaccination (A/Beijing/262/95) between older women (n = 297, age, 76.7 ± 6.9) and older men (n = 172, age, 76.3 ± 7.6). Vertical line indicates antibody titer as expressed by [1 + Log_2 (HI titer/10)]. Data, mean ± SE (From Shinkai et al., unpublished data).

11.3.2 Postmenopausal Women

After menopause, blood estrogen levels drop dramatically in females, whereas androgen levels show a relatively smaller age-related decline in men (Figure 11.1). The gender difference in immune function does not seem to predominate in older people.

For example, a greater respiratory burst reaction was reported in women than in men (below the age of 55 years), but the difference was not seen in older subjects (over 65 years of age).[78] It has been recently noted that older women (mean age 76.3 years) and men (76.7 years) mounted similar levels of HI antibodies against influenza vaccine (Figure 11.2). In old age, significant gender differences in the incidence of autoimmune diseases disappear. In the case of rheumatoid arthritis, for example, the gender ratio for case incidence reaches a maximum of 3 or 4 to 1 during the reproductive years, decreasing thereafter to around 1:1 in old age.[82] However, as few studies have compared *in vivo* and *in vitro* immune function between older women and men, the extent of sexual dimorphism in immune function during old age cannot be verified.

Postmenopausal women have significantly fewer cells spontaneously secreting IFN-gamma and TNF-alpha than either men or premenopausal women,[81] suggesting that hormonal changes may contribute to the age-associated decline in immune reactivity of older women. There is no reduction in the number of PBMC that respond to PHA stimulation by secreting IFN-gamma and IL-2 in postmenopausal women.[81] Thus, aging may be associated with a decline in the activation state, rather than in the frequency of available cytokine-producing cells.

Higher levels of catabolic cytokines such as IL-6, IL-1beta, and TNF-alpha are often found in older people, and this may influence both muscle mass and neuroendocrine dysregulation.[83] Considering gender differences in the development of the syndrome of frailty, Walston and Fried [84] speculated that low levels of both estrogen and androgens in older women led to increased levels of catabolic cytokines, and this in turn accelerated the development of the syndrome of frailty in women of advanced age. Supporting data include the following observations:[84]

- Withdrawal of estrogen leads to increased levels of monocytes and catabolic cytokines in postmenopausal women; estrogen exerts a protective effect by blocking the secretion of TNF-alpha at the level of the monocyte.
- Testosterone reduces the amount of IL-6 produced by monocytes as well as inhibiting anti-DNA antibody production; there is evidence that testosterone may help, in part, by checking an increased level of catabolic cytokines in men.

11.4 Exercise-Induced Immunomodulatory Hormones

Changes in the distribution and function of immune cells with exercise may reflect neurohormonal responses to exercise. Thus, it is important to see how neurohormonal responses age, and to explore how gender and training affect aging of the neurohormonal response to exercise.

11.4.1 Catecholamines, Cortisol, and Beta-Endorphin

At the onset of exercise, signals activating the motor cortex to initiate muscle contraction may, in a parallel fashion, activate higher endocrine centers, causing a release of hormones and mobilization of extramuscular fuel ("central command").[85] During continuous exercise, feedback signals from the exercising muscles can intensify these hormonal changes (the "exercise pressor reflex").[85,86] Among the exercise-induced hormones are several immunomodulatory hormones that potentially influence the function and trafficking of immune cells.[87,88] Activation of the sympathoadrenal system in response to exercise results in increased levels of plasma catecholamines (epinephrine and norepinephrine); these hormones have marked physiological effects on heart rate, vasomotor tone, and, ultimately, on blood flow through lymphoid tissues and leukocyte circulation patterns. Stimulation of the hypothalamic–pituitary axis during exercise results in the secretion of adrenocorticotropic hormone (ACTH) and, in turn, causes a release of glucocorticoids into the circulation; the glucocorticoids have potent immunosuppressive effects on cytokines, macrophages, monocytes, and NK cells, and also induce redistribution of immune cells. Other hormones, such as the anterior pituitary hormone beta-endorphin, are also actively secreted as a consequence of sustained moderate exercise.

11.4.2 Aging of Hormone Responses

Aging has been associated with an augmentation of plasma norepinephrine levels at rest[89-91] and in response to a variety of challenges.[89,90,92-94] Such findings have led to a general perspective that aging may result in increased sympathetic nervous system activity. However, an assessment of age-associated changes in sympathetic nervous system response to certain types of stress may be confounded by age-related differences in aerobic fitness and adiposity.[94-97] Age differences are largely abolished if young and elderly subjects are first matched for maximal oxygen intake per unit of body mass and are then exercised at the same relative work rate.[98] In general, at any given fraction of aerobic power, the effect of strenuous exercise on catecholamine response is either the same in an older person as in someone younger,[99] or is less marked in the older person.[100]

Cortisol is an integral part of the hypothalamic–pituitary–adrenal (HPA) axis response to stress. Earlier studies on the effects of aging on basal cortisol levels and/or cortisol responses to stimulation tests concluded that, in humans, aging does not seem to be associated with changes in the basal activity of the HPA axis or in its ability to respond to challenge.[101-103] Recent evidence, however, has challenged this view: a 24-h study[104] has now demonstrated higher cortisol levels in older than in younger adults. In both men and women, mean cortisol levels increased 20 to 50% between 20 and 80 years of age.[104] The diurnal rhythmicity of cortisol secretion was preserved in old age, but the relative amplitude was dampened, and the timing of the circadian elevation was advanced.[104] The level of the nocturnal nadir increased progressively with aging in both sexes, suggesting etiological involvement with the sleep disorders commonly seen in the elderly. Laughlin and Barrett-Connor[105] reported blood cortisol levels obtained between 7:30 and 11:00 a.m. from 857 men and 735 nonestrogen-using, postmenopausal women; values increased progressively (20% overall) with age in both men and women between 50 and 89 years of age. The age-related decrease in HPA axis sensitivity to glucocorticoid feedback suppression may be causally related to the increased level of plasma cortisol in the elderly.[106,107]

11.4.3 Gender Difference in Hormone Responses

Recent studies[108-110] have demonstrated sexual dimorphism in neuroendocrine responses to various physiological stresses, such as hypoglycemia and cognitive testing. Women show a smaller sympathetic nervous activity in response to exercise. Davis et al.[111] found that women (mean age 28 years) had a smaller catecholamine response to prolonged moderate exercise (90-min cycle ergometer exercise at 80% anaerobic threshold) than did men matched for age, body mass index, nutrient intake, and physical fitness level. Ettinger et al.[112] noted that, in response to static hand grip exercise (30% maximal voluntary contraction to exhaustion), women (mean age 39 years) showed smaller increases in both blood pressure and muscle sympathetic nerve activity assessed by microneurography when compared with men (35 years). Gender difference in the sympathetic nervous response to a bout of exercise may change with advancing age; however, as yet no reports document responses in the elderly. Matsukawa et al.[113] have examined gender difference in age-related changes in resting muscle sympathetic nerve activity (MSNA) in healthy subjects, and found that the MSNA was lower in women than in men among those aged <30 years ($P = 0.0012$), 30 to 39 years ($P = 0.0126$), and 40 to 49 years ($P = 0.0462$), but activity was similar in women and men who were aged 50 to 59 years ($P = 0.191$, NS) and >60 years ($P = 0.1739$, NS), suggesting that gender differences were attenuated with aging.

In 50- to 89-year-old community dwelling adults, basal cortisol levels were 10% higher in women than in men.[105] Furthermore,[104,114] women have a greater cortisol response to stressful events than do men and their response persists for a longer period. One study,[111] however, reported that plasma cortisol levels increased similarly in young women and men in response to prolonged moderate exercise. Overall, given that aging is associated with elevated cortisol level in both genders, older women may have more alterations in their HPA axis, possibly underlying in part their greater susceptibility to senile osteoporosis, sarcopenia, and depression.[84]

Goldfarb et al.[115] reported that, independently of menstrual phase, women (26.8 years) cycling at 80% $\dot{V}O_{2max}$ had a similar beta-endorphin response to men (26.4 years); however, at 60% $\dot{V}O_{2max}$, beta-endorphin levels were slightly lower than in men. Again, no paper has documented gender difference in beta-endorphin response to a bout of vigorous exercise in the aged.

11.4.4 Hormone Responses to Exercise Training in the Aged

In both sexes the main determinant of hormone response to a given bout of exercise is the fraction of maximal oxygen intake utilized.[85,116] Thus, training at any age decreases the amount of hormone released at a given absolute intensity of effort. However, conditioning also permits exercise to a higher peak work rate, and may thus increase the hormone concentration reached during a prolonged bout of all-out exercise.[85,116] This is true both for catecholamines and for pituitary hormones.[116-118] Since epinephrine clearance is identical in trained and untrained subjects, the higher plasma epinephrine levels found in trained subjects during maximal exercise indicates that physical training increases the capacity to secrete adrenomedullary hormones (the so called "sports adrenal medulla").[119] The increased capacity to secrete epinephrine seems to be a long-term adaptation to training.[85,120]

Responses of the HPA axis to exercise training were first compared between trained and untrained elderly groups. Heuser et al.[121] found that cortisol responses to human coroticotropin-releasing hormone (hCRH) were significantly greater in endurance athletes (mean age 57 years); ACTH responses also tended to be larger in well-trained individuals. In contrast, Struder et al.[122] reported that cortisol responses to combined corticotropin, luteinizing hormone, and thyrotropin-releasing hormone challenge did not differ between elderly distance runners (mean age 69.9 years) and sedentary individuals (69.1 years). A consistent finding was that basal cortisol and ACTH levels did not differ between trained subjects and sedentary controls. Early longitudinal experiments showed no change in cortisol secretion with 20 minutes of graded exercise to 80 to 90% $\dot{V}O_{2max}$ before and after 9- to 10-week endurance training.[123] However, a recent prospective study has shown that after a 10-week heavy resistance training, 62-year-old subjects demonstrated a significant decrease in resting cortisol along with a significant increase in total testosterone in response to exercise stress.[124] Thus, results to date have been inconsistent, suggesting that future study should take into account the substantial diurnal variation in HPA axis activity.

Overall, exercise training in later life reduces the magnitude of catecholamine and pituitary hormone responses to a given bout of exercise, and increases the resistance to physical stress. Given that stress hormones are in general immunosuppressive, appropriate exercise training may be beneficial for the aging immune system, raising the threshold level of immunosuppressive (i.e., strenuous and/or prolonged) physical exercise.

11.5 Immune Responses to Exercise in the Aged

Exercise influences natural immunity, T and B cell functions, and cytokine responses through hemodynamic changes and by means of the earlier mentioned immunomodulatory hormones secreted in response to physical stress. The magnitude of the effects on the immune system reflects the intensity, duration, and chronicity of the exercise (Figure 11.3).[87,125,126]

11.5.1 Acute Responses to a Bout of Exercise

Unfortunately, no data are available on gender differences in immune response to acute exercise in the elderly. Limited data show that, in general,

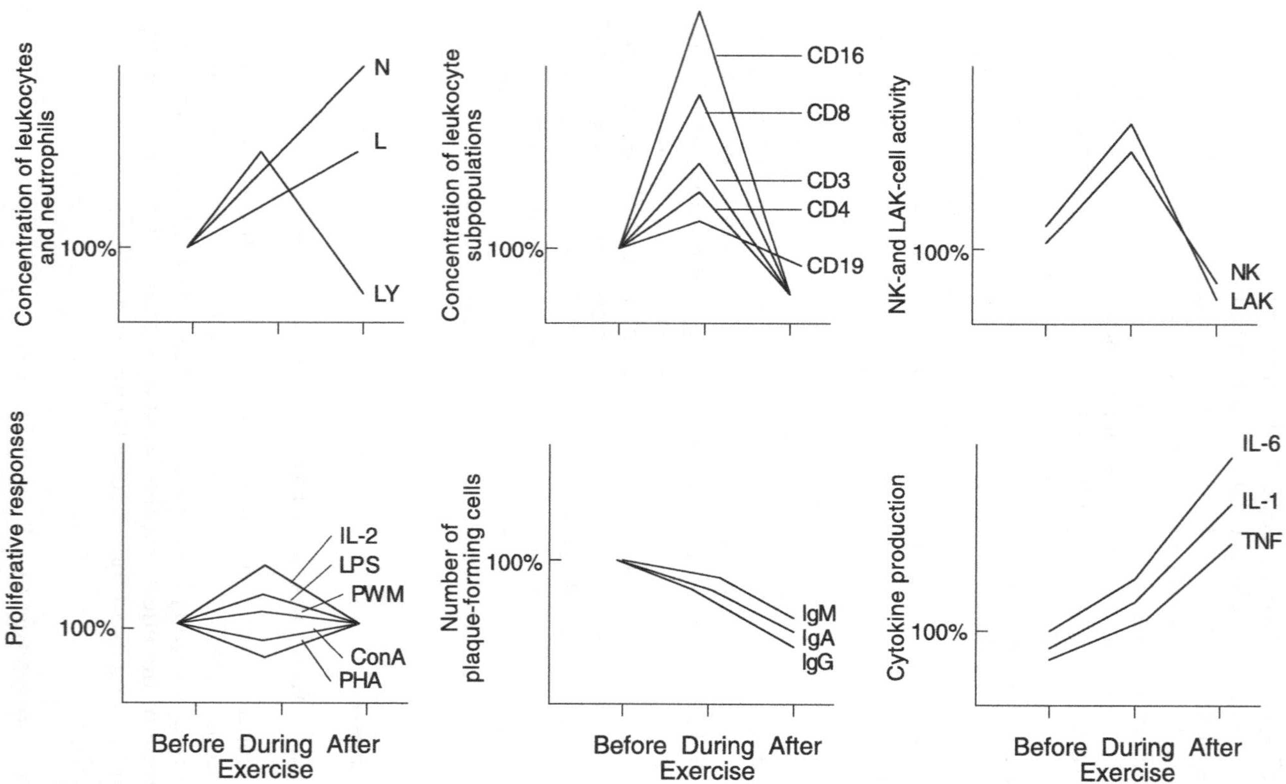

FIGURE 11.3

Schematic representation of major immunological changes that occur in humans in relation to acute physical exercise. Abbreviations: N, neutrophils; L, leukocytes; LY, lymphocytes; LAK, lymphokine-activated killer; NK, natural killer; IL-2, interleukin 2; LPS, lipopolysaccharide; PWM, pokeweed mitogen; Con A, concanavalin A; PHA, phytohemagglutinin; TNF, tumor necrosis factor. (Reprinted from *Immunol. Today*, 15(8), Hoffman-Goetz, L. and Pedersen, B.K., Exercise and the immune system: a model of stress response? 382–387, Copyright 1994, with permission from Elsevier Science.)

a single bout of moderate exercise is well tolerated by the elderly, but strenuous exercise may lead to greater postexercise immunosuppression in the peripheral blood of older adults relative to young individuals. The results seem to imply that older adults should adopt a more cautious approach to strenuous exercise.

Fiatarone et al.[127] found an immediate rise of NK activity to 202% of normal when nine active older women (mean age 71 years) completed a maximal cycle ergometer test. The average response did not differ greatly from the 231% peak of NK activity which they had seen in eight young active women (30 years), nor were there any age-related differences in the responsiveness of the NK cells to IL-2, although there was more interindividual variation of response in the older subjects. Mazzeo et al.[128] examined PHA-induced lymphocyte proliferation at rest and immediately after a 20-min supine cycle ergometer exercise at 60% of peak capacity both in young (mean age 23 years) and elderly (69 years) male groups. Although pre-exercise PHA responsiveness was significantly lower for elderly vs. young subjects, immediately after exercise elderly subjects showed less suppression of proliferation (9% decrease) than did young subjects (22% decrease), suggesting that the extent of immunosuppression from a single bout of exercise differed across age groups. Shinkai et al.[35] compared the immune responses to a short triathlon event (1.5 km swimming, 54.8 km cycling, and 13.4 km running) between nine young (mean age 24.3 years) and nine older (49.3 years) male athletes. Baseline immunological data showed no significant differences between these two groups. Age differences in monocytosis and lymphopenia were found immediately after the race, and lymphocyte mitogenesis also differed immediately and for 8 days after the race. The magnitude of the monocytosis was much greater in the young group (320% increase relative to the baseline data) vs. the older group (110% increase). In contrast, a postexercise lymphopenia was more profound in the older group (45 vs. 36% decrease in the young group), and a suppressed lymphocyte mitogenesis to ConA and PWM was observed only in the older group. The responses of NK cells and activity were comparable in the two groups.

Strenuous exercise increases concentrations of various proinflammatory and antiinflammatory cytokines, naturally occurring cytokine inhibitors, and chemokines.[43] Given that aging is associated with increased inflammatory activity, strenuous exercise may induce the cytokine cascade more markedly in aging adults than in young peers.

11.5.2 Immune Responses to Exercise Training in the Aged

11.5.2.1 Cross-Sectional Studies

Cross-sectional studies have shown that, regardless of gender, the fit elderly who engage in regular endurance exercise over a long period (i.e., for multiple years) have an increased per-cell function of both T cells (as assessed by mitogenesis to lectins or anti-CD3, and cytokine production) and NK cells, but circulating leukocyte and lymphocyte subset counts are similar when compared with age- and sex-matched controls.

Nieman et al.[129] studied exceptionally active, highly conditioned elderly women, 65 to 84 years of age, with an aerobic power 67% greater than age-matched sedentary subjects. The active group had retained 56% greater lymphocyte proliferative response to PHA, and 54% greater NK cell activity than their sedentary peers. However, the two groups had similar leukocyte and lymphocyte subset counts, indicating that functional activities per-cell were greater in the well-trained individuals. Findings were also compared with data on young college women, tested approximately 12 weeks later; the initially sedentary elderly subjects had a much lower T cell functional capacity than the young females, but no significant difference in NK cell activity.

Shinkai et al.[32] examined resting immune function in 17 elderly male runners, 16 young sedentary controls, and 19 elderly male controls (mean ages 63.8, 23.6, and 65.8 years, respectively). The previously described age-related differences were again demonstrated. The elderly runners, who had an aerobic power 33% greater than that of elderly controls, retained superior T cell function with respect to both lymphocyte proliferative responses to PHA and PWM, and cytokine production of IL-2, IFN-gamma, and IL-4. However, other aspects of immune function (circulating leukocyte and lymphocyte subset counts, NK cell activity, lymphocyte responsiveness to allogenic antigens, and IL-1beta production) did not differ between the elderly runners and their sedentary peers.

They further examined whether benefits could be anticipated in middle-aged and age-advanced male runners (Table 11.1).[35] When compared with young controls, data for groups in the sixth and eighth age decades showed substantial changes in the major leukocyte and lymphocyte subset counts (Tables 11.2 and 11.3). A shift from naive ($CD45RA^+$) to memory ($CD45RO^+$) T cell-types was clearly demonstrated in the older groups. The age-associated changes in circulating immune cells did not differ significantly between the two older groups, except that the $CD3^-CD56^+$ NK cell number was further increased in the oldest age group. There were no significant differences in circulating immune cell counts between runners and sedentary controls in the older age groups. However, both groups of older runners exhibited significantly greater responsiveness of lymphocyte to PHA and PWM relative to their respective sedentary control groups (Figure 11.4). Runners in the sixth decade had slightly higher per-cell activity of NK cells compared with age-matched controls.

Benefits of regular physical activity may also be seen in moderate exercisers. Gueldner et al.[130] found that lymphocytes from active older women (mean age 71.5 years) who had engaged in long-term moderate exercise (more than 15 years for more than half of them) exhibited a higher responsiveness to anti-CD3 stimulation *in vitro* than did age- and sex-matched inactive controls (72.5 years), thus suggesting a possibility that even moderate exercise

TABLE 11.1

Physical Characteristics of Five Test Groups (All Males)

Group	Age (years)	Height (cm)	Body Mass (kg)	Body Mass Index (kg/m^2)	Sum of 7 Skinfolds (mm)	Waist/Hip Ratio	% Body Fat	$\dot{V}O_{2max}$ (mL/kg/min)
20C (n = 14)	23.0 ± 0.7	169 ± 1	66.2 ± 2.1	23.2 ± 0.7	126 ± 14	0.86 ± 0.02	22.1 ± 2.3	38.7 ± 1.5
50C (n = 14)	54.4 ± 0.9	167 ± 1	64.4 ± 1.9	23.1 ± 0.6	129 ± 11	0.94 ± 0.02	19.9 ± 1.1	31.0 ± 1.2
50R (n = 16)	55.2 ± 0.7	165 ± 1	61.1 ± 1.7	22.4 ± 0.5	93 ± 5	0.88 ± 0.01[a]	17.5 ± 0.9	42.2 ± 1.3[b]
70C (n = 14)	74.1 ± 0.9	164 ± 2	57.8 ± 2.6	21.5 ± 0.9	108 ± 9	0.94 ± 0.02	17.0 ± 1.4	28.5 ± 1.7
70R (n = 12)	74.3 ± 1.2	162 ± 2	58.9 ± 1.8	22.4 ± 0.5	105 ± 5	0.93 ± 0.01	15.6 ± 1.3	34.4 ± 1.2[a]
Age effect	$p<0.001$	0.107	0.032	NS	NS	0.001	0.112	<0.001

Note: Age effect, one-way ANOVA applied on data for three control groups. 20C, 50C (R), and 70C (R) represent control (runner) groups aged 20s, 50s, and 70s, respectively. Data, mean ± SE. (From Shinkai et al.,[35] with permission).

[a] $p<0.01$ vs. respective age-matched control group.
[b] $p<0.001$ vs. respective age-matched control group.

TABLE 11.2

Leukocyte Subset Concentrations in Peripheral Blood Samples of Runners and Controls

Group	Total WBC (mm^{-3})	Neutrophiles (mm^{-3})	Eosinophils (mm^{-3})	Basophils (mm^{-3})	Monocytes (mm^{-3})	Lymphocytes (mm^{-3})
20C (n = 14)	6430 ± 420	2930 ± 280	210 ± 40	50 ± 10	660 ± 60	2570 ± 130
50C (n = 14)	5260 ± 290	3100 ± 260	150 ± 30	50 ± 7	320 ± 40	1640 ± 60
50R (n = 16)	4680 ± 320	2730 ± 390	140 ± 20	40 ± 4	320 ± 40	1640 ± 100
70C (n = 14)	5200 ± 270	2870 ± 190	160 ± 30	40 ± 6	400 ± 50	1730 ± 110
70R (n = 12)	4750 ± 250	2660 ± 170	130 ± 20	40 ± 4	320 ± 30	1600 ± 110
Age effect	$p = 0.020$	NS	NS	NS	<0.001	<0.001

Note: Age effect, one-way ANOVA applied on data for three control groups; 20C, 50C (R), and 70C (R) represent control (runner) groups aged 20s, 50s, and 70s, respectively. Data, mean ± SE. (From Shinkai et al.,[35] with permission).

TABLE 11.3

Lymphocyte Subset Concentrations in Peripheral Blood Samples of Runners and Controls

Group	$CD3^-CD56^+$ cells (mm^{-3})	$CD3^+CD56^+$ cells (mm^{-3})	$CD3^+CD56^-$ cells (mm^{-3})	$CD19^+$ cells (mm^{-3})	$CD4^+$ cells (mm^{-3})	$CD8^+$ cells (mm^{-3})
20C (n = 14)	290 ± 40	60 ± 7	1830 ± 90	240 ± 30	1010 ± 70	720 ± 70
50C (n = 14)	320 ± 40	80 ± 20	980 ± 60	130 ± 20	710 ± 50	310 ± 40
50R (n = 16)	360 ± 60	50 ± 10	1000 ± 80	120 ± 20	660 ± 50	300 ± 40
70C (n = 14)	430 ± 60	70 ± 10	970 ± 60	120 ± 40	640 ± 60	340 ± 40
70R (n = 12)	410 ± 70	70 ± 10	880 ± 90	90 ± 20	550 ± 60	320 ± 60
Age effect	$p = 0.040$	NS	<0.001	0.006	<0.001	<0.001

Note: Age effect, one-way ANOVA applied on data for three control groups; 20C, 50C (R), and 70C (R) represent control (runner) groups aged 20s, 50s, and 70s, respectively. Data, mean ± SE. (From Shinkai et al.,[35] with permission).

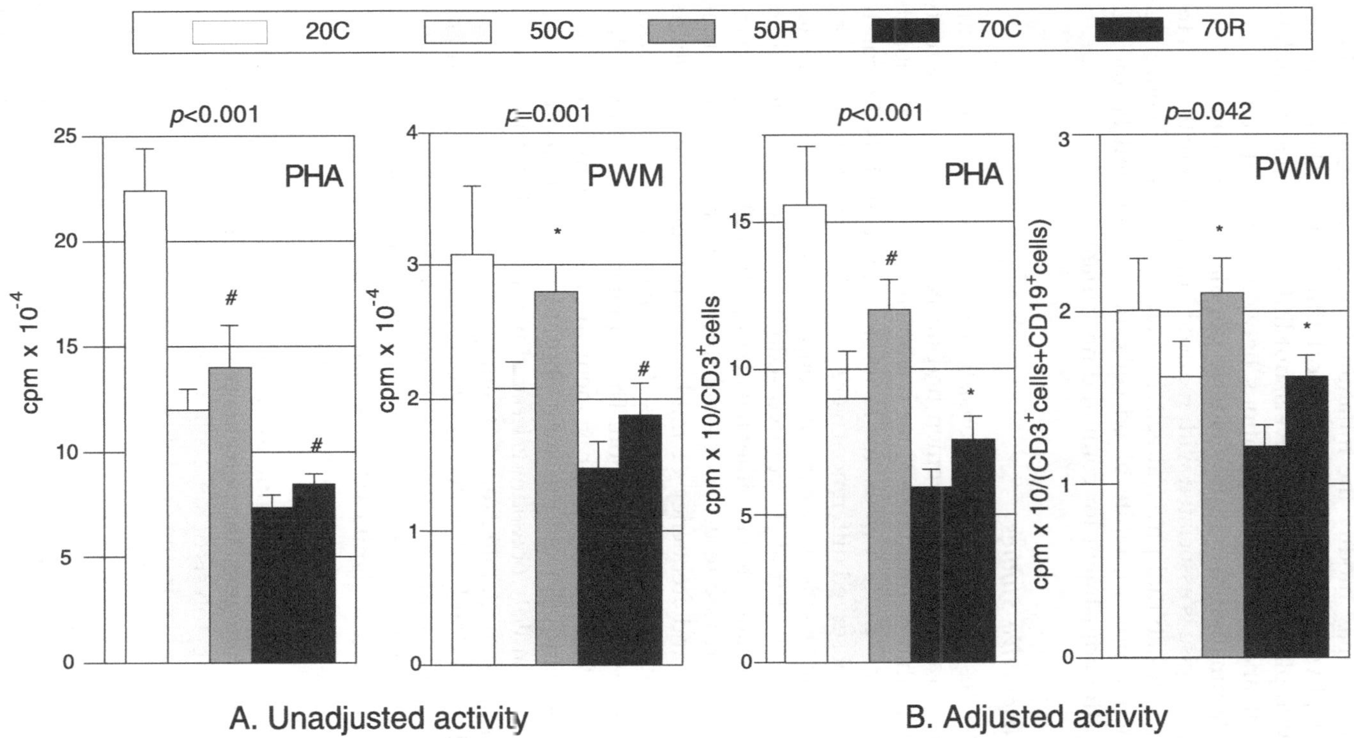

FIGURE 11.4
Comparison of lymphocyte proliferative response to mitogens (PHA, PWM) among elderly runners, and young and elderly controls. Unadjusted activity (A) and adjusted activity (B) on a per respective major responding cell in peripheral blood mononuclear cell suspension. 20C, 50C, and 70C represent control groups aged 20s, 50s, and 70s, respectively. R, runner group. Data are expressed as mean ± SE. *p* values, age effect. $^{\#}p<0.1$, $^{*}p<0.05$ vs. respective age-matched control group. (From Shinkai et al.,[35] with permission).

training can modulate the aging of immune function if it is carried out appropriately on a long-term basis.

Physical activity may modify the inflammatory process. Cross-sectional studies[131-134] of physical activity and physical fitness have shown inverse associations with plasma fibrinogen levels, but little is known about elderly subjects. Recent analysis[135] of associations between physical activity and markers of inflammation in a healthy elderly population has demonstrated that increased exercise is associated with reduced inflammation; those in the higher quartiles of habitual physical activity had lower plasma concentrations of C-reactive protein, white blood cells, fibrinogen, and Factor VIII activity, even after adjustment for confounding variables.

11.5.2.2 Prospective Studies

Prospective studies have reported inconsistent results. Crist et al.[136] found that moderately trained elderly women had an NK cell cytotoxic activity 33% greater than that of untrained elderly women. Their group of subjects trained moderately, 3 times a week, for 16 weeks. However, it is difficult to know whether the observed differences were present before the women were assigned to exercise or sedentary control groups. Nieman et al.[129] conducted a randomized controlled trial. Thirty-two sedentary, elderly women, 67 to 85 years of age, were allocated to either a walking (30 to 40 minutes, 5 days/week at 60% of heart rate reserve) or a calisthenic group (who undertook the same duration and frequency of mild range-of-motion and flexibility movements, keeping their heart rates close to resting levels). Thirty subjects completed the 12 weeks of intervention. The walking group improved their $\dot{V}O_{2max}$ by 12.6%, without any improvement in NK cell activity or T cell function. Another study[137] from the same laboratory showed an increase in NK cell activity for mildly obese middle-aged women as they engaged in a 15-week program of moderate exercise training.

Woods et al.[138] randomly allocated previously sedentary older men and women (mean age 65 years) to either a 6-month moderate aerobic exercise group or flexibility/toning control group. After the training period, the exercised group exhibited a significant 20% increase in $\dot{V}O_{2max}$, whereas the flexibility-control group had a smaller insignificant increase (9%). There were no intervention-induced changes in leukocyte and lymphocyte subsets. Both groups exhibited a small intervention-induced increase in the T cell proliferative response to mitogens; the percentage change was higher in the exercised group. NK cell cytolysis of K562 cells tended to increase in the exercised group, with little change in the flexibility controls.

Two studies have reported the effect of strength training on immune function in the elderly. Rall et al.[139] examined the effects of 12 weeks of progressive resistance training on *in vivo* and *in vitro* immune parameters in a controlled study involving eight subjects with rheumatoid arthritis, eight healthy young (20 to 30 years), and eight healthy elderly (65 to 80 years) individuals and age-matched controls. The trained subjects exercised at 80% of their

1-repetition maximum, performing eight repetitions per set, three sets per session twice a week. Training did not induce any changes in peripheral blood mononuclear cell subsets, IL-1beta, TNF-alpha, IL-6, IL-2, or prostaglandin E_2 production, lymphocyte proliferation, or delayed type hypersensitivity response in any of the training groups compared with control subjects. Flynn et al.[140] found that, in women aged 67 to 87 years, 10 weeks of resistance training did not influence such resting immune measures as lymphocyte subset number, lymphocyte proliferative response to mitogen, and natural cell-mediated cytotoxicity, although the subjects substantially improved their strength (148% increase in 8-repetition maximum).

Previous prospective studies did not concur, nor did they support the view that regular exercise training improves immune function in the healthy elderly. Possible reasons include a lower intensity of exercise training, and other differences in subject characteristics. In addition, all of the prospective exercise interventions were of much shorter duration than the period for which the subjects in the cross-sectional studies had engaged in exercise training. As regards subject characteristics, Paw et al.[141] examined the effects of 17 weeks of physical exercise plus enriched foods on the development of a delayed hypersensitivity skin test response against seven recall antigens in frail older men and women. Nonexercising subjects showed an average decline of 0.5 responses and a larger decline in the summed diameters of all positive skin responses than did the exercising subjects, indicating that only exercise may prevent or slow the age-related decline in immune response.

11.6 Conclusions

Human immune function undergoes adverse changes with aging. The T cells, which have a central role in cellular immunity, show the largest age-related differences in distribution and function. The underlying causes include thymus involution and continuous attrition caused by chronic antigenic overload. Immune function is apparently sexually dimorphic; women have more vigorous immunologic activity than do men, thus reducing their risks of infection. However, the same mechanisms make women more susceptible to various autoimmune diseases. The sexual dimorphism in immune function may become less apparent with aging, although it persists into later life, and may contribute in part to the greater incidence of frailty in women of advanced age. In both sexes exercise training in later life reduces the magnitude of catecholamine and pituitary hormone responses to a given bout of exercise, and increases the resistance to physical stress. The immune responses to acute exercise and training have not been studied extensively in the elderly. However, limited data suggest that, regardless of gender, a long-term (i.e., multiple-year) effect of exercise could modulate the normal course of aging in the immune system beneficially in later life, and that physical exercise may relieve the increased inflammatory activity seen in old age. Short-term (i.e., less than six months) moderate aerobic exercise or strength training seems to have neither detrimental nor positive effects on selected indices of immune function.

References

1. Miller, R.A., Aging and immune function, *Int. Rev. Cytol.*, 124, 187–215, 1991.
2. Ben-Yehuda, A. and Weksler, M. E., Immune senescence: mechanisms and clinical implications, *Cancer Invest.*, 10, 525–531, 1992.
3. Shephard, R. J. and Shek, P. N., Exercise, aging, and immune function, *Int. J. Sports Med.*, 16, 1–6, 1995.
4. Ben-Yehuda, A. and Weksler, M. E., Host resistance and the immune system, *Clin. Geriatr. Med.*, 8, 701–711, 1992.
5. Effros, R. B. and Walford, R. L., Infections and immunity, in *Aging and the Immune Response*, Goidl, E. A., Ed., Marcel Dekker, New York, 1987, 45–65.
6. Makinodan, T., James, S. J., Inamizu, T., et al., Immunologic basis for susceptibility to infection in the aged, *Gerontology*, 30, 279–289, 1984.
7. Omer, Y. and Shoenfeld, Y., Aging and autoantibodies, *Autoimmunity* 1, 141–149, 1988.
8. Ligthart, G. J., Radl, J., Corberand, J. X., et al., Monoclonal gammopathies in human aging: increased occurrence with age and correlation with health status, *Mech. Ageing Dev.*, 52, 235–243, 1990.
9. Radl, J., Age-related monoclonal gammapathies: clinical lessons from the aging C57BL mouse, *Immunol. Today*, 11, 234–236, 1990.
10. Ershler, W. B., The influence of an aging immune system on cancer incidence and progression. *J. Gerontol.*, 48, B3–B7, 1993.
11. Ferguson, F. G., Wikby, A., Maxson, P., et al., Immune parameters in a longitudinal study of a very old population of Swedish people: a comparison between survivors and nonsurvivors. *J. Gerontol.*, 50A, B378–B382, 1995.
12. Lehtonen, L., Eskola, J., Vainio, O., and Lehtonen, A., Changes in lymphocyte subsets and immune competence in very advanced age, *J. Gerontol.*, 45, M108–M112, 1990.
13. Wayne, S. J., Rhyne, R. L., Garry, P. J., et al., Cell-mediated immunity as a predictor of morbidity and mortality in subjects over 60, *J. Gerontol.*, 45, M45–M48, 1990.
14. Cannon, J. G. and St. Pierre, B. A., Gender differences in host defense mechanisms, *J. Psychiatr. Res.*, 31, 99–113, 1997.
15. Legato, M. J., Gender-specific physiology: how real is it? How important is it? *Int. J. Fertil.*, 42, 19–29, 1997.
16. Schuurs, A. H., and Verheul, H. A., Effects of gender and sex steroids on the immune response, *J. Steroid Biochem.*, 35, 157–172, 1990.
17. Silva, J. A. P., Sex hormones and glucocorticoids: interactions with the immune system, *Ann. N. Y. Acad. Sci.*, 876, 102–117, 1999.
18. George, A. J. T. and Ritter, M. A., Thymic involution with aging: obsolescence or good housekeeping? *Immunol. Today*, 17, 267–272, 1996.

19. Mackall, C. L., Fleisher, T. A., Brown, M. R., et al., Age, thymopoiesis, and $CD4^+$ T-lymphocyte regeneration after intensive chemotherapy, *N. Engl. J. Med.*, 332, 143–149, 1995.
20. Franceschi, C., Motta, L., Valensin, S., et al., Do men and women follow different trajectories to reach extreme longevity? *Aging Clin. Exp. Res.*, 12, 77–84, 2000.
21. Utsuyama, M., Kasai, M., Kurashima, C., et al., Age influence on the thymic capacity to promote differentiation of T cells: induction of different composition of T cell subsets by aging thymus, *Mech. Ageing Dev.*, 58, 267–277, 1991.
22. Utsuyama, M., Hirokawa, K., Kurashima, C., et al., Differential age-change in the numbers of $CD4^+CD45RA^+$ and $CD4^+CD29^+$ T cell subsets in human peripheral blood, *Mech. Ageing Dev.*, 63, 54–68, 1992.
23. Mazzeo, R. S., Aging, immune function, and exercise: hormonal regulation, *Int. J. Sports Med.*, 21 Suppl. 1, S10–S13, 2000.
24. Gelato, M. C., Aging and immune function: a possible role for growth hormone, *Horm. Res. (Basel)*, 45, 46–49, 1996.
25. LeRoith, D., Yanowski. J., Kaldjian, E. P., et al., The effects of growth hormone and insulin-like growth factor I on the immune system of aged female monkeys, *Endocrinology*, 137, 1071–1079, 1996.
26. Khorram, O., Vu, L., and Yen, S. S. C., Activation of immune function by dehydroepiandrosterone (DHEA) in age-advanced men, *J. Gerontol.*, 52A, M1–M7, 1997.
27. Yen, S. S. C., Morales, A. J., and Khorram, O., Replacement of DHEA in aging men and women. Potential remedial effects, *Ann. N.Y. Acad. Sci.*, 774, 128–142, 1995.
28. Olsen, N. J. and Kovacs, W. J., Gonadal steroids and immunity, *Endocr. Rev.*, 17, 369–384, 1996.
29. Lamberts, S. W. J., Annewieki, B., and Aat-Jan, L., The endocrinology of aging, *Science*, 278, 419–424, 1997.
30. Erkeller-Yuksel, F. M., Deneys, V., Yuksel, B., et al., Age-related changes in human blood lymphocyte subpopulations, *J. Pediatr.*, 120, 216–222, 1992.
31. Sansoni, P., Cossarizza, A., Brianti, V., et al., Lymphocyte subsets and natural killer cell activity in healthy old people and centenarians, *Blood*, 82, 2767–2773, 1993.
32. Shinkai, S., Kohno, H., Kimura, K., et al., Physical activity and immune senescence in men, *Med. Sci. Sports Exerc.*, 27, 1516–1526, 1995.
33. Ligthart, G., Corberand, J. X., Geertzen, H. G. M., et al., Necessity of the assessment of health status in human immunogerontological studies: evaluation of the SENIEUR protocol, *Mech. Ageing Dev.*, 55, 89–105, 1990.
34. Paoli, P. De., Battistin, S., and Santini, G. F., Age-related changes in human lymphocyte subsets: progressive reduction of the CD4 CD45R (suppressor inducer) population, *Clin. Immunol. Immunopathol.*, 48, 290–296, 1988.
35. Shinkai, S., Konishi, M., and Shephard, R. J., Aging and immune response to exercise, *Can. J. Physiol. Pharmacol.*, 76, 562–576, 1998.
36. Gillis, S., Kozak, R., Durante, M., and Weksler, M. E., Immunological studies of aging. Decreased production of and response to T cell growth factor by lymphocytes from aged human, *J. Clin. Invest.*, 67, 937–942, 1981.
37. Murasko, D. M., Weiner, P., and Kaye, D., Decline in mitogen induced proliferation of lymphocytes with increasing age, *Clin. Exp. Immunol.*, 70, 440–448, 1987.

38. Nagel, J. E., Chopra, R. K., Chrest, F. J., et al., Decreased proliferation, interleukin 2 synthesis, and interleukin 2 receptor expression are accompanied by decreased mRNA expression in phytohemagglutinin-stimulated cells from elderly donors, *J. Clin. Invest.*, 81, 1096–1102, 1988.
39. Negoro, S., Hara, H. Miyata, S., et al., Mechanisms of age-related decline in antigen-specific T cell proliferative response: IL-2 receptor expression and recombinant IL-2 induced proliferative response of purified Tac-positive T cells, *Mech. Ageing Dev.*, 36, 223–241, 1986.
40. Holbrook, N. J., Chopra, R. K., McCoy, M. T., et al., Expression of interleukin 2 and the interleukin 2 receptor in aging rats, *Immunology*, 120, 1–9, 1989.
41. Lucey, D. R., Clerici, M., and Shearer, G. M., Type 1 and type 2 cytokine dysregulation in human infectious, neoplastic and inflammatory diseases, *Clin. Microbiol. Rev.*, 9, 532–562, 1996.
42. Shearer, G. M., Th1/Th2 changes in aging, *Mech. Ageing Dev.*, 94, 1–5, 1997.
43. Pedersen, B. K., Bruunsgaard, H., Ostrowski, K., et al., Cytokines in aging and exercise, *Int. J. Sports Med.*, 21 Suppl. 1, S4–S9, 2000.
44. Fagiolo, U., Cossarizza, A., Scala, E., et al., Increased cytokine production in mononuclear cells of healthy elderly people, *Eur. J. Immunol.*, 23, 2375–2378, 1993.
45. Ridker, P. M., Cushman, M., Stampfer, M. J., et al., Inflammation, aspirin, and the risk of cardiovascular disease in apparently healthy men, *N. Engl. J. Med.*, 336, 973–976, 1997.
46. Ross, R., Atherosclerosis — an inflammatory disease, *N. Engl. J. Med.*, 342, 115–126, 1999.
47. Bruunsgaard, H., Andersen-Ranberg, K., Jeune, B., et al., A high plasma concentration of TNF-alpha is associated with dementia in centenarians, *J. Gerontol.*, 54A, M357–M364, 1999.
48. Huberman, M., Sredni, B., Stern, L., et al., IL-2 and IL-6 secretion in dementia: correlation with type and severity of disease, *J. Neurol. Sci.*, 130, 161–164, 1995.
49. Ferrucci, L., Harris, T. B., Guralnik, J. K., et al., Serum IL-6 level and the development of disability in older persons, *J. Am. Geriatr. Soc.*, 47, 639–646, 1999.
50. Mooradian, A. D., Reed, R. L., Osterweil, D. et al., Detectable serum levels of tumor necrosis factor alpha may predict early mortality in elderly institutionalized patients, *J. Am. Geriatr. Soc.*, 39, 891–894, 1991.
51. Rink, L., Cakman, I., and Kirchner, H., Altered cytokine production in the elderly, *Mech. Ageing Dev.*, 102, 199–209, 1998.
52. 51) Castle, S., Uyemura, K., Wong, W., et al., Evidence of enhanced type 2 immune response and impaired upregulation of a type 1 response in frail elderly nursing home residents, *Mech. Ageing Dev.*, 94, 7–16, 1997.
53. Paganelli, R., Quinti, I., Fagiolo, U., et al., Changes in circulating B cells and immunoglobulin classes and subclasses in a healhy aged population, *Clin. Exp. Immunol.*, 90, 351–354, 1992.
54. Franceschi, C., Monti, D., Sansoni, P., et al., The immunology of exceptional individuals: the lesson of centenarians, *Immunol. Today*, 16, 12–16, 1995.
55. Albright, J. W. and Albright, J. F., Soluble receptors and other substances that regulate proinflammatory cytokines in young and aging humans, *J. Gerontol.*, 55A, B20–B25, 2000.
56. Hara, H., Negoro, S., Miyata, S., et al., Age-associated changes in proliferative and differentiative response of human B cells and production of T cell-derived factors regulating B cell functions, *Mech. Ageing Dev.*, 38, 245–258, 1987.

57. Scribner, D. J., Weiner, H. L., and Moorhead, J. W., Anti-immunoglobulin stimulation of murine lymphocytes. V. Age-related decline in Fc receptor-mediated immunoregulation, *J. Immunol.*, 121, 377–382, 1979.
58. Haq, J. A. and Szewczuk, M. R., Differential effect of aging on B-cell immune responses to cholera toxin in the inductive and effector sites of the mucosal immune system, *Infect. Immunity*, 59, 3094–3100, 1991.
59. Buckley, C. E., Buckley, E. G., and Dorsey, F. C., Longitudinal changes in serum immunoglobulin levels in older humans, *Fed. Proc.*, 33, 2036–2039, 1974.
60. Emanuelli, G., Lanzio, M., Anfossi, T., et al., Influence of age on polymorphonuclear leukocytes *in vitro*: phagocytic activity in healthy human subjects, *Gerontology*, 32, 308–316, 1986.
61. Inamizu, T., Chang, M.-P., and Makinodan, T., Influence of age on the production and regulation of interleukin-1 in mice, *Immunology*, 55, 447–455, 1985.
62. Rudd, A. G. and Banerjee, D. K., Interleukin-1 production by human monocytes in aging and disease, *Age Ageing*, 18, 43–46, 1989.
63. Krishnaraj, R. and Svanborg, A., Preferential accumulation of mature NK cells during human immunosenescence, *J. Cell. Biochem.*, 50: 386–391, 1992.
64. Facchini, A. E., Mariani, E., Mariani, A. R., et al., Increased number of circulating Leu11+ (CD16) large granular lymphocytes and decreased NK activity during human aging, *Clin. Exp. Immunol.*, 68, 340–347, 1987.
65. Murasko, D. M., Nelson, B. J., Silver, R., et al., Immunologic response in an elderly population with a mean age of 85, *Am. J. Med.*, 81, 612–618, 1986.
66. Ligthart, G. J., Schuit, H. R. E., and Hijmans, W., Natural killer cell function is not diminished in the healthy aged and is proportional to the number of NK cells in the peripheral blood, *Immunology*, 68, 396–402, 1989.
67. Rukavina, D., Laskarin, G., Rubesa, G., et al., Age-related decline of perforin expression in human cytotoxic T lymphocytes and natural killer cells, *Blood*, 92, 2410–2420, 1998.
68. Klein, S. L., The effects of hormones on sex differences in infection: from genes to behavior, *Neurosci. Biobehav. Rev.*, 24, 627–638, 2000.
69. Butterworth, M., McClellan, B., and Allansmith, M., Influence of sex in immunoglobulin levels, *Nature*, 214, 1224–1225, 1967.
70. Lichtman, M. A., Vaughan, J. H., and Hames, C. G., The distribution of serum immunoglobulins, anti-gamma-G globulins ("rheumatoid factors") and antinuclear antibodies in white and Negro subjects in Evans County, Georgia, *Arthritis Rheuma.*, 10, 204–215, 1967.
71. Struve, J., Aronsson, B., Frenning, B., et al., Intramuscular vs. intradermal administration of a recombinant hepatitis B vaccine: a comparison of response rates and analysis of factors influencing the antibody response, *Scand. J. Infect. Dis.*, 24, 423–429, 1992.
72. Sweet, R. L., Blankfort-Doyle, M., Bobbie, M. O., et al., The occurrence of chlamydial and gonococcal salpingitis during the menstrual cycle, *J. Am. Med. Assoc.*, 255, 2062–2064, 1986.
73. Cohen, M. S., Britigan, B. E., French, M., et al., Preliminary observations on lactoferrin secretion in human vaginal mucus: variation during the menstrual cycle, evidence of hormonal regulation, and implications for infection with *Neisseria gonorrhoeae*, *Am. J. Obst. Gynecol.*, 157, 1122–1125, 1987.
74. Leibovici, L., Alpert, G., Kalter-Leibovici, O., et al., Risk factors for recurrence of symptomatic urinary tract infection in young women, *Isr. J. Med. Sci.*, 25, 110–111, 1989.

75. Inman, R. D., Immunologic sex differences and the female preponderance in systemic lupus erythematosus, *Arthritis Rheum.*, 21, 849–852, 1978.
76. Bain, B. J. and England, J. M., Normal hematological values: sex difference in neutrophil count, *Br. Med. J.*, 1, 306–309, 1975.
77. Bain, B. J. and England, J. M., Variations in leucocyte count during menstrual cycle, *Br. Med. J.*, 2, 473–475, 1975.
78. Alvarez, E. and Maria, C. S., Influence of the age and sex on respiratory burst of human monocytes, *Mech. Ageing Dev.*, 90, 157–161, 1996.
79. Choong, M. L., Ton, S. H., and Cheong, S. K., Influence of race, age and sex on the lymphocyte subsets in peripheral blood of healthy Malaysian adults, *Ann. Clin. Biochem.*, 32, 532–539, 1995.
80. Bizzarro, A., Valentini, G., Di Martino, G., et al., Influence of testosterone therapy on clinical and immunological features of autoimmune diseases associated with Klinefelter's syndrome, *J. Clin. Endocrinol. Metab.*, 64, 32–36, 1987.
81. Verthelyi, D. and Klinman, D. M., Sex hormone levels correlate with the activity of cytokine-secreting cells *in vivo*, *Immunology*, 100, 384–390, 2000.
82. Masi, A. T., Incidence of rheumatoid arthritis: do the observed age–sex interaction patterns support a role of androgenic–anabolic (AA) steroid deficiency in its pathogenesis? *Br. J. Rheumatol.*, 33, 697–699, 1994.
83. Fried, L. P. and Walston, J. M., Frailty and failure to thrive, in *Principles of Geriatric Medicine and Gerontology*, 4th ed., Hazzard, W. R., Blass, J. P. Ettinger, W. H., et al., Eds, New York, McGraw-Hill, 1998.
84. Walston, J. and Fried, L. P., Frailty and the older man, *Med. Clin. North Am.*, 83, 1173–1194, 1999.
85. Kjaer, M., Regulation of hormonal and metabolic responses during exercise in humans, *Exerc. Sport Sci. Rev.*, 19, 161–184, 1991.
86. Rowell, L. B. and O'Leary, D. S., Reflex control of the circulation during exercise: chemoreflexes and mechanoreflexes, *J. Appl. Physiol.*, 69, 407–418, 1990.
87. Hoffman-Goetz, L. and Pedersen, B. K., Exercise and the immune system: a model of the stress response? *Immunol. Today*, 15(8), 382–387, 1994.
88. Shinkai, S., Watanabe, S., Asai, H., et al., Cortisol response to exercise and postexercise suppression of blood lymphocyte subset counts, *Int. J. Sports Med.*, 17, 597–603, 1996.
89. Barnes, R. F., Raskind, M., Gumbrecht, G., et al., The effect of age on the plasma catecholamine response to mental stress in man, *J. Clin. Endocrinol. Metab.*, 54, 64–69, 1982.
90. Lehmann, M. and Keul, J., Age-associated changes of exercise-induced plasma catecholamine responses, *Eur. J. Appl. Physiol. Occup. Physiol.*, 55, 302–306, 1986.
91. Poehlman, E. T., MacAuliffe, and Danforth, Jr., E., Effects of age and levels of physical activity on plasma norepinephrine kinetics, *Am. J. Physiol.*, 258, E256–E262, 1990.
92. Young, J. B., Rowe, J. W., Pallotta, J. A., et al., Enhanced plasma norepinephrine responses to upright posture and oral glucose administration in elderly human subjects, *Metabolism*, 29, 532–539, 1980.
93. Palmer, G. J., Ziegler, M. G., and Lake, C. R., Response of norepinephrine and blood pressure to stress increases with age, *J. Gerontol.*, 33, 482–487, 1978.
94. Fleg, J. L., Tzankoff, S. P., and Lakatta, E. G., Age-related augmentation of plasma catecholamines during dynamic exercise in healthy males, *J. Appl. Physiol.*, 59, 1033–1039, 1985.

95. Hagberg, J. M., Seals, D. R., Yerg, J. E., et al., Metabolic responses to exercise in young and older athletes and sedentary men, *J. Appl. Physiol.*, 65, 900–908, 1988.
96. Gustafson, A. B. and Kalkhoff, R. K., Influence of sex and obesity on plasma catecholamine response to isometric exercise, *J. Clin. Endocrinol. Metab.*, 55, 703–708, 1982.
97. Schwartz, R. S., Jaeger, J. F., and Veith, R. C., The importance of body composition to the increase in plasma norepinephrine appearance rate in elderly men, *J. Gerontol.*, 42, 546–551, 1987.
98. Kastello, G. M., Sothmann, M. S., and Murthy, V. S., Young and old subjects matched for aerobic capacity have similar noradrenergic responses to exercise, *J. Appl. Physiol.*, 74, 49–54, 1993.
99. Jensen, E. J., Espersen, K., Kanstrup, I.-L., et al., Exercise-induced changes in plasma catecholamines and neuropeptide Y: relation to age and sampling times, *J. Appl. Physiol.*, 76, 1269–1273, 1994.
100. Kohrt, W. M., Spina, R. J., Ehsani, A. A., et al., Effects of age, adiposity, and fitness level on plasma catecholamine responses to standing and exercise, *J. Appl. Physiol.*, 75, 1828–1835, 1993.
101. Blackman, M. R., Elahi, D., and Harman, S. H., Endocrinology and aging, in *Endocrinology*, DeGroot, L. J., Ed., Saunders, Philadelphia, 1994, 2702–2730.
102. Seeman, T. E. and Robbins, R. J., Aging and hypothalamo–pituitary–adrenal response to challenge in humans, *Endocr. Rev.*, 15, 233–260, 1994.
103. Urban, R. J. and Veldhuis, J. D., Hypothalamo-pituitary concomitants of aging, in *Endocrinology of Aging*, James, R. and Sowers, J.V.F., Eds., Raven Press, New York, 1988, 41–74.
104. Cauter, E. V., Leproult, R., and Kupfer, D., Effects of gender and age on the levels and circadian rhythmicity of plasma cortisol, *J. Clin. Endocrinol. Metab.*, 81, 2468–2473, 1996.
105. Laughlin, G. A. and Barrett-Connor, E., Sexual dimorphism in the influence of advanced aging on adrenal hormone levels: the Rancho Bernardo study, *J. Clin. Endocrinol. Metab.*, 85, 3561–3568, 2000.
106. Wilkinson, C. W., Peskind, E. R., Raskind, M. A., Decreased hypothalamic–pituitary–adrenal axis sensitivity to cortisol feedback inhibition in human aging, *Neuroendocrinology*, 65, 79–90, 1997.
107. Boscaro, M., Paoletta, A., Scarpa, E., et al., Age-related changes in glucocorticoid fast feedback inhibition of adrenocorticotropin in man, *J. Clin. Endocrinol. Metab.*, 83, 1380–1383, 1998.
108. Frankenhauser, M., Dunne, E., Lundberg, U., Sex differences in sympathetic-adrenal medullary reactions induced by different stressors, *Psychopharmacology*, 47, 1–5, 1976.
109. Diamond, M. P., Jones, T., Caprio, S., et al., Gender influences counterregulatory hormone responses to hypoglycemia, *Metabolism*, 42, 1568–1572, 1993.
110. Amiel, S. A., Maran, A., Powrie, J. K., et al., Gender differences in counterregulation to hypoglycemia, *Diabetologia*, 36, 460–464, 1993.
111. Davis, S. N., Galassetti, P., Wasserman, D. H., et al., Effects of gender on neuroendocrine and metabolic counterregulatory responses to exercise in normal man, *J. Clin. Endocrinol. Metab.*, 85, 224–230, 2000.
112. Ettinger, S. M., Silber, D. H., Collins, B. G., et al., Influences of gender on sympathetic nerve responses to static exercise, *J. Appl. Physiol.*, 80, 245–251, 1996.

113. Matsukawa, T., Sugiyama, Y., Watanabe, T., et al., Gender difference in age-related changes in muscle sympathetic nerve activity in healthy subjects, *Am. J. Physiol.*, 275, R1600–R1604, 1998.
114. Seeman, T. E. and Robbins, R. J., Aging and hypothalamic–pituitary–adrenal response to challenge in humans, *Endocr. Rev.*, 15, 233–260, 1994.
115. Goldfarb, A. H., Jamurtas, A. Z., Kamimori, G. H., et al., Gender effect on beta-endorphin response to exercise, *Med. Sci. Sports Exerc.*, 30, 1672–1676, 1998.
116. Shephard, R. J., *Aging, Physical Activity, and Health*, Human Kinetics, Champaign, IL, 1997, 175.
117. Farrell, P. A., Kjaer, M., Bach, F. W., and Galbo, H., Beta-endorphin and adrenocorticotropin response to supramaximal treadmill exercise in trained and untrained males, *Acta Physiol. Scand.*, 130, 619–625, 1987.
118. Kjaer, M., Farrell, P. A., Christensen, N. J., et al., Increased epinephrine response and inaccurate glucose regulation in exercising athletes, *J. Appl. Physiol.*, 61, 1693–1700, 1986.
119. Kjaer, M., Christensen, N. J., Sonne, B., et al., The effect of exercise on epinephrine turnover in trained and untrained man, *J. Appl. Physiol.*, 59, 1061–1067, 1985.
120. Kjaer, M., Adrenal medulla and exercise training, *Eur. J. Appl. Physiol.*, 77, 195–199, 1998.
121. Heuser, I. J. E., Wark, H-. J., Keul, J., et al., Hypothalamic–pituitary–adrenal axis function in elderly endurance athletes, *J. Clin. Endocrinol. Metab.*, 73, 485–488, 1991.
122. Struder, H. K., Hollmann, W., Platen, P., et al., Hypothalamic–pituitary–adrenal–gonadal axis function after exercise in sedentary and endurance trained elderly males, *Eur. J. Appl. Physiol.*, 77, 285–288, 1998.
123. Sidney, K. H. and Shephard, R. J., Growth hormone and cortisol: age differences, effects of exercise and training, *Can. J. Appl. Sports Sci.* 2, 189–193, 1978.
124. Kraemer, W. J., Hakkinen, K., Newton, R. U., et al., Effects of heavy-resistance training on hormonal response patterns in younger vs. older men, *J. Appl. Physiol.*, 87, 982–992, 1999.
125. Moldoveanu, A. I., Shephard, R. J., and Shek, P. N., The cytokine response to physical activity and training, *Sports Med.*, 31, 115–144, 2001.
126. Tvede, N., Kappel, M., Halkjaer-Kristensen, J., et al., The effect of light, moderate and severe bicycle exercise on lymphocyte subsets, natural and lymphokine activated killer cells, lymphocyte proliferative response and interleukin 2 production, *Int. J. Sports Med.*, 14, 275–282, 1993.
127. Fiatarone, M. A., Morley, J. E., Bloom, E. T., et al., The effect of exercise on natural killer cell activity in young and old subjects, *J. Gerontol. Med. Sci.*, 44, M37–M45, 1989.
128. Mazzeo, R. S., Rowland, J., Rajkumar, C., et al., Effect of a single bout of exercise on immune function in young and elderly subjects, *Med. Sci. Sports Exerc.*, 28 (suppl.), S93, 1996.
129. Nieman, D. C., Henson, D. A., Gusewitch, G., et al., Physical activity and immune function in elderly women, *Med. Sci. Sports Exerc.*, 25, 823–831, 1993.
130. Gueldner, S. H., Poon, L. E., La Via, M., Virella, G., Michel, Y., Bramlett, M. H., Noble, C. A., and Paulling, E., Long term exercise patterns and immune function in healthy older women. A report of preliminary findings, *Mech. Ageing Dev.*, 93, 215–222, 1997.

131. Cushman, M., Yanez, D., Psaty, B. M., et al., Association of fibrinogen and coagulation factors VII and VIII with cardiovascular risk factors in the elderly: the cardiovascular health study, *Am. J. Epidemiol.* 143, 665–676, 1996.
132. Elwood, P., Yarnell, J., Pickering, J., et al., Exercise, fibrinogen, and other risk factors for ischaemic heart disease. Caerphilly prospective heart disease study, *Br. Heart J.*, 69, 183–187, 1993.
133. Lakka T. A., Salonen, J. T., Moderate to high intensity conditioning leisure time physical activity and high cardiorespiratory fitness are associated with reduced plasma fibrinogen in eastern Finnish men, *J. Clin. Epidemiol.*, 46, 1119–1127, 1993.
134. Connelly, J., Cooper, J., Meade, T., Strenuous exercise, plasma fibrinogen, and factor VII activity, *Br. Heart J.*, 67, 351–354, 1992.
135. Geffken, D. F., Cushman, M., Burke, G. L., et al., Association between physical activity and markers of inflammation in a healthy elderly population, *Am. J. Epidemiol.*, 153, 242–250, 2001.
136. Crist, D. M., Mackinnon, L. T., Thompson, R. F., et al., Physical exercise increases natural cellular-mediated tumor cytotoxicity in elderly women, *Gerontology*, 35, 66–71, 1989.
137. Nieman, D. C., Nehlsen-Cannarella, S. L., Markoff, P. A., et al., The effects of moderate exercise training on natural killer cells and acute upper respiratory tract infections, *Int. J. Sports Med.*, 11, 467–473, 1990.
138. Woods, J. A., Ceddia, M. A., Wolters, B. W., et al., Effects of 6 months of moderate aerobic exercise training on immune function in the elderly, *Mech. Ageing Dev.*, 109, 1–19, 1999.
139. Rall, L.C., Roubenoff, R., Cannon, J.G., et al., Effects of progressive resistance training on immune response in aging and chronic inflammation, *Med. Sci. Sports Exerc.*, 28, 1356–1365, 1996.
140. Flynn, M. G., Fahlman, M., Braun, W. A., et al., Effects of resistance training on selected indexes of immune function in elderly women, *J. Appl. Physiol.*, 86, 1905–1913, 1999.
141. Paw, M. J., de Jong, N. D., Kloek, G.C., et al., Immunity in frail elderly: a randomized controlled trial of exercise and enriched foods, *Med. Sci. Sports Exerc.*, 32, 2005–2011, 2000.

12

Conclusions: Implications for Health and Society

Roy J. Shephard

CONTENTS

12.1 Introduction

The material reviewed in this book has demonstrated that the aging process causes a substantial deterioration in various components of functional capacity, with superimposed effects of both gender and habitual physical activity. This final chapter reviews certain implications of these findings for health and society. Critical issues are the extent of functional impairment and disability, resulting losses of productivity and the onset of dependency in elderly women

0-8493-1027-X/02/$0.00+$1.50

and men, associated economic costs, and the potential of reversing dependency by an appropriate exercise regimen.

12.2 Extent of Functional Impairment and Disability

12.2.1 Functional Impairment

Aging of the various biological systems in itself progressively reduces functional capacity (Chapter 5). The individual's maximal oxygen intake declines progressively (Chapter 4) until it is no longer sufficient to sustain prolonged aerobic activity,[22,59] muscle strength decreases (Chapter 6) until it becomes insufficient to open jars, carry even light loads, or lift the body mass from a chair or toilet seat,[6] and flexibility becomes insufficient to climb steps, enter a car, climb into a bath or even clothe oneself unaided. Some 20% of those over the age of 60 years attribute their difficulty in undertaking simple activities to "old age" as opposed to some specific medical condition.[92] Most women begin their adult lives with lower maximal aerobic power and much lower strength than men, but the rate of aging of most functions tends to be similar for both sexes, so women are inherently more vulnerable to functional impairment and disability before they die.

In Canada, by the age of 65 years, 37% of women and 31% of men have noted some limitations in their physical activity.[28] As early as 55 years of age, 2% of men and 10% of women are unable to carry their groceries, and in those over the age of 80 years, the prevalence of this particular handicap rises to 20% of men and 30% of women.[81]

In Britain, 2.1 million men and 5.2 million women out of a population of approximately 60 million are unable to walk on a level surface at a pace of 4.8 km/h; on a moderate slope, the number who cannot maintain this pace increase to 5.6 million men and 11.7 million women. Furthermore, this total includes 81% of all men and 92% of all women aged 65 to 74 years.[80] Likewise, in the U.S., the National Health Interview Survey[88] has noted that substantial fractions of those over the age of 55 years have difficulty in walking 0.4 km or in carrying a load of 11 kg (Table 12.1). Although the British survey reported that difficulty in maintaining a fast walking pace was more common in women than in men, in the U.S. a slightly larger proportion of men were disadvantaged in terms of their ability to walk at a speed of their own choice. Nevertheless, many more women than men had difficulty in carrying a moderate load. By the age of 80 to 84 years, 31 to 57% of men and 54 to 70% of women indicated that they were unable to do heavy housework (Table 12.2), although here the gender difference may reflect the allocation of domestic tasks rather than intrinsic differences in functional ability.[11] Men also had the advantage in tasks requiring muscular strength. Thus, by the age of 80 to 84 years, 12 to 15% of men and 17 to 31% of women

TABLE 12.1

Percentages of U.S. Citizens Who Have Worked Since the Age of 45 Years, but Who in 1984 Had Difficulty (D) or Were Unable (U) either to Walk a Distance of 0.4 km, or to Carry a Load of 11 kg

	Walking 0.4 km				Carrying 11 kg			
	M		F		M		F	
Age (yr)	D	U	D	U	D	U	D	U
55–59	12.3	5.0	11.6	3.5	12.6	5.8	22.9	9.1
60–64	17.0	7.9	15.4	3.8	15.8	8.0	31.0	8.7
65–69	20.1	9.4	16.8	5.6	19.9	7.9	33.8	9.3
70–74	23.3	8.7	23.1	7.5	25.6	10.2	40.8	10.7

Source: U.S. National Center for Health Statistics (1987), Aging in the eighties: Ability to perform work-related activities. Data from the supplement on aging to the National Health Interview Survey, U.S., 1984. Advanced Data from Vital and Health Statistics, No. 136, DHS Publication PHS87-1250 (Hyattsville, MD: U.S. Public Health Services).

TABLE 12.2

Percentages of Three Elderly Populations with Limitations of Specific Abilities during the Ninth Decade of Life

	Age 80–84 yr						Age >85 yr					
	Men			Women			Men			Women		
Ability	EB	NH	RI	EB	NH	RI	EB	NH	RI	EB	NH	RI
Heavy housework	57	31	43	70	54	56	74	53	68	89	56	69
Climbing stairs	15	12	12	31	12	17	29	10	16	50	30	26
Walking across room	12	8	10	23	9	15	22	10	17	38	31	22
Bed to chair	4	1	8	14	8	9	11	5	8	22	14	9
Use of toilet	3	2	6	12	5	8	12	1	7	19	8	10

Based on data for three U.S. populations: east Boston (EB), New Haven (NH), and rural Iowa (RI).

Source: Coroni-Huntley, J., Brock, D.B., Ostfeld, A.M., et al.,[11] Established populations for epidemiological studies of the elderly: Resource data book. U.S. Public Health Service, National Institute on Aging, Washington, D.C., 1986.

were unable to climb stairs, 8 to 12% of men and 9 to 23% of women were unable to walk across a room unaided, and 1 to 8% of men and 8 to 14% of women were unable to rise from a chair or bed.[11,48] Nevertheless, differences in the prevalence of poor function between the locations that were studied (East Boston vs. New Haven vs. rural Iowa) were almost as great as gender differences seen at any given location.

In Japan, no significant gender differences in an index of self-care and mobility were seen in a sample of 752 elderly people living at home.[24]

When interpreting functional changes, it is often difficult to disentangle what is a consequence of normal aging from the effects of disuse and chronic disease. One U.S. study estimated that as much as half of age-related decline in functional capacity was self-imposed, due to an accumulation of body fat and a failure to take adequate physical activity.[32] The prevalence of inactivity among the elderly can be illustrated by a statistic of Guralnik and associates;[23] by the age of 65 to 74 years, 41% of American men and 53% of American women never walk as far as 1.6 km without taking a rest; among those over the age of 85 years, the corresponding figures are 49% and 59%. In the U.S., chronic fatigue is associated with a lack of fitness even in middle-aged individuals.[37] Likewise, in Denmark, Avelund et al.[5] noted a substantial inverse relationship between levels of habitual physical activity and the loss of functional capacity. Poor performance on a stepping test was associated with tiredness in 75-year-old women[5] and with a limitation of mobility in men.

It remains less clear whether benefits of regular physical activity are due simply to an impact on functional capacity.[26,46] Regular exercise may also have a less direct impact on function, enhancing mood state, preventing chronic disease, or (in cross-sectional studies) simply serving as a marker of the absence of disease.

12.2.2 Disability

Disability is a major problem for senior citizens. The U.S. National Center for Health Statistics[88] estimated that 15% of the elderly still living in the community suffered from some type of disability. Other reports have suggested that as many as 40 to 50% are limited in either the amount or type of activity that they can undertake.[87] In some of those who report "disability," the problem is relatively minor, but about a third are confined to their homes.[39,46] More than 1.5 million U.S. residents live in nursing homes; a similar number have accepted sheltered living arrangements or receive home care or day-care services, and as many as an additional 5 million receive extensive informal care from family and friends.[57] Institutionalization almost invariably leads to deterioration in quality of life, with quality inversely related to the extent of dependency.[55] There are also heavy economic costs to be borne either by the individual or by society.

In Canada, 83% of adults aged 75 to 84 years and 89% of those over the age of 85 years report some type of disability that limits their mobility or agility.[82] Approximately 64% of those over the age of 85 years consider themselves to be severely disabled.[29]

On average, an elderly American man is affected by some type of disability for 10.8 years; in women the period of disability is as much as 14 years.[79] During the final year of life, almost total disability is common. The gender difference in the period of disability is well recognized in many developed societies.[13] In part, it reflects the greater average age at death of women, and in part it is due to a faster progression from disability to death in men than in women.[66] Other factors influencing gender differences in the length of disability include the lower initial functional capacity of women,[70] problems that women encounter in attending rehabilitation programs,[85] and differential effects of lifestyle and chronic disease.[47] It remains unclear how far gender differences in symptom reporting,[18,38,42,53] coping skills,[67] willingness to use assistive devices,[14] social opportunities, and physical demands also contribute to the greater reported disability in women.

A tendency for women to report more disability than men after control for physical abilities was noted in one study of community-dwelling seniors aged 65 to 97 years.[12] Women also showed a lower quality of life than men in the year following hospital admission for congestive heart failure,[10] despite controlling data for clinical and socioeconomic variables. On the other hand, the commonly anticipated female over-reporting of morbidity is not always observed.[45] A recent British survey concluded that, although women over the age of 60 years experienced functional impairment more commonly than men, there were no gender differences in self-assessments of health.[3] Merrill et al.[50] compared self-reports with objective measures of disability, concluding that both men and women generally reported their levels of disability accurately. Other investigators found no gender differences in the extent of emotional distress among 369 older adults with severe rheumatoid arthritis,[16] or in the quality of life for men and women with severe mental illness[49] or cancer.[20] The steep increase of unemployment among heavy industrial workers in recent years appears to have increased mental and somatic symptoms among older men, which may be one reason why previously observed gender differences in the reporting of ill health are no longer seen.[41]

The extent of disability reported in any given situation depends on the functional demands made on the individual, extent of support offered by family and friends, environmental adaptations available, and coping mechanisms adopted.[84] One person may show only minimal radiographic changes in key joints, yet complain of severe disability from osteoarthritis; another may have severe radiographic lesions, yet report little disability. Hachisuka et al.[25] concluded that, in Japan, elderly women who had sustained a stroke faced greater physical demands than men because they received less family support when undertaking the activities of daily living. In consequence, they were more likely to perceive a disability. In Sweden, men aged 76 years were more likely than their female peers to show dependency in cooking, bathing, and dressing.[78]

In one survey of Canadian seniors, a surprisingly large 85% of those who reported limitations of physical activity also indicated that they were either "very happy" or "pretty happy" with their situation.[28] Likewise, various medical complaints accounted for only about a third of age-related deterioration in the quality of life among a 76-year-old cohort in Göteborg, Sweden.[21]

If the life of a frail elderly person is sustained by heroic surgical and medical treatment, there may be a major discrepancy between the calendar life span and the disability-free life span. Although an age-related loss of function can in itself cause disability, chronic disease is the usual source of impairment. The apparent prevalence of various disease conditions varies according to the diagnostic criteria applied. For example, aging is inevitably associated with a progressive increase in blood pressure, but when a certain arbitrary level of pressure is surpassed, hypertension is diagnosed; the proportion of individuals regarded as hypertensive depends largely on the cut-off pressure and the care taken to avoid a transient, anxiety-related increase of pressure.[93] Similarly, when the age-related decrease in bone mineral content reaches an arbitrary figure, clinical osteoporosis is diagnosed. The likelihood of developing various disabling conditions differs substantially between women and men (Chapter 5).

One early British study identified the main causes of disability as arthritis and rheumatism (36%), pulmonary conditions (17%), strokes and paralysis (15%), blindness and failing sight (14%), circulatory conditions (14%), cardiac conditions and abnormal blood pressure (13%), the sequelae of accidents (10%), and neurological problems (5%). In consequence, function was limited by problems such as muscular weakness, joint stiffness, breathlessness, tremor or spasticity, and disorders of balance.[30] In Canada,[27,82] the main health problems of senior citizens have been listed as arthritis and rheumatism (affecting 46% of men and 63% of women), hypertension (33% of men and 43% of women), "heart trouble" (28% of men and 24% of women), respiratory problems (26% of men and 23% of women), and diabetes mellitus (9% in both sexes). The experience of U.S. senior citizens is somewhat similar, with 50% reporting arthritis, 39% hypertension, 30% hearing disability, 20% deformity or orthopedic problem, 15% sinus problems, 10% visual problems, and 9% diabetes.[88] Many elderly people have multiple disorders, and it is then difficult to assess the contribution of specific conditions to the reported level of disability.

In young and middle old age, the main causes of disability are chronic disease and a restriction of mobility, but in the oldest old mental deterioration and a loss of the special senses become important sources of impairment.[62] For the 76-year-old participants in the Göteborg study, the main factors limiting health-related quality of life were anginal pain, urinary incontinence, and locomotor and mental disorders.[21]

12.3 Implications of Age-Related Functional Losses for Productivity and Dependency

12.3.1 Productivity

In theory, the loss of functional capacity with aging might limit the working ability of older adults, and such concerns have sometimes been advanced as arguments against the recruitment, promotion, and continuing employment of older individuals.[69] However, in practice it is uncommon to find clear examples of situations where a limitation of maximal aerobic power or muscle strength has specifically compromised the productivity of older workers. A Danish telephone survey[54] found 15% of employees reporting a reduced work ability relative to their peers. The handicap was moderate in 7% and considerable in 8% of individuals, but problems were not necessarily attributed to physical limitations. The proportion of individuals with a handicap increased from 10% of the youngest cohort to 20% of men and 21% of women aged more than 45 years. A second study from Denmark found that the only physical predictor of continuing employment in older age groups was (in women only) the absence of musculo-skeletal problems affecting the knee joints.[44] In Finland, the likelihood of continuing employment was similar in women and men, and the physical demands of the job apparently had little influence.[68] Among Finnish pensioners, 50% of men and 70% of women were considered to retain a good working ability.[86]

There are many possible reasons why the functional consequences of aging have such a limited impact upon industrial productivity.[74] Firstly, in developed societies automation is such that very few occupations now demand high levels of oxygen transport or muscular strength. Even in those occupations where physical demand remains potentially high, inefficient management, union restrictions, a lack of tools or supplies, or the absence of a key colleague may be the real factors that limit productivity, rather than any age-related loss of functional capacity.[71]

Secondly, functional capacity ranges widely within a given age and gender category, so that a well-endowed older female worker who has maintained her personal fitness may have a maximal aerobic power matching or exceeding that of a sedentary young man.[75] Sometimes, the physical demands of the occupation itself serve to conserve aerobic fitness or muscular strength, although even in "heavy" work the intensity of effort is now rarely sufficient to have an appreciable training effect.[2]

Self-selection is a third factor reducing the number of problems. People choose heavy work if they are well endowed physically and, if a task is physically demanding, employers also tend to select those with a good physique. After recruitment, there is also a substantial "healthy worker effect": those with inadequate working capacity change jobs or take early retirement.[31,36] Seniority rules may also give an older worker the right to remain in a "heavy" job category while undertaking a specific task that makes only limited physical demands.

Finally, technical problems encountered by a work-site ergonomist may have exaggerated the physical demands of a given job. The true energy cost may be substantially less than has been claimed, because energy expenditures have been measured only during the heaviest segment of a day's work, or the pace of activity has been artificially accelerated while the measurements were made. Furthermore, the experience of an older worker may increase mechanical efficiency and thus reduce the energy cost of a particular occupational task. Much energy expended at a given work station may arise from displacement of body mass; the experienced worker then learns how to minimize such movement, and a low body mass can further diminish this cost both in women and men.[19]

The end result is that, in most occupations with substantial physical demand, there is little justification for requiring the retirement of older employees on the grounds of poor productivity. In self-paced work, the output of an elderly employee may be a little less that that of a fit young individual. But often, the slower rate of production in the older person is offset by the effects of experience and a differing work ethos, so the quality of work is greater than in a younger employee. The main handicap of the older employee arises not from a decrease in functional capacity, but rather from an accumulation of wage and vacation benefits; such benefits give a lower productivity per dollar expended, even if the physical output per hour is the same as or greater than that of a younger person.

If ill health is sufficient to make substantial inroads into an individual's functional capacity, many employees are willing to accept early retirement, provided that adequate financial provision is made for their retirement years.[31,36] The other alternative is to work part time, since the tolerated fraction of the maximal rate of working is much larger for a four-hour than for an eight-hour day.[8]

12.3.2 Dependency

The causes of dependency and institutionalization in advanced age are varied (Chapter 5). In some people, the precipitating event is the loss of social support, for example, as a daughter moves to a distant location or a husband dies. In others, there is a catastrophic event such as a stroke, a fall with hip fracture, the onset of blindness, or a progressive loss of mental competency. But in many seniors, the cause of dependency appears to be simply a progressive loss of functional capacity, so that they are no longer able to undertake either the instrumental activities of daily living, or the basic necessities such as feeding, personal toilet, and dressing.

The minimum physical capacity needed in order to live independently varies greatly with the extent of social and environmental support. Some people with congestive heart failure may have an aerobic power of less than 10 ml/[kg·min] and yet manage to live on their own. Based on such observations, it has been suggested that the threshold maximal oxygen intake for independence was probably in the range 12 to 14 ml/[kg·min].[72] One more recent study found that the optimal "cut-point" between a high and low level of function was a maximal aerobic power of 18 ml/[kg·min].[52] Another recent empirical study of 85-year-old individuals (Chapter 5) found that the maximal aerobic power compatible with full independence was 17.7 ml/[kg·min] in men and 15.4 ml/[kg·min] in women.[59] Similar data showing the thresholds of muscle strength and flexibility needed to maintain the independence of elderly populations should be collected.

The national economic burden arising from 10 to 15 years of partial or total dependency is extremely high. One U.S. analysis set the cost of institutional care at U.S. $38,000 per person per year.[65] In Japan, the cost of geriatric care was estimated at 6.8158 trillion yen (about U.S. $70 billion), with 80% of this cost coming from the public purse.[34] Moreover, the per capita cost of geriatric medical and hospital care is increasing rapidly, in part because the medical inflation rate is far outpacing the consumer price index, and in part because inappropriate and excessive treatment is provided at an advanced age.[9] A study from the Netherlands found that, during the final year of life, medical costs increased more than 27-fold in those under the age of 65 years, and some 4.7-fold in those over the age of 65.[89] In the U.S., the costs of Medicare and Medicaid for those over the age of 65 years were $20, $42, and $87 billion in 1975, 1980, and 1985, respectively.[60] By 1993, annual expenditures were U.S. $8704 for each elderly recipient.[65] Health economists thus show considerable interest in the potential to prevent and reverse functional limitations, disability, and dependency by an appropriate regimen of regular physical activity.

12.4 Potential to Reverse Functional Limitations by an Enhanced Lifestyle

A major part of the age-related loss of functional capacity, with the associated social and economic costs of prolonged disability, is due to adoption of an inappropriate lifestyle. One study of 574 Alameda County residents aged 65 to 102 years found that heavy drinking, cigarette smoking, and physical inactivity were all significant predictors of frailty.[83] Age- and gender-adjusted associations between disability and alcohol abuse were also seen in a prospective study of 3481 Baltimore residents.[4] Prevention and/or reversal of functional limitations thus seem likely consequences of adopting a more healthy lifestyle. Cohort differences in the quality of life between the original Framingham cohort and their offspring over the age span of 55 to 70 years may reflect, in part, the fact that the offspring are physically more active, with a much lower prevalence of cigarette smoking.[1] Enhanced treatment of chronic conditions is a further likely reason why disability at any given age is less in the current generation of seniors than in earlier cohorts.[7] Likely measures to reverse the consequences of a poor lifestyle include an increase of habitual physical activity, the control of body mass, and cessation of cigarette smoking. In contrast, it seems unlikely that cumulative cardiac and hepatic damage from an excessive consumption of alcohol can be reversed by abstinence in old age.

12.4.1 Increase of Habitual Physical Activity

Differences of functional capacity between master athletes and the general population,[35] as well as the substantial training responses of elderly populations,[72] suggest the value of an appropriate regime of regular physical activity as a means of enhancing function in the elderly. Although regular exercise has only a small impact upon the inherent rate of aging,[35,72] a 3-month progressive training program can augment maximal aerobic power and muscle strength by as much as 20% — the equivalent of up to 20 years' reversal in these aspects of functional aging.[72]

Some economists have suggested that any extension of life span regular exercise would have an adverse impact on societal costs, because expenditures on pensions and health care would then be paid over a longer period.[91] However, there are at least three important reasons to reject this conclusion. Firstly, healthy individuals are able to retire later than those who have become sick; they thus make a larger contribution to society over the course of their careers. Secondly, the main social costs associated with aging are incurred in the final year of life, as heroic attempts are made to prolong the survival of sedentary and severely disabled individuals.[9,17] Regular physical activity decreases the risk of chronic disease and thus the scope for heroic treatment; it increases healthy life expectancy.[17] Further, if the medical costs incurred in extreme old age are a concern, the remedy is not to forbid exercise, but rather to curtail the use of public funds for unwarranted medical and surgical attempts at prolonging human life.[17] Finally, there is little evidence that regular physical activity prolongs survival into advanced old age. What it does is to avert *premature* death, at a time when an individual is contributing to society rather than drawing upon its resources. The survival curves for active and sedentary individuals converge around the age of 80 years and, in advanced old age,[58,61] the very active person may even have a slightly shorter calendar life expectancy than the sedentary resident of a nursing home.[43]

Whether an increase of habitual physical activity can reduce dependency depends in part on the most common causes of disability and institutionalization. Robine and Ritchie[64] attributed all of the normally observed loss of disability-free life expectancy to specific medical conditions, the main causes being circulatory diseases, locomotor disorders, and respiratory disorders. Plainly, regular physical activity can postpone a general debility by as much as 20 years. It can also reduce the likelihood of the various medical problems noted by Robine and Ritchie, although the magnitude of these benefits is less clearly established. Some forms of physical activity such as seniors' walking groups provide a source of social support which can help to counter the loss of a significant caregiver; in the active individual, this benefit is augmented by an enhanced mood state and thus a better perceived health for any given level of function.[56] Regular exercise also has a positive effect on the risks of cardiac catastrophe,[63] stroke,[77,90] hypertension,[15] and debilitating congestive failure.[73] Objective changes are harder to demonstrate in chronic respiratory disease but, again an exercise program can have substantial subjective effect upon functional capacity.[51] Finally, regular physical activity has some influence on a number of other important aspects of personal lifestyle, reducing obesity and curtailing cigarette smoking.

Cross-sectional associations between physical fitness and the ability to undertake the activities of daily living do not establish which of these variables is cause and which effect. However, one empirical study demonstrated a substantial correlation between the extent of dependency among seniors and the levels of habitual physical activity reported at an age of 50 years.[76] Other longitudinal investigations have had similar findings. Kaplan et al.[33] noted that the loss of functional ability among seniors over a 6-year interval was associated with initial responses to a five-item inventory of habitual physical activity. LaCroix et al.[40] reported that individuals 65 years and older who reported frequent walks, gardening, or vigorous exercise when they were first examined had, relative to their sedentary peers, a much greater likelihood of maintaining their ability to walk 800 m and to climb up and down a flight of stairs without assistance over a 4-year interval.

It thus seems reasonable to conclude that a regular program of physical activity will do much to counteract the terminal disability observed in sedentary seniors, enhancing the quality-adjusted life span without increasing the numbers of individuals who reach extreme old age.

12.4.2 Control of Body Mass

The accumulation of body fat with age is commonly due to a small decrease in daily physical activity, with no change in food intake.[70] Conversely, an increase in physical activity is the method of choice for reducing body fat content and body mass. Regular physical activity helps to avert the depression of resting metabolism and mood state associated with dieting, and it also increases the likelihood that tissue lost during a period of negative energy balance will be fat rather than lean tissue.[70]

The control of body fat is important in avoiding many of the chronic diseases that have an adverse effect upon function in old age. However, a reduction in body mass also has a more immediate impact upon functional capacity. After adjusting for other health behaviors, LaCroix et al.[40] found that the loss of mobility in a 4-year prospective study of subjects 65 years of age and older was significantly linked to a body mass index at the 80th percentile or higher. The muscle force and aerobic power required to undertake many of the tasks important to the independence of an elderly person (for example, rising from a chair or climbing a flight of stairs) are almost directly proportional to an individual's body mass. Thus, a 10% reduction in body mass will effectively increase muscle strength and maximal aerobic power by some 10%, equivalent to a 10-year reversal of the effects of aging. Further, the elimination of body heat, and thus the tolerance of physical effort in warm weather, is facilitated by a reduction in superficial body fat.

12.4.3 Cessation of Cigarette Smoking

Cessation of smoking contributes to the avoidance of many of the chronic diseases that have an adverse effect upon functional capacity in the elderly. In addition, smoking has more direct negative effects upon the performance of aerobic work: it blocks the oxygen-carrying capacity of haemoglobin and increases the work of breathing (Chapter 9). LaCroix et al.[40] noted an impact of smoking on the loss of mobility in their 4-year prospective study of adults >65 years of age. Together, the physiological and pathological problems associated with smoking can reduce effective peak aerobic power by 10% or more and, conversely, the aerobic power is likely to be increased by 10%, or the equivalent of 10 years of aging, after successful cigarette withdrawal.

12.4.4 Overall Impact of Lifestyle

The cumulative influence of regular physical activity, control of body mass, and cessation of smoking can bring about a 40% increase in aerobic power, the equivalent of approximately 40 years of aging, sufficient to correct the functional problems encountered in most frail elderly men and women.

12.5 Conclusions

In both men and women, aging leads to a loss of function, disability, and a poor quality of life, with substantial social and economic costs. Women have a longer period of disability and poor quality life than men. Regular physical activity postpones the likely age of dependency in both sexes, increasing quality-adjusted life expectancy without greatly extending calendar life span. Such benefits can be augmented further by control of obesity and cessation of smoking. In many people, the problems of frailty and dependency currently encountered during advanced old age could be avoided by adopting a prudent lifestyle, reminiscent of that to which humans have adapted over the many centuries of their existence.

References

1. Allaire, S.H., LaValley, M.P., Evans, S.R., et al., Evidence for decline in disability and improved health among persons aged 55 to 70 years: the Framingham heart study, *Am. J. Publ. Health*, 89, 1678–1683, 1999.
2. Allen, J.G., Aerobic capacity and physiological fitness of Australian men, *Ergonomics*, 9, 485–494, 1966.
3. Arber, S. and Cooper, H., Gender differences in health in later life: the new paradox? *Soc. Sci. Med.*, 48, 61–76, 1999.
4. Armenian, H.K., Pratt, L.A., Gallo, J., et al., Psychopathology as a predictor of disability: a population-based follow-up study in Baltimore, Maryland, *Am. J. Epidemiol.*, 148, 269–275, 1998.

5. Avlund, K., Schroll, M., Davidsen, M., et al., Maximal isometric muscle strength and functional ability in daily activities among 75-year-old men and women, *Scand. J. Med. Sci. Sports*, 4, 32–40, 1994.
6. Bassey, E.J., Fiatarone, M.A., O'Neill, E.F., et al., Leg extensor power and functional performance in very old men and women, *Clin. Sci.*, 82, 321–327, 1992.
7. Bergstrom, U., Book, C., Lindroth, Y., et al., Lower disease activity and disability in Swedish patients with rheumatoid arthritis in 1995 compared with 1978, *Scand. J. Rheumatol.*, 28, 160–165, 1999.
8. Bonjer, H.J., Relationship between physical working capacity and allowable caloric expenditure, in *International Colloquium on Muscular Exercise and Training*, Rohmert, W., Ed., Gentner Verlag, Darmstadt, Germany, 1968, 86–98.
9. Chassin, M.R., Kosecoff, J., Park, R.E., et al., Does inappropriate use explain geographic variations in the use of health care services? *JAMA*, 258, 2533–2537, 1987.
10. Chin, M.H. and Goldman, L., Gender differences in 1-year survival and quality of life among patients admitted with congestive heart failure, *Med. Care*, 36, 1033–1046, 1998.
11. Coroni-Huntley, J., Brock, D.B., Ostfeld, A.M., et al., Established populations for epidemiological studies of the elderly: Resource data book. U.S. Public Health Service, National Institute on Aging, Washington, D.C. 1986.
12. Daltroy, L.H., Larson, M.G., Eaton, H.M., et al., Discrepancies between self-reported and observed physical function in the elderly: the influence of response shift and other factors, *Soc. Sci. Med.*, 48, 1549–1561, 1999.
13. Dunlop, D.D., Hughes, S.L., and Manheim, L.M., Disability in activities of daily living: patterns of change and a hierarchy of disability, *Am. J. Publ. Health*, 87, 378–383, 1997.
14. Edwards, N.I. and Jones, D.A., Ownership and use of assistive devices, *Age and Ageing*, 27, 463–468, 1998.
15. Fagard, R. and Tipton, C.M., Physical activity, fitness and hypertension, in *Physical Activity, Fitness and Health*, Bouchard, C., Shephard, R.J., and Stephens, T., Eds., Human Kinetics Publishers, Champaign, IL, 1994, 633–655.
16. Fifield, J., Reisine, S., Sheehan, T.J., et al., Gender, paid work, and symptoms of emotional distress in rheumatoid arthritis patients, *Arthr. Rheum.*, 39, 427–435, 1996.
17. Fries, J.F., *Aging Well*, Addison-Wesley, Reading, MA, 1980.
18. Gijsbers-van Wijk, C.M., Huisman, H., and Kolk, A.M., Gender differences in physical symptoms and illness behavior. A health diary study, *Soc. Sci. Med.*, 49, 1061–1074, 1999.
19. Godin, G. and Shephard, R.J., Body weight and the energy cost of activity, *Arch. Environ. Hlth.*, 27, 289–293, 1973.
20. Greimel, E.R., Padilla, G.V., and Grant, M.M., Gender differences in outcomes among patients with cancer, *Psycho-Oncol.*, 7, 197–206, 1998.
21. Grimby, G. and Svanborg, A., Morbidity and health-related quality of life among ambulant elderly citizens, *Aging (Milano)*, 9, 356–364, 1997.
22. Guralnik, J.M., LaCroix, A.Z., Abbott, R.D., et al., Maintaining mobility in late life, *Am. J. Epidemiol.*, 137, 845–857, 1993.
23. Guralnik, J.M., LaCroix, A.Z., Everett, D.F., et al., Aging in the eighties: the prevalence of comorbidity and its association with disability. Advance Data from Vital and Health Statistics, National Center for Health Statistics, Hyattsville, MD, 1989.

24. Hachisuka, K., Saeki, S., Tsutsui, Y., et al., Gender-related differences in scores of the Barthel index and Frenchay activities index in randomly sampled elderly persons living at home in Japan, *J. Clin. Epidemiol.*, 52, 1089–1094, 1999.
25. Hachisuka, K., Tsutsui, Y., Furusawa, K., et al., Gender differences in disability and lifestyle among community-dwelling elderly stroke patients in Kitakyushu, Japan, *Arch. Phys. Med. Rehabil.*, 79, 998–1002, 1998.
26. Hawkins, W.E. and Duncan, T., Structural equation analysis of an exercise/sleep health practices model on quality of life of elderly persons, *Percept. Mot. Skills*, 72, 831–836, 1991.
27. Health and Welfare Canada, The Canada Health Survey, Health and Welfare Canada, Ottawa, Ontario, 1982.
28. Health and Welfare Canada, The Active Health Report on Seniors, Health and Welfare Canada, Ottawa, Ontario, 1989.
29. Health and Welfare Canada, Aging and Independence: Overview of a National Survey, Health and Welfare Canada, Ottawa, Ontario, 1993.
30. Hunt, A., *The Elderly at Home*, Her Majesty's Stationery Office, London, 1978.
31. Huuhtanen, P. and Piispa, M., Attitudes on work and retirement by occupation, in *Aging and Work*, Ilmarinen, J., Ed., Institute for Occupational Medicine, Helsinki, Finland, 1993, 152–156.
32. Jackson, A.S., Beard, E.F., Wier, L.T., et al., Changes in aerobic power of men ages 25–70 years, *Med. Sci. Sports Exerc.*, 27, 113–120, 1995.
33. Kaplan, R.M., Feeny, D.A., and Revicki, D.A., Methods for assessing relative importance in preference-based outcome measures, *Qual. Life Res.*, 2, 467–475, 1993.
34. Katsunama, H., Japan, in *Principles and Practice of Geriatric Medicine,* Pathy, M.S.J., Ed., John Wiley & Sons, Chichester, U.K., 1998, 1549–1559.
35. Kavanagh, T., Mertens, D.J., Matosevic, V., et al., Health and aging of master athletes, *Clin. Sports Med.*, 1, 72–88, 1989.
36. Kilbom, Å., Blatzari, L., Ilmarinen, J., et al., Aging and retirement: an international comparison, in *Aging and Work,* Ilmarinen, J., Ed., Institute for Occupational Health, Helsinki, Finland, 1993, 54–62.
37. Kohl, H.W., Moorefield, D.L., and Blair, S.N., Is cardiorespiratory fitness associated with general chronic fatigue in apparently healthy men and women? *Med. Sci. Sports Exerc.*, 19, S56 (Abstr.), 1987.
38. Kroenke, K. and Spitzer, L., Gender differences in the reporting of physical and somatoform symptoms, *Psychosom. Med.*, 60, 150–155, 1998.
39. Kunkel, S.R. and Appelbaum, R.A., Estimating the prevalence of long-term disability for an aging society, *J. Gerontol.*, 47, S253–S260, 1992.
40. LaCroix, A.Z., Guralnik, J.M., Berkman, L.F., et al., Maintaining mobility in later life. II. Smoking, alcohol consumption, physical activity, and body mass index, *Am. J. Epidemiol.*, 137, 858–869, 1993.
41. Lahelma, E., Martikainen, P., Rahkonen, O., et al., Gender differences in ill health in Finland: patterns, magnitude and change, *Soc. Sci. Med.*, 48, 7–19, 1999.
42. Leijon, M., Hensing, G., and Alexanderson, K., Gender trends in sick-listing with musculoskeletal symptoms in a Swedish county during a period of rapid increase in sickness absence, *Scand. J. Soc. Med.*, 26, 204–213, 1998.
43. Linsted, K.D., Tonstad, K., and Kuzma, J., Self-report of physical activity and patterns of mortality in Seventh-Day Adventist men, *J. Clin. Epidemiol.*, 44, 355–364, 1991.

44. Lund, T. and Borg, V., Work environment and self-rated health as predictors of remaining in work 5 years later among Danish employees 35–59 years of age, *Exp. Aging Res.*, 25, 429–434, 1999.
45. Macintyre, S., Ford, G., and Hunt, K., Do women "over-report" morbidity? Men's and women's responses to structured prompting on a standard question on long standing illness, *Soc. Sci. Med.*, 48, 89–98, 1999.
46. Manton, K.G., Epidemiological, demographic and social correlates of disability, *Millbank Q.*, 67 (Suppl. 2:1), 13–58, 1989.
47. Manton, K.G., Demographic trends for the aging female population, *J. Am. Med. Womens Assoc.*, 52, 99–105, 1997.
48. Manton, K.G., Corder, L.S., and Stallard, E., Disability and mortality among the oldest-old: implications for current and future health and long-term care service needs, *J. Gerontol. Soc.*, 48, S153–S166, 1993.
49. Mercier, C., Peladeau, N., and Tempier, R., Age, gender and quality of life, *Commun. Mental Hlth. J.*, 34, 487–500, 1998.
50. Merrill, S.S., Seeman, T.E., Kasl, S.V., et al., Gender differences in the comparison of self-reported disability and performance measures, *J. Gerontol.*, 52, M19–M26, 1997.
51. Mertens, D.J., Shephard, R.J., and Kavanagh, T., Long-term exercise for chronic obstructive lung disease, *Respiration*, 35, 96–107, 1978.
52. Morey, M.C., Pieper, C.F., and Coroni-Huntley, J., Is there a threshold between peak oxygen uptake and self-reported physical functioning in older adults? *Med. Sci. Sports Exerc.*, 30, 1223–1229, 1998.
53. Neitzert, C.S., Davis, C., and Kennedy, S.H., Personality factors related to the prevalence of somatic symptoms and medical complaints in a healthy student population, *Br. J. Med. Psychol.*, 70, 93–101, 1997.
54. Nielsen, J., Employability and workability among Danish employees, *Exp. Aging Res.*, 25, 393–397, 1999.
55. Noro, A. and Aro, S., Health-related quality of life among the least dependent institutional elderly compared with the noninstitutional elderly population, *Qual. Life Res.*, 5, 355–366, 1996.
56. North, T.C., McCullagh, P., and Tran, Z.V., Effect of exercise on depression, *Ex. Sport Sci. Rev.*, 18, 379–416, 1990.
57. Ouslander, J.G., Nursing home care, in *Principles of Geriatric Medicine and Gerontology,* Hazzard, W.R., et al., Eds., McGraw Hill, New York, 1994.
58. Paffenbarger, R.S., Hyde, R.T., Wing, A.L., et al., Some interrelations of physical activity, physiological fitness, health and longevity, in *Physical Activity, Fitness and Health,* Bouchard, C., Shephard, R.J., and Stephens, T., Eds., Human Kinetics, Champaign, IL., 1994, 119–133.
59. Paterson, D.H., Cunningham, D.A., Koval, J.J., et al., Aerobic fitness in a population of independently living men and women aged 55–86 years, *Med. Sci. Sports Exerc.*, 31, 1813–1820, 1999.
60. Pawlson, L.G., Health care implications of an aging population, in *Principles of Geriatric Medicine and Gerontology,* Hazzard, W.R., et al., Eds., McGraw Hill, New York, 1994, 167–176.
61. Pekkanen, J., Marti, B., Nissinen, A., et al., Reduction of premature mortality by high physical activity: A 20-year follow-up of middle-aged Finnish men, *Lancet,* i, 1473–1477, 1987.

62. Pope, A.M. and Tarlov, A.R., *Disability in America: Towards a National Agenda for Prevention*, Institute of Medicine, National Academy Press, Washington, D.C., 1991.
63. Powell, K.E., Thompson, P.D., Caspersen, C.J., et al., Physical activity and the incidence of coronary heart disease, *Ann. Rev. Publ. Hlth.*, 8, 253–287, 1987.
64. Robine, J.M. and Ritchie, K., Healthy life expectancy: evaluation of global indicator of change in population health, *Br. Med. J.*, 302, 457–460, 1991.
65. Rowland, D., Medicaid at 30, *JAMA*, 274, 271–273, 1995.
66. Sauvaget, C., Tsuji, L., Aonuma, T., et al., Health-life expectancy according to various functional levels, *J. Am. Geriatr. Soc.*, 47, 1326–1331, 1999.
67. Schwartz, C.E., Teaching coping skills enhances quality of life more than peer support: results of a randomized trial with multiple sclerosis patients, *Health Psychol.*, 18, 211–220, 1999.
68. Seitsamo, J. and Martikainen, R., Changes in capability in a sample of Finnish aging workers, *Exp. Aging Res.*, 25, 345–352, 1999.
69. Shephard, R.J., Assessment of occupational fitness in the context of human rights legislation, *Can. J. Sport Sci.*, 14, 74–84, 1990.
70. Shephard, R.J., *Aerobic Fitness and Health*, Human Kinetics Publishers, Champaign, IL., 1994.
71. Shephard, R.J., Worksite health promotion and productivity, in *Worksite Health Promotion Economics*, Kaman, R.L., Ed., Human Kinetics Publishers, Champaign, IL, 1995, 147–174.
72. Shephard, R.J., *Aging, Physical Activity and Health*, Human Kinetics Publishers, Champaign, IL, 1997.
73. Shephard, R.J., Exercise for patients with congestive heart failure, *Sports Med.*, 23, 75–92, 1997.
74. Shephard, R.J., Age and physical work capacity, *Exp. Aging Res.*, 25, 331–343, 1999.
75. Shephard, R.J., Exercise and training in women, Part 1. Influence of gender on exercise and training responses, *Can. J. Appl. Physiol.*, 25, 19–34, 2000.
76. Shephard, R.J. and Montelpare, W.J., Geriatric benefits of exercise as an adult, *J. Gerontol.*, 43, M86–M90, 1988.
77. Shinton, R. and Sagar, G., Lifelong exercise and stroke, *Br. Med. J.*, 307, 231–234, 1993.
78. Sonn, U., Grimby, G., and Svanborg, A., Activities of daily living studied longitudinally between 70 and 76 years of age, *Disabil. Rehabil.*, 18, 91–100, 1996.
79. Spirduso, W., *Physical Dimensions of Aging*, Human Kinetics Publishers, Champaign, IL, 1995.
80. Sports Council and Health Education Authority, The Allied Dunbar National Fitness Survey: the Main Findings, Sports Council and Health Education Authority, London, 1992.
81. Statistics Canada, *General Social Survey*, Statistics Canada, Ottawa, Ontario, 1985.
82. Statistics Canada, *Health and Activity Limitations Survey*, Statistics Canada, Ottawa, Ontario, 1986.
83. Strawbridge, W.J., Shema, S.J., Balfour, J.L., et al., Antecedents of frailty over three decades in an older cohort, *J. Gerontol.*, 53, S9–S16, 1998.
84. Svänborg, A., Ecology, aging and health in a medical perspective, in *Aging and Technological Advances*, Robinson, P.K., Livingston, J., and Birren, J.E., Eds., Plenum Press, New York, 1985, 159–168.

85. Tardivel, J., Gender differences in relation to motivation and compliance in cardiac rehabilitation, *Nursing Crit. Care*, 3, 214–219, 1998.
86. Tuomi, K., Järvinen, E., Eskelinen, L., et al., Effect of retirement on health and work ability among municipal employees, *Scand. J. Work Environ. Health*, 17 (Suppl. 1), 75–81, 1991.
87. U.S. Department of Health and Human Services, Disability Survey 72. U.S. Department of Health and Human Services, Washington, D.C., 1981.
88. U.S. National Center for Health Statistics, *Prevalence of Selected Chronic Conditions, United States, 1986–88*, Vital Statistics 10, No. 182, Hyattsville, MD, 1993.
89. van Vliet, R.C. and Lamers, L.M., The high costs of death: should health plans get higher payments when members die? *Med. Care*, 36, 1451–1460, 1998.
90. Wannamethee, G. and Shaper, A.G., Physical activity and stroke in British middle-aged men, *Br. Med. J.*, 304, 597–601, 1992.
91. Warner, K.E., Selling health promotion to corporate America: uses and abuses of the economic argument, *Health Ed. Q.*, 14, 39–55, 1987.
92. Williamson, J.D. and Fried, L.P., Characterization of older adults who attribute functional decrements to "old age," *J. Am. Geriatr. Soc.*, 44, 1429–1434, 1996.
93. Young, M.A., Rowlands, D.B., Stallard, T.J., et al., Effect of environment on blood pressure, *Br. Med. J.*, 286, 1235–1236, 1983.

Index

H

I

J

L

M

N

O

P

Q

R

S

T

V

W

X

For Product Safety Concerns and Information please contact our
EU representative GPSR@taylorandfrancis.com Taylor & Francis
Verlag GmbH, Kaufingerstraße 24, 80331 München, Germany